Collective Trauma and the Psychology of Secrets in Transnational Film

Collective Trauma and the Psychology of Secrets in Transnational Film advances a methodological line of inquiry based on a fresh insight into the ways in which cinematic meaning is generated and can be ascertained. Premised on a critical reading strategy informed by a metapsychology of secrets, the book features analyses of internationally acclaimed films—Guillermo del Torro's *Pan's Labyrinth,* Andrey Zvyagintsev's *The Return,* Jee-woon Kim's *A Tale of Two Sisters,* and Alejandro Amenábar's *The Others.* It demonstrates how a rethinking of the figure of the secret in national film yields a new vantage point for examining heretofore unrecognized connections between collective historical experience, cinematic production, and a transnational aesthetic of concealment and hiding.

Deborah Lynn Porter was trained as a Sinologist and has published on Chinese fiction, myth, and cultural history spanning two millennia. She teaches at the Jackson School of International Studies where she chairs the Master's Program in International Studies and codirects the online Integrated Social Sciences degree program. She is now preparing a monograph-length analysis of Chinese cultural patterns along the same lines advanced in this book.

Routledge Advances in Film Studies

For a full list of titles in this series, please visit www.routledge.com.

49 **Early Race Filmmaking in America**
Edited by Barbara Tepa Lupack

50 **Film Text Analysis**
New Perspectives on the Analysis of Filmic Meaning
Edited by Janina Wildfeuer and John A. Bateman

51 **The Camera-Eye Metaphor in Cinema**
Christian Quendler

52 **Surveillance in Asian Cinema**
Under Eastern Eyes
Edited by Karen Fang

53 **US Youth Films and Popular Music**
Identity, Genre, and Musical Agency
Tim McNelis

54 **The Cinematic Eighteenth Century**
History, Culture, and Adaptation
Edited by Srividhya Swaminathan and Steven W. Thomas

55 **The Contemporary Femme Fatale**
Gender, Genre and American Cinema
Katherine Farrimond

56 **Film Comedy and the American Dream**
Zach Sands

57 **Ecocinema and the City**
Robin L. Murray and Joseph K. Heumann

58 **Collective Trauma and the Psychology of Secrets in Transnational Film**
Deborah Lynn Porter

Collective Trauma and the Psychology of Secrets in Transnational Film

Deborah Lynn Porter

Routledge
Taylor & Francis Group
LONDON AND NEW YORK

First published 2018 by Routledge

2 Park Square, Milton Park, Abingdon, Oxfordshire OX14 4RN
52 Vanderbilt Avenue, New York, NY 10017

Routledge is an imprint of the Taylor & Francis Group, an informa business

First issued in paperback 2020

Library of Congress Cataloging-in-Publication Data
CIP data has been applied for.

ISBN: 978-0-8153-7175-5 (hbk)
ISBN: 978-0-367-59303-2 (pbk)

Typeset in Sabon
by codeMantra

Docendo discimus

Contents

List of Figures

Acknowledgments

This project was exciting for me pedagogically and intellectually. It culminates a shift in my academic focus away from Chinese pre-Imperial (221 B.C.) culture to contemporary cinema, even though I see these in conversation with each other. I have the good fortune of being surrounded by generous family, friends, colleagues, and students, and I am so very grateful for all that our interactions contributed to the process of research, reflection, and writing. Simone Porter inspired the pedagogical orientation of the project; her intellectual curiosity, enthusiasm for new perspectives, and the ease with which she absorbed the interpretive position advanced herein convinced me that others may also like to be exposed to the frameworks. Tam Morgan, Laura Skosey-LaLonde, Judith, and Dr William Whitson listened with ceaseless patience as I regaled them with the twists and turns of my paths of investigation. Eve Golden warmly and perspicaciously offered incisive editorial questions, comments, and suggestions, which sharpened considerably the articulation of my argument.

The Jackson School of International Studies is an ideal place for sharing intellectual fare; I appreciate working among peers whose research significantly shaped my thinking about collective memory, cultural production, and social science research. Professors Glennys Young, Hwa-sook Nam, and Elena Campbell graciously read drafts of chapters related to their specific area studies expertise and offered important linguistic corrections; any remaining errors are my responsibility. Finally, I want to express deep gratitude to the students with whom I had the privilege to explore these brilliant films and uncover their embedded lessons.

Art Resources, New York, has kindly granted permission to reproduce Andrea Mantegna's *The Lamentation of Christ*, Julius Schnorr Carolsfeld's *Sacrifice of Isaac*, Andrei Rublev's *Icon of the Trinity of the Old Testament Trinity*, and William Shakespeare Burton's *The Wounded Cavalier.* The Victoria and Albert Museum of London has also generously permitted reproduction of William Morris's "Blackthorn" design.

Note on Romanization Systems Used for Russian and Korean Film Analyses

Russian words are transcribed according to ALA-LC (Library of Congress) Romanization without Diacritics [*Russkii iazyk*].

Korean words are transcribed according to the McCune-Reischauer system.

1 New Psychoanalytical Tools for Social Science Inquiry[1]

As beloved an art form as it is, film has more to tell us than it is commonly given credit for. But this is changing. The upsurge of film and visual culture studies in the social sciences over the last two decades is just one example. This book is another. In it, I use film to explore collective experience, specifically traumatic experience and collective memory. The analytic technique I demonstrate here is the culmination of ten years of developing a course in the Jackson School of International Studies at the University of Washington.

My course, *Putting the World on the Couch: Psychoanalysis and International Studies,* started out as a survey of how social science scholarship and psychoanalysis engage each other and of the new areas of research that have emerged out of that cross-fertilization.[2] Film was my point of entrée into collective memory formation processes.

Film serves a teaching function in the world at large, not only among scholars;[3] see, for example, Sam Wineburg, Susan Mosborg, Dan Porat, and Ariel Duncan's investigation of how people learned about the Vietnam War.[4] It has become an important object of social science research precisely because of this expanded role as an "influential source of historical information and perspective across family generations."[5] In fact, some scholars have argued that since the end of World War II, cinema has been our dominant source of historical memory; in this view, it functions as a "prosthetic" memory for collective experience.[6]

My students quickly came to appreciate the opportunity that cultural artifacts offer for exploring collective aspects of trauma and memory formation that are often too diffuse or unwieldy to be studied in the world at large. But the more we explored, the more I felt the need for a clear exploratory strategy. What perspectives, what knowledge, would best enable my students to cull from these rich resources insights about collective memory formation? How should I even talk about ways to do this? Ultimately, the course developed into an effort to teach this expanded vision of cineliteracy, and that is the organizing principle of this book.

The Puzzle of Collective Memory

Before we can take full advantage of film's capacity to refract and comment on collective memories of traumatic experience, we need to have a clear grasp of what collective memory is. This is a challenge. There is no consensus among scholars on such central perplexities as how collective memory is formed or transmitted, to say nothing of "the unfathomability of traumatic experience" and how that is represented and interpreted.[7]

Sociologist Maurice Halbwachs is considered the founder of collective memory studies. He argues that groups have collective memories, which are manifested through social frameworks such as families, religious organizations, and schools.[8] Because these institutions are the channels through which experience can be recollected and expressed, Halbwachs reasons, an individual's understanding of herself and her past is strongly linked to the institutional, or group, consciousness. This view also allows Halbwachs to account for the way the meanings of memory can change over time. He contends that the memories a person maintains may vary from context to context—that is, say, of family, class, or religion—and that these variants may be held simultaneously.[9]

Halbwachs's work has catalyzed an avalanche of research, but he does not give much attention to the physical and mental realities of memory or to the relationship between individual and collective memory. Individual memory involves neurological and cognitive processes that have no known equivalents in groups and appears therefore to be constitutionally distinct from collective processes. Another indication of the complexity of these issues is the fact that there is more than one kind of individual memory: "procedural" memory stores bodily skills and habitual movements, "semantic" memory stores the fund of knowledge that is acquired mentally through conscious learning, and "episodic" memory processes autobiographical experience.[10] Halbwachs does not address these distinctions.

At the same time, however, Halbwachs's recognition of the linguistic basis of collective memory establishes a kinship between it and its individual counterpart. Language is certainly a collective phenomenon, and the new assumption is that it is central to both individual and collective memory processes.[11] Workers in the field have compared the language used in individual and collective accounts of traumatic developments and identified congruencies in the ways memories take narrative form; the congruencies reflect a system through which "institutions vested with authority, including 'stories, myths and images' but extending to the church and the law, articulate memory."[12]

This is a helpful concept for investigating how a film represents collective memory. It allows us to link concrete elements of a filmic representation to the language of cultural memory. Sensitivity to how memories of violence may be expressed through tropes of vengeance in film,[13] or how concepts of justice or compassion are signaled through rhetorical devices and images,[14] for example, gives form to the amorphous concept of memory analysis. Nonetheless, while these approaches have refined our ability to identify the "what" of what is shared among individual and collective memories, they leave open the question of "why."

To answer, we must explain why past experiences and the affects associated with them are preserved; we must also account for the processes by which these experiences are articulated—the processes that lead, or do not lead, to their discursive production and transmission.[15] Such accounts, however, often end up derailed, mired once more in the relationship between individual memories of trauma and collective experience of the same event. Questions about how to balance out "memories of individual suffering in theory and 'on the ground'," and collective memory processes that "exceed those of relations between individuals,"[16] still dominate the discussion.[17]

New Tools for Collective Memory Research

I teach in my classes, and will demonstrate here, some analytic tools that break down the binary division in collective memory research. They exemplify a psycholinguistic approach that permits the "analysis of specificity and particularity of discourses and practices" while also ensuring that these specifics and particulars are not divorced from the collective structures and institutions from which they are drawn. They are built on the work of Hungarian-French philosopher and psychoanalyst Nicolas Abraham, and of Abraham in conjunction with his colleague Maria Torok,[18] who theorizes about *how the linguistic surround informs awareness in individuals.*

Abraham and Torok's model of the mind focuses distinctively on *breakdowns of signification*, that is, on apparent losses of intelligibility in language. They thought that the psyche is naturally inclined to growth and expansion, which it accomplishes by feeding on, digesting, *and naming* the life experiences that people confront in development. Abraham believed that the impersonal and programmatic quality of the classical Freudian formulation involving predetermined and universal "drives" or "instincts" denies the uniqueness of individual lives.[19]

The processing of experience into language, in Abraham's view, is what ultimately gives us the power to think about it. But young children's mastery of language depends for a crucial developmental period on the linguistic surround provided by their parents, and the parents' own past experiences, conscious or not, will have imparted an affective charge to their speech and so to the words that they offer their children. Thus, Abraham and Torok argue, mental organization is not only a dynamic response to a subject's predictable lived experience but also a conceptual structure that is passed down in families. The authors postulate that when the words necessary to name a child's experience are overly laden with affect or content that is unavailable or unwelcome to the parent's awareness, the words that the child needs may be (consciously or unconsciously) withheld or transmitted to the child with an affective burden that is beyond the child's capacity to process. The child may or may not consciously perceive the parent's discomfort, but in either case, the necessary linguistic tools are not made available. The processing and naming of the child's experience fail, and a void is left in their stead. In this way, the unconscious linguistic distortions and repressions embodied in the parent's speech are reconstructed in the child's.

Abraham believed that traumatic experience interrupts or overwhelms a person's capacity to process it into language, leaving behind fragments of personal history of which the person can neither think nor speak. Inaccessible to awareness, these fragments remain present in the person's psyche and language only as an absence. Yet they *do* remain present, and in their absence may be felt, seen, and passed on to linguistic heirs. More about that in a moment.

This view disallows the idea that the so-called "real" world is a transparent, intentional, and objective correlate of subjective lived experience—an idea that, according to Abraham, discounts the role of the unconscious in shaping and informing conscious experience. He maintains that "reality" is experience that demands to be accommodated; it is experience that agitates the psyche toward the process of psychic expansion that Nicholas Rand calls *self-fashioning*.[20] Self-fashioning is a system of assimilation and adaptation that continues throughout life, which Abraham understood to be *the* organizing or sensemaking principle of the psyche. But the readiness of a child's psyche to digest and assimilate new experience is determined by the degree to which a parent's unconscious (in the form of words) enables or inhibits it. Self-fashioning, therefore, even while it grapples with "the stuff of our own lives,"[21] is influenced by parental sagas transmitted by the fact of absence and is the product of an infinitely regressed family history.

This idea, that the linguistic surround colors how people process and name experience, is of course not novel to Abraham and Torok; indeed, it was a premise of Halbwachs's understanding of collective memory. Kali Tal demonstrates it from a different perspective, showing how the linguistic surround created by the sharing and retelling of individual trauma narratives penetrates "the vocabulary of the larger culture where, she claims, they become tools for the construction of national myths."[22]

The same idea has been central to the development of individual memory theories, especially with regard to the transgenerational familial transmission of memory through silence; this is in stark contradistinction to Halbwachs's idea, which understood memory formation as a function of *overt* expression of individuals that was shaped by and within a collective.[23] Affects in general, and transgenerational trauma in particular, are thought by many theorists to be transmitted by the same psycholinguistic mechanisms.[24] Bruce Bradfield demonstrated that parents' "unformulated experience" influences their children's development.[25] Other studies indicate that children and grandchildren of Holocaust survivors differentiate less completely from their parents than other children: They see themselves as protectors of their parents rather than vice versa and so tend to inhibit their own impulses to establish independence and autonomy.[26] Nanette Auerhahn and Dori Laub's work has shown that "knowledge of psychic trauma weaves through the memories of several generations," passed on by parents and internalized as an unconscious organizing principle.[27] Studies of transgenerational transmission of private trauma attest to silent "cooperative communication" patterns that exist among family members and are governed by unspoken rules of silence.

Similar patterns have been observed in the transmission of historical traumas. For example, Rachel Lev-Wiesel saw transgenerational traumatic responses across three generations after forced relocations in 1940s Israel and Palestine, and after immigrations from Morocco to Israel following World War II; Hatsantour Karenian et al. investigated the transgenerational effects of the Turkish genocide of Armenians in 1915, building upon earlier work in which third-generation survivors were found to exhibit more pathological symptoms than the second generation; and Teresa Evans-Campbell established transmission among American Indian/Native Alaska communities with a multilevel framework of historical trauma.[28]

To the limited extent that trauma researchers have taken the psychological processing of trauma into account, they have tended to explain its inaccessibility with *dynamic repression*. Dynamic repression implies the banishment of affects (desire, hatred, envy, and the like) that arise predictably in the course of psychosexual development but are rejected in compliance with parental or social prohibitions (either from without or as internalized standards).[29] Abraham and Torok, however, reject the notion that repression has only one structure. They postulate that repressive structures, like internal conflicts, reflect the particular conditions in which they arise. They are a response not to invariant or universal stresses but to the specific challenges encountered in individual lives—"the particularity of any individual's life story, the specificity of texts, and the singularity of historical situations."[30] Abraham and Torok's theories emerged out of their clinical work on the transgenerational impact of the Holocaust and the suffering of its survivors; their patients caused them to question the reigning concepts that explain the etiology of trauma disorders. The old psychoanalytic paradigms did not appear to account adequately for the wide range of symptoms observed in the children and grandchildren of Holocaust survivors.[31]

Abraham and Torok theorize that some situations are experienced as so shameful that they are concealed from awareness.[32] *Preservative repression* is what the authors called the process of keeping a shameful experience out of consciousness. They identify shame as a silent force, an independent entity that impacts psychic development within families. They do not explain explicitly why they single out shame (as opposed to other responses to trauma) to play such a dominant role in preservative repression; they arrived at this conclusion inductively, through the evidence of their patients' language. The result of this kind of shame, however, is a secret.

Abraham and Torok use the word *secret* idiosyncratically to refer to content that is preserved unconsciously at the same time that it is banished from linguistic circulation. In their usage, a secret

> is not primarily a hushed up fact, a covert plot, a private feeling, or confidential knowledge kept from others. "Secret" is not synonymous with "hidden," "unknown," or "latent," even in the Freudian sense of a person's unconscious or repressed desires, apt to reappear only in opaque, symptomatic compromise formations. In Abraham and Torok's sense, *the secret is a trauma* [emphasis added] whose very occurrence and devastating emotional consequences are entombed and thereby consigned to internal silence, albeit unwittingly, by the sufferers themselves.[33]

By this definition, a secret may be transmitted across generations and into the unwitting custody of a child. Recall that the child, in his own pursuit of linguistic and psychic growth, struggles to decipher a parent's unsatisfactory communication. In the case of a secret, she will fail. But in the process, she will recognize not only that something is missing—that there is something unnamed going on to which she is not privy—but that something must be protected; otherwise, why is it hidden?

This is a powerful hypothesis that links "certain states of mental disarray, hitherto resistant to analysis, to the concealment of a secret"[34] and explains "how influences *outside* [emphasis added] an individual's lived experience can determine her or his psychic development."[35] In other words, the "invisible" psychic presence of one person's shameful experience may account for certain kinds of mysterious behavior in others—such as the enigmatic and incongruent characters whose filmic lives I will analyze later. I will concentrate on the secret psychic configurations that are established "when a shameful and therefore unspeakable experience must be barred from consciousness or simply 'kept secret.'"[36]

Abraham and Torok call such powerful absences *phantoms*. Their *theory of the phantom*—that is, that an individual's identity may be influenced by the unwitting inheritance of someone else's secret—is a challenge to the sovereignty of dynamic repression as the organizing principle of traumatic memory and an alternative entry into the matter of individual versus collective memory in general. The possibility that secrets, and the linguistic distortions they exact, may endure over generations obviates unsatisfactory timeworn distinctions between individual and collective memory, and identifies unspoken family (collective) history as a generative force of individual identity. Phantom theorists maintain that it is in *preservative* repression that we discover how our psyches are organized by the "psychological implant in us of our ancestor's secrets."[37]

Phantoms do not occur only on the individual level. They can also be created and transmitted silently through a society, for example, in response to social catastrophe.[38] This is a useful perspective on social movements, ideological currents, and political motives. It suggests "the existence within an individual of a collective psychology comprised of several generations"; moreover, it expands the parameters of psychopathology and opens a new vantage point for investigating memory formation. It brings the idea and importance of secrets to the forefront of collective memory analysis. In short, to the extent that "unsettling disruptions in the psychic life of one person can adversely and unconsciously affect someone else,"[39] phantom production occurs where individual and societal memory coincide.

Backward Reading

But even as the phantom is defined by concealment, it reveals. It reveals how an individual memory is shaped by family memory, which is shaped by a family's implication in a (shame generating) collective experience. It provides a structure for interpreting memory constructed in intimate and larger contexts. Furthermore, it resolves a perennial vexation in the interpretive analysis of traumatic memory as represented in cultural artifacts such as literature, art, and cinema: the idea that trauma, by its very definition, overpowers the human capacity to describe or represent. How does one interpret an artifact produced in the wake of an experience that is a priori "unspeakable"?

Here, I will lay out a methodology that obviates this philosophical dead-end. It is applicable in situations of both individual and collective human suffering, and is based on another concept developed by Abraham.

Abraham trained in philosophy at the Sorbonne after emigrating to France from Hungary in the late 1930s. He worked in poetry and translation before turning to psychoanalysis. His attempts to establish a methodology for studying the relationship between phenomena and the unconscious[40] led to his *theory of the symbol*, which I will delineate in detail later. As he became more deeply engaged in clinical practice, he and Maria Torok found this theory helpful for understanding their patients' sometimes inexplicable behavior. From this emerged a body of work investigating how silenced shameful experience impacts upon on an individual and his or her descendants. (When I discuss the theory of the symbol later, I refer to Abraham alone as its author; when I discuss theories relating to secrets, I refer to Abraham and Torok together.)

Recall that Abraham and Torok's model of the mind focuses on *breakdowns* of signification, that is, on apparent losses of intelligibility in language. I say "apparent" because they argued not only that such breakdowns *are in fact* intelligible but also that they are markers of crucial experiences of which we are not consciously aware. The obstacles that at first frustrate interpretation, they held, are the very clues that ultimately enable it. This paradox is the starting point for the method of film analysis that I teach. Confounding conventional notions of truth, illusion, and authorial intention as it does, it is a powerful tool for exploring the complexities of human motivation.

Abraham sees the subjective meaning of *all* phenomena as a product of the digestive process of processing and naming that I described earlier; subjective meaning is therefore, in his view, intrinsically linguistic. He came to construe the speech and behavior of his patients as phenomenal by-products (*worldly objects,* he calls them) of the psychic agitation that motivates growth and expansion in all of us. This vision transcends the differences that have long separated phenomenological investigation,[41] sociological research, and clinical psychoanalysis.[42] *Symbols* are what Abraham calls the phenomena—that is, the linguistic traces—that result from the breakdowns of the self-fashioning process; he believes that they stand for something and that that something can be identified, investigated, and understood. Specifically, he believes, they point to the affective disturbance responsible for interrupting the self-fashioning process. Esther Rashkin elucidates Abraham's choice of terminology and some of its implications:

> For the Greeks, the *symbolon* was a piece of pottery or earthenware that was broken in two prior to someone's (usually a warrior's) voyage. One of the two pieces remained at the site of departure while the other was carried by the traveler and "voyaged" with him. Upon his return (often many years later), the traveler's piece of pottery served as a sign of recognition and as proof of his identity when it was rejoined with its complement. The word "symbol" referred to each of the two pieces together (from the Greek *symballo* = to put together). An initial statement of Abraham's theory of the symbol can be extrapolated from these two meanings. When we read a text we read its symbols. We read fragments of semantic or phonetic elements that, if joined to their missing parts, would signify something (a drama, a scene, or simply a lexical or phonetic element) that must for some reason be kept hidden or out of circulation.[43]

Ordinary language supposes the successful replacement of an object with a word that simultaneously marks its absence and substitutes for it; *symbolic language*, in Abraham's sense, points to failures of this process, points at which the successful substitution cannot be made.

The existence of a secret is manifested symptomatically in incongruent speech and inexplicable behavior; this very incomprehensibility, in Abraham and Torok's view, is the pointer to a concealed traumatic experience. My analyses will demonstrate what such secrets look like and the kind of symptoms they may produce. They will also show how symptoms may be reconstituted to reveal this unconscious dimension of a subject's experience and its hidden source.

Secrets are reconstructed by *anasemic,* or "backward," reading,[44] a technique that allows us to identify symbolic language, that is, the fragmented linguistic patterns that are produced by breakdowns in the processes of psychic assimilation and are thus inconsistent with the other productions of what Abraham calls a "unifying" conscious self.[45] Once these patterns are delineated, it is possible to reunite the lexical fragments with their absent complements. As in a jigsaw puzzle, the "jagged edges" that pinpoint and demarcate symbolic language not only mark the fact of a missing piece, but they also reveal what that piece must look like.

Rashkin, an expert on Abraham and Torok's theories who has applied them to the analysis of literature and film, offers an example of backward reading. She asks us to imagine a story about mail delivery in which the word "post" never appears—not in *post*al, not in *post*man, not in *post* office. Why and how should this be? In her example, it is because the writer is profoundly uncomfortable with the word "pillar," which is associated with some terrible episode in his past—a theft, perhaps, as Rashkin suggests, or we ourselves might even imagine a death. The word "pillar" is thus prohibited from consciousness, along with all its synonyms, the word "post" being one of them. Even though "post" in this story would connote mail and not columns, its affective contamination is sufficient to forbid it in its own form, and the hypothetical writer is forced away from it and to associated but uncontaminated words like the "letters, dispatches, stamps, parcels" that Rashkin mentions. These, she says, are "the 'words that hide,' the cryptonyms of the secret word 'pillar.' Each one carries secreted within it, through a process of lexical and phonetic encrypting ... the word that cannot be said."[46]

Thus, we rediscover the context, hitherto unintelligible, out of which the symbol was torn. Paradoxically, our ability to reconstruct the piece implied by the jagged edge relies on our ability literally to "read" the absence that defines it, that is, to understand how lexical strategies of avoidance are symbolic in both form and meaning. This is what gives Abraham's understanding the value it has for psychoanalytic, sociological, historical, and filmic inquiry.

Phantoms are the psycholinguistic residuum of secrets that may be seen in individuals, in cultural artifacts, and in society. Study of the phantom phenomenon in film is a way to access collective memory where it contacts the individual. In sum, I posit that unspeakable traumatic secrets give rise to a characteristic representation in filmic narrative, that this process is unconsciously intended to obscure awareness and comprehension of the secrets, and that it nonetheless systematically generates and uncovers the very meaning it purports to suppress. In their elaboration of this process, Abraham and Torok give social science research an important tool, and I believe that the film analyses in this book will help to prove that.

Collective History and Cinematic Representation

I have chosen the four films I will analyze in this book as case studies of collective trauma and collective memory formation: Guillermo del Toro's *Pan's Labyrinth* (*El fauno de labertino*), a fantastical 2003 account of a young girl's experience in post-Civil War Franquist Spain; *The Return* (*Vozvrashcheniye*), Andrey Zvyagintsev's elegiac 2003 account of an enigmatic father-son reunion; *A Tale of Two Sisters* (*Janghwa, Hongryeon*), Kim Jee-woon's sophisticated 2004 evocation of psychological horror; and, finally, *The Others*, Alejandro Amenábar's 2001 gothic sleeper hit about a woman and her children on Jersey Island in 1945.[47] Each of these films received extensive critical and popular acclaim, both in their countries of origin and internationally, and they have accrued considerable academic attention as well, fueled by their vibrant "after-life" on Internet cinema sites.[48] This familiarity across a wide spectrum of viewers made them compelling subjects for classroom analysis. Their diverse provenance, moreover, encouraged the transnational and transcultural perspective that is the very lifeblood of the Jackson School.

All belong to the category that I have come to call *phantom films*. That is, each has a protagonist whose enigmatic representation (as I will show) is driven by a secret concealed within the filmic idiom. Reconstruction of that secret will be our entrée into collective trauma. It is only after reconstructing this hidden meaning that we will be able to read the films' commentaries on collective memory and history. I will claim that the films model the fact of preservative repression and how it is transmitted. In examining this process, we will be extending Abraham and Torok's work to a new medium. They dealt explicitly with the familiar language of speech, but, as I will show, their principles apply to other idioms as well. The language of film is visual, but here too, the breakdown of signification is a marker of trauma—its concealment and its revelation.

One of the traumas that weighs on these films was caused by the dramatic increase in the proliferation of new forms of international exchange—a phenomenon referred to as *globalization*.[49] The collective memory processes we see in them deal with the swallowing of national identity by an increasingly global culture, and the language whose breakdown we will follow is in some sense a visual language.[50] Hollywood, the dominant producer of the early film industry, greatly influenced which cinematographic techniques spread to become the paradigms for production efforts elsewhere.[51] The result was a visual lingua franca, the first grammar for international cineliteracy.[52]

A national film is a film made outside of Hollywood, out of its own society. National films are understood to be offshoots of Hollywood paradigms; they share a common language with it, but they also possess an individual language based on their own culture.[53] However, the advent of globalization increased Hollywood's purchase on modes of expression and imposed a greater cultural homogeneity. At best, the global paradigm suppresses the national films; more intensely, it leaves them out.[54] The products of some national cinemas represent reactions to globalization in that they manifest breakdowns of national systems of signification that once were meaningful but no longer serve as adequate representations of (national) existence. This visual breakdown of meaning is analogous to the personal linguistic breakdowns in Abraham and Torok's model, and the films we will explore will evidence both. We will see preservative repression in action, both in individual characters and their disordered behavior and speech, and in the filmic idiom itself, both of which express the affective chaos produced when language and experience do not align. This gap between them reflects a memory that globalization increasingly dominates and suppresses as unworthy.[55]

The breakdown in signification can be seen in the contraposition of two languages: the globalized Hollywood visual language, in which all national directors are literate, and the language derivative of national cinematic paradigms, which had been cultivated before the global visual language became so ruthlessly dominant. The relationship between these two cinematic languages reconstructs the colonization of national memory by a global visual language. This category of film is called "transnational" because it represents a form of cinematic expression in which national consciousness (and collective memory construction) is represented in the fact of their suppression and dissolution—a traumatic loss that is enshrined, and revealed, in preservative repression.[56]

Film scholars have categorized these four films as examples of transnational cinema because they illustrate how national films critique global visual language to reflect the way it "flattens" national experience. Through their visual language, they demonstrate resistance against the displacement of the nation as a viable marker of (collective) identity.[57] The films deploy global cinematic language paradoxically to interrogate the fixity of borders and they use the revealed inconsistencies to represent traumatic collective experience and its memory. Thus, Del

Toro merges the fantastical and the real in *Pan's Labyrinth*. He relies on familiar phantasmagoric tropes of children's literature to refract global "visuality" and, in this "transnational and transcultural context," to challenge memories of the Spanish civil war;[58] the gothic-inspired *A Tale of Two Sisters* also deploys global cinematic features to represent national memory as fractured and illegible;[59] in *The Others,* the visual structuring of time and space challenges notions of temporal reality to comment on subjective and collective perceptions of effaced historical memory;[60] and the journey undertaken by the father and sons in *The Return* has been interpreted as a "creation of a new structure of belonging and cultural knowledge."[61]

Filmic Language and Speech

Filmic language by itself, however, can take us only so far. The actual language in film has meaning too. I will demonstrate how the language of the nations, whose unraveling the films allegorize, establishes and communicates a linguistic surround that transmits a collective traumatic experience. I read the national languages of these films as a third vernacular that must be reconciled with the national and global filmic languages that, hybridized together, characterize transnational films. And I will show how the imagery of both cinematic languages can be translated into the distinct national speech of each film.

Cinematographic language cannot be separated from the words that it denotes; the more we can translate what we see into language, the closer we can get to the secrets that language conceals. I will illustrate how fundamentally, cinematography can be clarified by linguistic investigation of the visual film. Film images alone do not yield access to the event that must be hidden from view; they must be contextualized within the national language. For example, I will show how the fairy-tale imagery with which del Toro cryptically communicates Ofelia's ancestral secret tells us even more about her haunting when it is read "in Spanish." Similarly, the imagery of Zvyagintsev's film, translated into Russian, reveals startling overlaps with del Toro's, although the two works could not be more different. Demonstrations such as these support Abraham and Torok's belief, and my own, that experience is essentially linguistic.

I will argue that these four films represent a specific subset of transnational cinema. Characterized by lexical networks that both conceal and reveal shameful experience, they offer an alternative understanding of how national films express the experience of social disintegration. As we read the films backward, we will note the absences that define episodes of linguistic breakdown and so identify and decode the secrets that inform these characters' identities.

To reconcile an inherited symbol with its absent-complement is to hear what had to be silenced. The uncovering of an encrypted secret, however, while it may do much to advance our understanding of a character's behavior, is not the end of the story. An analysis of this kind "brings to the fore still other enigmas or fragments that demand solution or completion."[62]

That is because—as per Abraham and Torok—the solution to these riddles lies not in the individual characters themselves but in their family histories. These transgenerational, transmitted secrets become accessible when the films' symbols are transported "across the silence inherited by a character and rejoin[ed] to a missing part of that character's unspoken history."[63] The reunion of symbols with their absent complements points to the historical moment when they were silenced.

Each phantom film will be shown to implicate a specific social, cultural, political, and historical context as a causative agent for the formation of the intrapsychic secret inscribed within it. The secrets that are represented in phantom films were generated by the repressed collective memory of these histories: in this way, they are "coauthors" of the films that give them expression. The dialectic between auteur and society offers a more precise understanding of the processes by which shameful dramas can haunt individuals and society.[64]

Affective Temporality

Phantom films link breakdowns in national symbolic systems of signification to unutterable collective experience. Tracing each film's secret back several hundred years to the collective experience that generated the secret that it depicts brings into view new aspects of the films' meanings. Specifically, the experience of and response to globalization may be understood in terms of an affective temporality; phantom films situate globalization within a sequence of affective events.

The idea that twentieth-century globalization is a reiteration of other earlier interactive patterns among nations underlies the work of Ella Shohat and Robert Stam, who argue that multicultural media are organized by figures of speech reflecting how "people everywhere live under the shadow of 1492."[65] This view anticipates my understanding of affective temporality,[66] which I understand as correlative patterns between major sociopolitical experiences and shame. The authors explain that this date is

> a metonym for a series of inter-related historical processes; it looks like the conquest of the New World, the Edicts of Expulsion against the Jews and Muslims, the Inquisition against marranos, the Portuguese incursions along the west coast of Africa, and the Transatlantic slave trade.[67]

The authors claim that the convergence of these nation-building enterprises left an indelible impact on the historical consciousness of white

Europeans and entailed a specific lexicon that justified the "Europeanist" arc of political and social change. This eventually crystallized into a powerful set of narrative and rhetorical motifs grounded in notions of white European progress and cultural mastery over nature. Shohat and Stam term the epistemology and the narrative systems that emerged from it *Eurocentricism.*

They maintain that Eurocentrism's endurance is a function of its transmission—not as a "systematic philosophy," but rather as "an interlocking network of embedded narratives, buried premises, and submerged metaphors that have cumulatively shaped a broadly shared common sense."[68] Shohat and Stam believe that Eurocentrism is a cognitive structure of mind preserved in linguistic and tropical patterns; this resonates with my understanding of a phantom as a psychic structure that is also transgenerationally transmitted. The ubiquitous "Tropes of Empire" for which Shohat and Stam offer a taxonomy appear not infrequently in phantom films.

For example, the trope of "racial blood,"[69] which "historically signified religious affiliation" in Eurocentric discourse, figures significantly in *Pan's Labyrinth* and *The Others*. Shohat and Stam claim that migrations to Latin America in the wake of the Spanish Inquisition entailed the transmission of a "'Moorish Sephardi unconscious.'"[70] This may account for why lexical fragments dating from the Inquisition appear in the films of Mexican national del Toro and of the Chilean/Spanish Amenábar. In addition to signifying Jewish or Moorish affiliation, the blood trope points to problematic genealogies more generally—to illegitimacy, for example. On the other hand, binary spatial tropes in Eurocentric discourse, such as split-level contrasts between subterranean and terrestrial, say, or light and dark,[71] signify differently than in phantom films. Whereas in the former, spatial metaphors are deployed to self-proclaim an enlightened position, in phantom films, these tropes more consistently intimate an unconscious parallel underlying and subverting the surface meaning of the text.

Shohat and Stan make it clear that Eurocentric discourse is the language of Empire; phantoms originate in and are transmitted along family lines. Whereas Eurocentrism emanates from the manifest expansion of state power, the discourse of haunted lineages devolves on the repression of the historical moment when state power incurred shame for a family. The use of the family in film to resolve historical tensions is, of course, a recognized convention in national films;[72] a family's reaction to a historical event is often presented, or interpreted, as a paradigm of national experience. Families in phantom texts may similarly be seen as a paradigm of larger experience, but the experience is of a different order. Here, the family serves as a metonym for the larger public to which the secret must not be revealed and the concealed secret as a metonym for collective trauma.

Phantom films therefore reveal the impact of collective trauma on family communication systems. The films I analyze draw attention to how families in Spain, Russia, Korea, and England refashioned traumatic histories, and, to an extent, themselves, as obstacles to awareness of unutterable collective experience. Thus, the secret that haunts Ofelia originates in the Spanish Inquisition (officially established in 1478), which allowed the Roman Catholic Church to institutionalize cruel and socially divisive techniques for rooting out "blasphemers"; Ivan's secret in *The Return* connects to issues about legitimacy that underlay the reign of Ivan IV (r. 1547–1583); the secret that haunts Su-mi in *A Tale of Two Sisters* implicates the Japanese occupation of Korea, but it also points to a royal secret whose preservation is implicated in several historical traumas; and, finally, Amenábar's Grace Stuart is haunted by a secret pertaining to the English civil war, especially the regicide of King Charles I in 1649. Each of these films tacitly unfolds a scenario of an affective experience analogous to those attributed to globalization and why it triggered the production of these sixteenth and seventeenth collective secrets.

Phantom films model a process of memory formation informed by preservative repression—the competing needs to forget and to remember. If fragmented cinematic language represents an obstacle to reading national symbols, it is not because of globalization per se but rather because some collective shameful secret about the nation's origins that had to be kept from view *had been triggered in the context of globalization.* The recursive relationship between collective experience and the individual secrets that haunt the subjects of phantom films rehistoricizes the intolerance of differences beyond the realm of globalizing cinematic language to the time when national consciousness itself first emerged. The interdigitation of global and national cinematic language performs a preservative function that can be accessed only if we take seriously the national linguistic surround of the film itself.

Cinema-Specific Features of Phantom Films

Film is a highly suitable medium for phantom narratives, as the many different visual and auditory media that contribute to it are all available for concealment. In the close readings to follow, I will demonstrate this. But first, I want to make some general observations to situate my phantom-centered approach more concretely among other perspectives on cinematographic language.

Since its inception, film has been known as a supple medium, well suited to the peeling off of the layers that surround human motivation. Furthermore, there are "remarkable analogies between filmic language and the analytic idiom used to describe unconscious processes"; the shaping of subjectivity through patterned silences is central to the production of meaning in film.[73] Film scholars point out that cinema is unique among media and art forms in that its affective power lies in "a peculiar regime of presence and absence."[74] On the one hand, the "uncommon perceptual richness"[75] of the cinematic image is sometimes taken for a natural or transparent signifier capable of "direct perception without codification."[76] On the other hand, critics have pointed out that the movement of the camera can also reflect attentional shifts and "embody or represent processes of 'lived perception.'"[77] These different perspectives share an implicit acknowledgment that a film delivers the world to perception by the way it construes and communicates meaning.

However, Christian Metz, a French film theorist who pioneered the application of linguistic theory to cinema studies, criticizes this perspective as transcendental idealism. He argues that "consciousness of the world is not a matter of building a picture up from discrete elements of sense data" but rather the "naturalized result of a deeper process of codification."[78] In other words, it's the representational patterns in film that are fragments of already established social and other codes;[79] it is the codes, not direct perception, that make sense out of a film.[80] In this, Metz links cinema's meaning to the social communicative systems I alluded to earlier.

Metz accepted the assumption of psychoanalyst Jacques Lacan (and Sigmund Freud) that "the unconscious is 'structured like a language.'"[81] Thus, he understood conscious perceptions as inextricable from the language systems that we use to think about and express experience[82] and argued, as he did with regard to imagery, against the idea that consciousness is directly transparent. Metz relied on Lacan's view that the psyche is organized by only desire and its repression, and (without necessarily admitting the "only" in that formulation) this supports Metz's argument that the "sense" of conscious behavior may lie in unconscious patterns of established codes. Because consciousness cannot fully grasp or control the meaning of its own acts, to seek perfect phenomenological transparency is neither possible nor necessary. His interdisciplinary methodology anticipates my own approach to cinema analysis.

Specifically, Metz linked cinematographic techniques to grammatical principles that he claimed governed cinematic expression. The cinematic grammar is an outgrowth of unconscious symbolic grammars or patterns that are embedded in culture.[83] His conception of cinema as a language precipitated the critical awareness of cinematic paradigms connected to Hollywood that we saw relate to transnational film. I am most interested in the intersection between cinematic grammar and the unconscious linguistic systems and strategies that it deploys to communicate.

My interest shares terrain with another project of critical scholarship called *hauntology*, which sees in the figure of the ghost a symptom of personal or collective traumatic history;[84] this is a useful interdisciplinary tool in the humanities and social sciences because the ghost is such a versatile metaphor for "the ways in which memory and history, whether traumatic, nostalgic, or both, linger on within the 'living present.'" Ghosts have also been construed as a "figure of resistance for those who are unseen and unacknowledged."[85] Colin Davis, a literary theorist and specialist in hauntology studies, identifies "two strands of hauntology" distinguished by how they see "the status of the secret"[86] and suggests that in this, the history of hauntology may be demonstrating its own tenets. Davis identifies Abraham and Torok's work as the "unacknowledged source of hauntology" but notes that this foundation has been obscured—"virtually removed"—by scholars who approach *all* texts as haunted by the indeterminateness of language; this interpretive position is intellectually informed by the work of French philosopher Jacques Derrida.

Derrida was concerned with the phenomenological, philosophical, and linguistic issues that preoccupied Abraham and Metz. But whereas Metz directed his inquiry into the realm of cinema, and Abraham directed his into the realm of psychoanalysis, Derrida turned his focus to those structures of language that underlie the logic of European philosophy. Like Metz and Abraham, Derrida was interested in how experience comes to be perceived; however, like Abraham, Derrida was interested in uncovering the reason why language means what it means. Abraham's theory of the symbol offers an "emotionally based" explanation for the genesis of patterns that organize languages (and cultures that emanate from them). Derrida's theories postulate a gap that separates language in its use ("texts") from language in its pre-articulated potentiality.

Because the words mean something only by virtue of their relation to other words, Derrida views the actual deployment of language as a foreclosure on its infinitely varied potential meanings. To pay attention to the way texts can both support and undermine their apparent structural cohesion is to perceive that language is intrinsically an unstable representation of reality. Whereas the phantom in Abraham and Torok designates a secret that is unspeakable because it is a subject of shame and prohibition that had to be hidden from view, for Derrida, spectrality is a function of the incontrovertible illegibility of language's origins; what haunts are the ineluctable slippages that occur in language, which point to the limits of what we can know.[87] While ghosts are theorized by all hauntologists to explain gaps between linguistic systems and meaning, Abraham and Torok assert that the gaps point to a fixed or identifiable meaning (a concrete experience) that can be reconstructed, while Derrida's ghost figures "an ethical injunction" against such attempts.[88]

This distinction has deep implications for film criticism. The prevailing hauntological approach reveals a pronounced Derridian inflection. For example, there is a tendency to interpret a character's incongruous speech and acts as an echo of the enduring inaccessibility of meaning.[89] Similarly, the trope of the ghostly return is commonly seen to represent the instability of "orders of knowledge" rather than a spectral communication per se. Spectrality reflects "what has yet to be understood";[90] it is a function of the impossibility of (linguistic) certainty.

Abraham and Torok view phantomatic haunting differently. Phantoms don't just show up, and they don't symbolize the inaccessibility of meaning. On the contrary, they return when a secret (here too an "order of knowledge" or "truth") is threatened with *exposure*, that is, accessibility to conscious awareness. These are ghosts who return to ensure that the subject remains blind to the obliterated traumatic act. They return, in other words, to lie. The "apparent 'revelations' articulated in speech and demeanor are by nature deceitful," and this deceit is "the entire purpose motivating" their presence.[91] Their returns enforce the unconscious obligation to perpetuate concealment of a specific family saga.

In the four films I analyze, haunting is represented by the cinematic trickery and "phantasmagoric deceptions"[92] that are clues to a phantom presence. These techniques recall the work of early film producer and cinema theorist George Méliès (1861–1938), who "located his enterprise within a long tradition of deceptive spectacle."[93] The centerpiece of Méliès's technique was his cinematic manipulation of the physical world. Some critique his execution and aesthetic as more invested in "self-conscious exteriority" than in immersion in character or plot.[94] I find, however, that his exposure of the illusion-generating machinery of cinematic representation has much in common with the compositional strategies of phantom films and illuminates them. For example, Méliès made frequent use of such "altered states of visual perception" as hallucinations and dreams.[95] He experimented with these and other early film "tricks" in his investigation of "the medium's pretension to reproduce reality."[96] Perhaps his most potent effect was the use of phantasmagoric images to confront the spectator with a "visual experience of things we know cannot be."[97]

Méliès was convinced of the capacity of phantasmagoric forms to represent the transition between states of mind.[98] His assurance derived from expertise in producing spectacular magic shows that relied on sleights of hand to induce doubt in perception. His paradoxical simultaneous invocation of the real and unreal calls into question the "distinction between reality and representation, fact and fantasy."[99] His manipulation of the boundaries between these distinctions, another competence deriving from his mastery of illusion, is self-referential; it gives the camera another lens for looking into the world and making sense of it.[100] Méliès's exploration of the illusions underlying the realist mimetic aesthetic reveals the uncanny location of fantasy at the interface of consciousness and unconsciousness.[101] These visual experiences confound expectable sensemaking the way confrontation by a *fantasy* confounds the ego.[102]

Following Abraham and Torok, I view fantasy as "a symptom in its own right: it is the representation of a psychic conflict seeking expression."[103] This is an extremely narrow definition in contrast with more prevalent psychoanalytic understanding of fantasies as "unfulfilled or unfulfillable desires arising chiefly along the path of instinctual development."[104] Abraham and Torok look for the meaning of fantasy in "its *specificity* and operational value"[105] (emphasis added). For them, the meaning of a fantasy is best elucidated by comparison with what it masks, namely, "reality."[106] If "reality" is the source of agitation propelling the psyche to expand,

> fantasy can be defined as all those representations, beliefs, or bodily states that gravitate toward the opposite effect, that is, the preservation of the [psychic] status quo. This definition does not address the contents or the formal characteristics of fantasy, only its function, a preventive and conservative [intrapsychic] function despite the highly innovative genius of fantasy, its vast field of action ... In our conception fantasy is essentially narcissistic; it tends to transform the world rather than inflict injury on the subject['s psyche]... [Fantasies symbolically] refer to a *secretly perpetuated* topography.[107]

Thus, in Abraham and Torok's definition, fantasy is a symptom of preservative repression. It refers to a specific psychic configuration produced to resist self-fashioning processes, and it emerges in response to the psyche's inability to accommodate experience that conflicts with unconscious obligations to conceal an event tainted by unutterable shame.

My four phantom films all tell stories about people who produce fantasies to exempt themselves from the psychic reorganization that would be necessary to accommodate a traumatic experience. They represent this cause-and-effect temporality through cinematographic distinctions between two separate mimetic contexts: one that represents the Abrahamian "reality" of psychic agitation and one that represents the preservative fantasy it triggers.

For example, temporal and spatial boundaries are established in the mises-en-scène that open *The Return* and *A Tale of Two Sisters*, which separate the narrative they contain from the narrative that follows them. Most critics of the films (including fans) note how this framing calls attention to the film's mode of storytelling, though their interpretations of its significance vary. I will demonstrate how these bracketed scenes establish a shot, zeroing in on a scene "in order to allow viewers to situate themselves before a particular event takes place."[108] Establishment shots install the "presence of the reality."[109] In phantom films, reality is always the affective context that seeks psychic accommodation. The narrow focus on this affective context tacitly calls attention to the words that are prohibited from the protagonists' consciousness.

What follows the mise-en-scène in both these films unfolds as a (fantasy) journey that underscores the psyche's need to extricate itself from uncomfortable processes. In the films of del Toro and Amenábar, what follows the initiatory scenes also represents psychic excursions, but the directors use a different technique to distinguish between "reality" and "fantasy." They open their films with the narration of a disembodied voice, which dissipates at the onset of the exposition and thereby signals a shift in focus to the new mimetic context.

The phantom films' juxtaposition of "reality" and "fantasy" parallels Méliès's techniques for calling attention to the "illusory nature of cinema's realist aesthetic." Perhaps even more compelling, the arrangement brings to mind a genre that he invented and called *actualités reconstituées*, a "recreation of current events to which the public has already been exposed via nonvisual media."[110] The oxymoronic context of this genre combines "contemporaneity and retrospection, which might be translated as 'old news,'"[111] which precisely captures the grammatical and semantic relation between the films' openings and the fantasies that follow. The opening scenes are an analogue of the "old news," that is, the shameful transgenerational family affair, the topic the film's representation (or one of the film's representations) conceals. They bracket information that is already "collectively" (unconsciously) known.

The fantasy, on the other hand, is the analogue to Méliès's "recreation" of the old news. It reconstructs the old news in such a way that the spectator can make sense of the representation as a whole. Yet whereas Méliès sought to imbue his reconstructions with historical authenticity,[112] a fantasy, by definition, all but denies it. Fantasies obfuscate beyond recognition any elements that might reveal the source of the disruption—at the same time that they symbolize them. In order to read—that is, to understand—a fantasy, we must acknowledge that reading means *re*reading; the fantasy itself is the rereading of an original "text." It is the affective information already bracketed in the film in a new context. It is a metanarrative.[113]

Del Toro and Kim make overt use of phantasmagoria in their representations of fantasy, while this is virtually absent in Zvyagintsev's and Amenábar's films. Yet Abraham and Torok enable us to recognize that all of these films are organized around the precipitation of a fantasy response to an experience that resists naming. In *Pan's Labyrinth,* it is Ofelia's mother's insistence that she call the sadistic Captain Vidal "father" that catalyzes her psychotic fantasies; in *The Return,* the boy Ivan's traumatic failure to complete a rite of passage is the trigger; for Bae Su-mi in *A Tale of Two Sisters*, the need to acknowledge the double death of her mother and younger sister is resisted by the fantasy of her younger sister's presence; and for Grace Stewart in *The Others*, the death of her husband Charles, who fought against the Nazis in World War II, is the "reality" that her fantasy of postmortem existence seeks to mask.

Phantom Films as Genre

Inasmuch as each of these films embeds a shameful secret, there are certain overlaps among them in technique, tone, and content.[114] While the presence of supernaturalisms—representations of spectralities or ghosts—in three of the four films may suggest that phantom films belong to the genre of horror, the films are linked more tightly by the consistency of their adherence to a singular cinematographic grammar whose sole communicative purpose is to conceal and reveal the secret that haunts it.

Their expressive idioms mimic the conflict at the core of every subject who is haunted by a family secret: the constant oscillation between an investigation of unconscious knowledge and the exertion of every psychic effort to conceal its existence.

All texts haunted by phantoms share these features. For example, Rashkin's analyses of French, American, and English short fiction have uncovered similar grammars in operation; fantasies occur in those texts too, though they are represented more often as short hallucinations or delusions as opposed to functioning as the text's organizing principle as they do in cinema. I will note in my individual analyses the remarkable overlaps among the lexical strategies deployed in the short story narratives and films to conceal secrets. But an even more compelling literary corollary for comparison is William Shakespeare's *Hamlet*.[115]

Hamlet is a tale about a prince who is unable to fulfill the task asked of him by the ghost of his dead father, who ruled Denmark. The ghost enjoins Hamlet to carry out vengeance against Claudius, Hamlet's father's brother, who married Hamlet's mother, Gertrude, upon his father's death. Claudius is a usurper, claims the ghost, and Hamlet's filial duty is to slay him and instate himself as the rightful leader of Denmark. The drama that unfolds depicts him as unable to enact the revenge and portrays him as feigning madness as a way to exempt himself from carrying out the task.

The enduring worldwide success of the drama is explained as an effect of its indecipherable staging of Hamlet's "failure to act."[116] I submit that a similar aesthetic accounts for the widely successful international reception of the phantom films I analyze; the protagonists of these films too have all been identified as enigmatic, while the films are praised for their "meticulous crafting," which both "expects and invites" deep reflection.[117] The question of the characters' motives explains their "lasting hold on our sympathies."[118]

Abraham has analyzed Hamlet's stymied comportment and argues that the latter's anguish over how "to be or not to be" is a symptom of phantomatic haunting. He insists that analysis of the drama should focus *first* on the ghost of Hamlet's father and only *then* on Hamlet, whose lack of agency is thereby construed as a response to the haunting.[119]

Abraham also elucidates how the ghost's request for vengeance is meant to distract Hamlet from conscious apprehension of the ghost's own concealed shameful acts (when alive). "Hamlet is not tormented by conflicts or desires of his own making but by the consequences of a shameful secret his father took to the grave. Hamlet's indecision is the result of events which happened to someone else."[120]

The protagonists of the films analyzed in this book are Hamlet's cinematic alter egos. I should not be misunderstood as suggesting that Shakespeare's drama *Hamlet* is a literary source of inspiration for these films, though at least one film intimates as much.[121] Rather, my point is that all protagonists are stymied like Hamlet; the source of their cinematic subjectivity is a psychic conflict that obstructs self-fashioning. Thus, we see an abundance of "Hamletisms,"[122] that is, enigmatic speech and acts that reverberate with his inexplicable failure to act. Like Hamlet, the protagonists of these films are "poetic entities that implicitly demand to be deciphered."[123] Like *Hamlet*, the films are literary embodiments of collective experience, whose depths we are invited to fathom.

Introducing the Films

The analyses that follow are case studies of four national films whose idioms are organized around the preservation of a secret. In each analysis, I will identify how the portraits of the protagonists cryptically point to an ancestral secret as the specific causative agent of the puzzling behavior and enigmatic subjectivities that are the films' central focus. I will delineate the symbolic lexicon embedded in each film that informs my reconstruction of the secret. Close reading of the relationships among words makes it possible to distinguish between two distinct levels of signification: the surface meaning and the shameful saga that the surface meaning is meant to hide. Having identified these lexical networks, I will use them to interpret other material and expressive components in the film.

I will also demonstrate the enormous potential of lexical analysis, which is unburdened by preconceived cultural significance, for uncovering meanings embedded in texts and cultural patterns, and for appreciating them as fragments of a sociohistorical context that extends beyond the film itself. I do not claim in these historical extensions that the strategy of backward reading can open up all texts; much less do I suggest that this approach alone explains "the meaning" of collective memory and history. Yet I believe that my linguistically grounded analyses will show that phantom films take us deep into the complex factors that drive human behavior over time.

The chapters are arranged in order of the complexity of the films' fantasy structures. I start with del Toro's *Pan's Labyrinth* in Chapter 2 because his phantasmagoria is the most explicit revelation of the four of a film's engagement with the realm of fantasy. I will illustrate how the lavish details of the phantasmagoria spell out the cause of Ofelia's hallucinations: the secret history of cuckolding unwittingly transmitted to her by the tailor who raised her. Tracing del Toro's symbolic representations of Ofelia's suffering backward through history, I am able to link it to broader sociohistorical patterns of silencing, in this case of ethnic (Jewish and Moorish) identity during the Spanish Inquisition. This reading enables a richer understanding of the film's postwar Franquist setting.

Zvyagintsev's award-winning film *The Return* (*Vozvrashchenie*), which I discuss in Chapter 3, is also about a child's inheritance of a secret about cuckoldry. The two films have dramatically distinct aesthetic sensibilities. Unlike del Toro, who relies on phantasmagoria to delineate Ofelia's fantasy, Zvyagintsev relies exclusively on the tripartite structure of the film's narrative segments to demarcate the distinction between "reality" and fantasy. Most critics have seen this dramatic confrontation between father and sons as a depiction of initiation into manhood. I do not reject that insight, but I will argue that the skills and wisdom that this father transmits to his sons pertain not so much to mature masculinity as to unconscious filial obligations to conceal a secret. Ultimately, this reading unveils the film as an allegory of a crucial period in the evolution of Russian collective identity, the reign of Ivan IV.

Kim's internationally hailed masterpiece *A Tale of Two Sisters*, which I analyze in Chapter 4, evokes the disarray and disjunction that occur when post-traumatic self-fashioning is thwarted by the unconscious need to preserve an ancestral secret. The fragmented, disrupted quality of Kim's narrative mimics Bae Su-mi's psychic disintegration. There is a startling psychoanalytic intuition in Kim's style, and it shows, especially in his depictions of the apparitions of Su-mi's fantasy. After reconstructing the secret that haunts Su-mi, her mother's abortion of a near-term fetus, I link this haunting to a collective but unarticulated Korean experience—namely the legacy of Japan's colonial sexual slavery policies. It is only once we have recognized the silenced and disguised intrapsychic drama embedded within the film that we can see how it comments on a larger historical drama.

Like the previous three films, Amenábar's *The Others*, the subject of Chapter 5, makes use of an idiom that points to an intrapsychic secret and the circumstances surrounding it as well as a symbolic lexicon that anchors it within collective sociohistorical frameworks. However, *The Others* is distinct in the way in which its metahistorical commentary ultimately blends back into the film via the silent and ghostly presence of the character whose perspective frames the final shot of the film. The entanglement of this figure—Victor, who I argue is a metaphor for England in 1945—in the secret that haunts Grace and her children reveals the film to be an allegory of England's collective denial of the regicide of Charles I (r. 1625–1649). Amenábar's focus on the processes of symptom formation at the juncture of the individual and the collective is astonishing in its precision and in its scope. It exemplifies the expansive possibilities that the concept of preservative repression affords to historical inquiry.

In Chapter 6, the Epilogue, I submit some insights culled from the previous four analyses and suggest some avenues for continued reflection. Phantom films testify to the powerful role of affect as a shaping force of historical events. The reconstruction of the secrets enabled me to move among different spaces and times along a historical vector shaped by a shameful experience. The movement reveals a trajectory of historical experience that unfolds as a result of two interacting evolutionary processes, biological and cultural.

This dialectical perspective is reinforced by the rich historical significance of the transcultural overlaps that link the films. While the structural similarities can be explained as a function of genre, the very link between shame and genre suggests that phantom structures have something to say about the evolution of literary forms, especially fiction (understood as "fantasy"). I briefly explore the implications of this with regard to the historical significance of the sixteenth and seventeenth centuries in the four phantom films and the fact that specific rulers and their reigns are singled out as generators of affect-laden historical vectors. I suggest that the anxiety over genealogical illegitimacy—as a result of cuckoldry or of religious identity—reflected in these shameful secrets may itself be the work of a phantom haunting a royal lineage. Finally, I note the use of religious symbols to point to the presence of hidden secrets in all four films and the possibility that religious discourse itself might be approached as symbolic of a secret in a family or institutional lineage.

Notes

1 This chapter's title pays sincere homage to Esther Rashkin's seminal and similarly entitled work "Tools for a New Psychoanalytical Literary Criticism: The Work of Abraham and Torok," *Diacritics* (1988): 31–52; revised as "Introduction" in *Family Secrets and the Psychoanalysis of Narrative* (Princeton, NJ: Princeton University Press, 1992).

2 Susannah Radstone, Janet Walker, and Noah Shenker, "Trauma Theory"; Susannah Radstone, Janet Walker, and Noah Shenker, "Introduction to Trauma Theory," *Oxford Bibliographies* (2013). See also idem., "Key Works in Trauma Theory and Film and Media Studies."

3 Robert Rosenstone, *Revisioning History: Film and the Construction of a New Past* (Princeton, NJ: Princeton University Press, 1995), and idem., "A History of What has not yet Happened," *Rethinking History* 4.2 (2000): 183–192 have discussed the positive openings for creative historical research offered by films but also raises the pitfalls of filmic historical reconstructions.

4 Sam Wineburg et al., "Common Belief and the Cultural Curriculum: An Intergenerational Study of Historical Consciousness," *American Educational Research Journal* 44.1 (2007): 40–76.
5 Jeremy D. Stoddard and Alan S. Marcus, "More Than 'Showing What Happened': Exploring the Potential of Teaching History with Film," *The High School Journal* 93.2 (2010): 83–90.
6 Russell Kilbourn, *Cinema, Memory, Modernity: The Representation of Memory from the Art Film to Transnational Cinema*, vol. 6 (New York: Routledge, 2013), 4, 6, 183.
7 Rashkin, "Introduction."
8 Maurice Halbwachs, *On Collective Memory* (Chicago, IL: The University of Chicago Press, 1992), 70–76.
9 Ibid., 70–76 *et passim.*
10 Endel Tulving, "Concepts of Memory," *The Oxford Handbook of Memory* (2000): 33–43; see also Jeffrey K. Olick and Joyce Robbins, "Social Memory Studies: From 'Collective Memory' to the Historical Sociology of Mnemonic Practices," *Annual Review of Sociology* 24.1 (1998): 105–140.
11 See Susan A. Crane, "Writing the Individual Back into Collective Memory," *The American Historical Review* 102.5 (1997): 1376; Endel Tulving, "Concepts of Memory," 33–44; James Wertsch, *Voices of Collective Remembering* (Cambridge: Cambridge University Press, 2002); Michael Rothberg, *Multidirectional Memory: Remembering the Holocaust in the Age of Decolonization* (Stanford, CA: Stanford University Press, 2009); Jeffrey Olick's work has been instrumental to my understanding as well: *The Politics of Regret: On Collective Memory and Historical Responsibility* (New York: Routledge, 2013) and idem., "Collective Memory: The Two Cultures," *Sociological Theory* 17.3 (1999): 333–348.
12 Susannah Radstone, "Reconceiving Binaries: The Limits of Memory," *History Workshop Journal* 59.1 (2005): 48–49. See also Wolf Kansteiner, "Finding Meaning in Memory: A Methodological Critique of Collective Memory Studies," *History and Theory* 41.2 (2002): 179–197, for a critique of collective memory scholarship; Kerwin Lee Klein, "On the Emergence of Memory in Historical Discourse," *Representations* 69 (2000): 127–150.
13 Michael Ignatieff, "Articles of Faith," Index on Censorship Wounded *Nation, Broken Lives—Truth Commissions and War Tribunals* 25:5 (1996): 121.
14 Martha Minow, *Between Vengeance and Forgiveness: Facing History after Genocide and Mass Violence* (Boston, MA: Beacon Press, 1998).
15 Radstone, "Reconceiving Binaries," 137.
16 Ibid., 146.
17 One reason why the binary endures may derive from the close associations between witnessing, testimony, and individual memory in studies of memory processes in post-conflict societies. Scholars have noted how the state uses a language of individual "suffering and recovery to tell the story of the struggle and redemption of a nation." This raises concerns that too much emphasis on individual memory precludes a view of how collective memory operates within structures of power inequalities. See Radstone, Ibid., 146, 148.
18 Nicolas Abraham and Maria Torok, *The Shell and the Kernel: Renewals of Psychoanalysis*, trans. Nicholas T. Rand, vol. 1 (Chicago, IL: University of Chicago Press, 1994).
19 Nicolas Rand, "Introduction," *The Shell and the Kernel*, 1.
20 Ibid., 14.

21 Rashkin, *Family Secrets*, 18.
22 Kali Tal, *Words That Hurt: Reading the Literature of Trauma* (Cambridge: Harvard University Press, 1996) frontispiece; cited in Radstone, "Reconceiving Binary," 146.
23 Habswachs, *Collective Memory*, 57, et passim.
24 Niko Besnier, "Language and Affect," *Annual Review, Anthropology* 19 (1990): 419–451.
25 Bruce Bradfield, "The Dissociation of Lived Experience: A Relational Psychoanalytic Analysis of the Intergenerational Transmission of Trauma," *International Journal of Psychoanalytic Self Psychology* 6.4 (2011): 531, 537–538.
26 Martin S. Bergmann and Milton E. Jucovy, eds., *Generations of the Holocaust* (New York: Columbia University Press, 1982); James Herzog, "World Beyond Metaphor: Thoughts on the Transmission of Trauma" in *Generations of the Holocaust*, 103–119; Nanette C. Auerhahn and Dori Laub, "Intergenerational Memory of the Holocaust," *International Handbook of Multigenrational Legacies of Trauma* (1998) 21–41; Irit Felsen, "Transgenerational Transmission of Effects of the Holocaust," *International Handbook of Multigenerational Legacies of Trauma* (1988): 43–68; and Judith Kestenberg, "Survivor-Parents and Their Children" in *Generations of the Holocaust* (New York: Columbia University Press, 1982).
27 Auerhahn and Laub, "International Memory," 22.
28 Bruce Bradfield, "The Dissociation of Lived Experience," 540. For other studies of transgenerational transmissions of trauma, see Rachel Lev-Wiesel, "Intergenerational Transmission of Trauma across Three Generations: A Preliminary Study," *Qualitative Social Work* 6.1 (2007): 75–94; and Hatsantour Karenian et al., "Collective Trauma Transmission and Traumatic Reactions among Descendants of Armenian Refugees," *International Journal of Social Psychiatry* 57.4 (2011): 327–337; Teresa Evans-Campbell, "Historical Trauma in American Indian/Native Alaska Communities: A Multilevel Framework for Exploring Impacts on Individuals, Families, and Communities," *Journal of Interpersonal Violence* 23.3 (2008): 316–338.
29 Sigmund Freud, *Five Lectures on Psychoanalysis* (New York: Norton, 1990), 21–25.
30 Rand, "Introduction," 1.
31 Many studies of the families of Holocaust survivors demonstrate a link between shame and the transmission of traumatic experience. For example, Jucovy found that "those parents who survived the Holocaust by participating actively as partisans or as ghetto fighters were more likely to tell children about their experiences than those parents who survived the death camps." Milton E. Jucovy, "Psychoanalytical Contributions to Holocaust Studies," *The International Journal of Psycho-Analysis* 73.2 (1992): 271.
32 Ibid., 28–29.
33 Nicholas Rand, "Editor's Note to 'New Perspectives in Metapsychology'" in *The Shell and the Kernel*, 99.
34 Ibid.
35 Ibid., 22.
36 Ibid.
37 Rand, "Introduction," 18.
38 Nicholas Rand, "Editor's Note" to "Secrets and Posterity," *The Shell and the Kernel*, 169.
39 Rashkin, *Unspeakable Secrets and the Psychoanalysis of Culture* (Albany, NY: SUNY Press, 2008), 166.

40 Rand, "Introduction," 3.
41 By this, I mean attempts to account for the formal structures of society in subjective terms. See Emile Durkheim, *The Rules of Sociological Method: And Selected Texts on Sociology and Its Method* (New York: Simon and Schuster, 2014), xxi, 20–50.
42 Rand, "Introduction," 3.
43 Rashkin, *Family Secrets*, 38–39.
44 Ibid., 41–47.
45 Abraham and Torok, *The Shell and the Kernel*, 93.
46 Rashkin, *Family Secrets*, 34–35.
47 *Pan's Labyrinth (El laberinto de fauno)*. Dir. Guillermo del Toro. Picturehouse (2006); New Line Home Entertainment (2007). DVD; *The Return* (*Vozvrashcheniye*). Dir. Andrey Zvyagintsev. Kino International (2004). DVD; *A Tale of Two Sisters* (*Janghwa Hongryeon*). Dir. Kim Jee-woon. IPictures Masulpiri Pictures. Tartan Asia Extreme (2006). DVD. *The Others*. Dir. Alejandro Amenábar. Miramax Lionsgate (2011). DVD.
48 I will reference the critical literature in each respective film analysis. *Pan's Labyrinth*'s worldwide box office sales grossed $87,041,569. *The Return* grossed $5,953,886. *A Tale of Two Sisters* was the first Korean horror film to be screened in American theaters; it grossed $72,541 in its limited release, and its domestic gross was the highest ever for a horror film. *The Others*' worldwide sales grossed $207,765,056. See Nash Information Services, www.thenumbers.com/movie. As for popular acclaim, the review aggregator Rotten Tomatoes reveals positive assessment of the films ranging from 83% (*The Others*) to 95% (*Pan's Labyrinth*, *The Return*).
49 The phenomenon of globalization has been studied as a postmodern consciousness, a mode of cultural production, and a site of international transaction. Whether shaped by uneven capital flows and the destabilization wrought by its inequity or the collapse of colonial systems and their replacement with forms of government—a new political order of globalization—that emerged from subaltern inclinations, globalization is understood as a force defined by oscillating flows—terrestrial, cultural, and psychic—between inner and outer territories that are marked by difference between the familiar and the unfamiliar. See Vicente Rodriguez Ortega, *Transnational Media Imaginaries: Cinema, Digital Technology and Uneven Globalization* (PhD dissertation, New York University, 2007), and Rob Wilson and Wimal Dissanayake, eds. *Global/Local: Cultural Production and the Transnational Imaginary* (Durham, NC: Duke University Press, 1996). Michael Hardt and Antonio Negri, *Empire* (Cambridge, MA: Harvard University Press, 2000) conceive political order of globalization as marked hybrid identities and expanding frontiers; Pheng Cheah, "Spectral Nationality: The Living on of the Postcolonial Nation in Neocolonial Globalization," *Boundary* 2.26 (Fall 1999): 225–252, examines the problem of subjectivity and its representation as legacies of a tradition that associates freedom with agency. See, for example, Homi K. Bhaba's concept of the "double and split time of national representation," which projects onto the nation the fragmented condition subjectivity. Homi K. Bhabha, "DissemiNation: Time, Narrative, and the Margins of the Modern Nation" in *Nation and Narration*, ed. Homi K. Bhabha (New York: Routledge, 1990), 297.
50 Elizabeth Ezra and Terry Rowden, "General Introduction: What Is Transnational Cinema?" in *Transnational Cinema: The Film Reader*, eds. Elizabeth Ezra and Terry Rowden (New York: Routledge, 2006) 1–11.

51 Will Higbee and Song Hwee Lim, "Concepts of Transnational Cinema: Towards a Critical Transnationalism in Film Studies," *Transnational Cinemas* 1.1 (2010): 7–21.
52 Ezra and Rowden, "General Introduction," 1–11.
53 Deborah Shaw, *The Three Amigos: The Transnational Filmmaking of Guillermo del Toro, Alejandro González Iñárritu, and Alfonso Cuarón* (Oxford: Oxford University Press, 2016), 8.
54 Ezra and Rowden, "General Introduction"; Higbee and Lim, "Concepts of Transnational Cinema."
55 Ibid., Chapter 3.
56 Arjun Appadurai was one of the earliest theorists to conceptualize the emergence of a new category of cinematic representation. See his "Disjuncture and Difference in the Global Cultural Economy," *Theory, Culture and Society* 7.2 (1990): 295–310. See also Stephen Crofts, "Concepts of National Cinema," *The Oxford Guide to Film Studies* (1998): 1–10; Tim Bergfelder, "National, Transnational or Supranational Cinema?: Rethinking European Film Studies," *Media, Culture & Society*, 27.3 (2005): 315–331; and Will Higbee and Song Hwee Lim, "Concepts of Transnational Cinema," 7–21.
57 Deborah Shaw, "Deconstructing and Reconstructing 'Transnational Cinema,'" *Contemporary Hispanic Cinema: Interrogating the Transnational in Spanish and Latin American Film* (2013): 54, calls them "paradigms of national cinema.
58 Roger Clark and Keith McDonald, "'A Constant Transit of Finding': Fantasy as Realisation in Pan's Labyrinth," *Children's Literature in Education* 41.1 (2010): 52–63.
59 Bliss Cua Lim, *Translating Time: Cinema, the Fantastic, and Temporal Critique* (Durham, NC: Duke University Press, 2009), analyzes Kim's reworking of the Japanese female ghost trope to reflect on Korean cultural reorganization in the wake of modernization.
60 Monika A. Szumilak, *Reconfiguring Spanish Subjects: Trans/Nationality and Technology in Spanish Narrative and Film after 1992*, PhD Dissertation, University of Michigan, 2005.
61 Lusin Dink, *Andrey Zvyagintsev: The Return, the Banishment, Elena: How Fathers Exile their Children* (PhD Dissertation, İstanbul Bilgi Üniversitesi, 2014), 25–35; for a similar perspective, see Tanja Franotović, "Exiles on the Road: The Role of Cinematic Journeys in the Creation of New Structures of Belonging and Cultural Knowledge," *Ars Aeterna* 1.1 (2009): 53–62.
62 Ibid.
63 Rashkin, *Family Secrets*, 162.
64 Rashkin, *Unspeakable Secrets*, 339.
65 Ella Shohat and Robert Stam, *Unthinking Eurocentrism: Multiculturalism and the Media* (New York: Routledge, 2014).
66 Ibid., 371.
67 Ibid., 364.
68 Ibid., 137.
69 Ibid.
70 Ibid., 140.
71 Ibid., 364 *et passim.*
72 See, for example, Sarah Harwood, *Family Fictions: Representations of the Family in 1980s Hollywood Cinema* (New York: St. Martin's Press, 1997), and Jyotika Virdi, *The Cinematic Imagination [sic.]: Indian Popular Films as Social History* (Newark: Rutgers University Press, 2003), for two excellent examples of analyses based on this premise.

73 Andrea Sabbadini, ed. *The Couch and the Silver Screen: Psychoanalytic Reflections on European Cinema* (New York: Routledge, 2003), 2.
74 Dominique Chateau and Martin Lefebvre, "Dance and Fetish: Phenomenology and Metz's Epistemological Shift," *October* 148 (2014): 122.
75 Ibid., 120.
76 Rand, "Introduction," 6.
77 Daniel Yacavone, "Film and the Phenomenology of Art: Reappraising Merleau-Ponty on Cinema as Form, Medium, and Expression," *New Literary History* 47.1 (2016): 171.
78 Ibid., 167.
79 Chateau and Lefebvre, "Dance and Fetish," 113.
80 Ibid., 129.
81 Joël Dor, *Introduction to the Reading of Lacan: The Unconscious Structured Like a Language* (New York: Other Press, LLC, 1998).
82 He famously theorized that the source of cinema's sense-giving consciousness is its representation of a psyche in what Lacan has termed the "imaginary" stage of psychic development. Metz compared the "situation of the film viewer to Lacan's description of the child looking at itself in the mirror, all the while, in an alienating fashion, (mis)identifying itself with its reflection as it moves towards becoming the subject of the unconscious." Christian Metz, *Le Signifiant Imaginaire: Psychanalyse et Cinéma*, vol. 1134 (Union Générale d'éditions, 1977), 62, 64, cited in Chateau and Lefebvre, "Dance and Fetish," 119, 129. Cf. Merleau-Ponty, for whom "the essence of cinematic art is not the indexical iconic character of the photographic image," as opposed to Bazin's realism, which emphasizes the "life-likeness" of imagistic information discussed in Yacavone, "Film and the Phenomenology of Art," 177.
83 Christian Metz, *Language and Cinema*, vol. 26 (Amsterdam: Walter de Gruyter, 1974), 163–180.
84 María del Pilar Blanco and Esther Peeren, "Introduction: Conceptualizing Spectralities" in *The Spectralities Reader: Ghosts and Haunting in Contemporary Cultural Theory,* eds. María del Pilar Blanco and Esther Peeren (New York: Bloomsbury, 2013), 2.
85 Murray Leeder, "Introduction" in *Cinematic Ghosts: Haunting and Spectrality from Silent Cinema to the Digital Era,* eds. María del Pilar Blanco and Esther Peeren (New York: Bloomsbury, 2015), 1.
86 Colin Davis, "État Présent: Hauntology, Spectres and Phantoms" in *The Spectralities Reader,* eds. Maria del Pilar Blanco and Esther Pereen (New York: Bloomsbury Publishing, 2013), 55.
87 Peter Buse and Andrew Stott, "Introduction: A Future for Haunting" in *Ghosts: Deconstruction, Psychoanalysis, History,* eds. Peter Buse and Andrew Stott (London: Macmillan, 1999), 11.
88 Colin Davis, "État Présent," 58. Jeffrey Mehlman, "The Floating Signifier": From Lévi-Strauss to Lacan," *Yale French Studies* 48 (1972): 13–37, esp. 19–20, 27–37.
89 Llyod Michaels, *The Phantom of the Cinema: Character in Modern Film* (Albany, NY: SUNY, 1998), 157, 16.
90 Colin Davis, *Haunted Subjects: Deconstruction, Psychoanalysis and the Return of the Dead* (New York, Springer, 2007), 11.
91 Ibid., 84.
92 Jordan Bear, "From Magician to Metal Brain: The Embodiment of Illusion in Early European Film Theory," *Studies in European Cinema* 5.1 (2008): 18.
93 Ibid.
94 Ibid., 18–19. Theorists also "mistrust[ed] the unmarked 'deceit' of many 'invisible' classical special effects"; Julie Turnock, *Plastic Reality: Special*

Effects, Art and Technology in 1970s U.S. Filmmaking (PhD Dissertation, University of Chicago, 2008), 10, n. 17.

95 Ibid., 21.

96 Elizabeth Ezra, *George Méliès* (Manchester: Manchester University Press, 2000), 55. See also Anna Powell, *Deleuze, Altered States and Film* (Edinburgh: Edinburgh University Press, 2007), 2–15, who offers a typology of films that induce altered states. Powell demonstrates how these films rely on a formal temporal grammar that stimulates speculative thought.

97 Joshua David Bellin, *Framing Monsters: Fantasy Film and Social Alienation* (Carbondale, IL: SIU Press, 2005), 14.

98 Ezra, *George Méliès*, 50.

99 Ibid., 51, 149.

100 Ibid.

101 Ibid. Powell, *Deleuze*, 72, discusses how the "hallucinating camera is disjunctive, shifting relation to the perceptions of characters. It does not attempt to record individual hallucinations but, rather, displays outward behavior objectively, without explaining enigmatic behavior."

102 Abraham and Torok, Ibid.; Powell, *Deleuze*, 72, discusses how the "hallucinating camera is disjunctive, shifting relation to the perceptions of characters. It does not attempt to record individual hallucinations but, rather, displays outward behavior objectively, without explaining enigmatic behavior."

103 Abraham and Torok, *The Shell and the Kernel*, 125.

104 Nicholas Rand, "Editor's Note," "Instruments of Therapy," 24–25.

105 Ibid.

106 Abraham and Torok, *The Shell and the Kernel*, 125.

107 Ibid.

108 Elizabeth Ezra, *George Méliès*, 44.

109 Ibid.

110 Ibid., 63.

111 Ibid.

112 Ibid.

113 Ibid., 72.

114 Lim, *Translating Time*, 12–13, 34–45.

115 William Shakespeare, *Hamlet* (New York: Norton, 1992).

116 R. A. Foakes, *Hamlet Versus Lear: Cultural Politics and Shakespeare's Art* (Cambridge: Cambridge University Press, 1993), 22. The first quote cites Foakes; the second, an assessment of the drama made by Victor Hugo, is cited in Foakes, Ibid., 14.

117 Lim, *Translating Time*, 239, *et passim*, approaches transnational cinema that is organized by the salience of "supernaturalisms"—ghosts and spectralities. She argues that they instantiate temporal multiplicity because a ghost introduces the legacy of someone else's life into the timeline of an individual subject. The confluence of different temporalities is understood by Lim as an implicit critique of the dominance of global visual language, whose legibility purports a shared present that denies or minimizes distinct (national) pasts.

118 Ibid.

119 "The Phantom of Hamlet or the Sixth Act, Preceded by the Intermission of 'Truth'" in *The Shell and the Kernel*, 187–205.

120 Nicholas Rand, "Editor's Note," "Secrets and Posterity: The Theory of the Transgenerational Phantom," 167.

121 We shall see below that Guillermo del Toro's *Pan's Labyrinth* suggests possible literary filiations.

122 Foakes, *Hamlet Versus Lear*, 21.
123 Rashkin, *Family Secrets*, 162. My suggestion that Abraham and Torok's concepts yield a way to break out of the dynamic repression binary mode of thinking about memory and representation shares an objective with Will Higbee, Saër Maty Bâ, and others who argue for the need to transcend binary, Eurocentric theoretical underpinnings of global film analysis and interpretation; *De-Westernizing Film Studies* (New York: Routledge, 2012), especially their "Introduction," 1–16.

Bibliography

A Tale of Two Sisters (*Janghwa Hongryeon*). Dir. Kim Jee-woon. IPictures Masulpiri Pictures. Tartan Asia Extreme (2006). DVD.

Abraham, Nicolas, and Maria Torok. *The Wolf Man's Magic Word: A Cryptonymy*. Vol. 37. University of Minnesota Press, 2005.

Abraham, Nicolas, Maria Torok. Trans. Nicholas Rand. *The Shell and the Kernel: Renewals of Psychoanalysis*. Vol. 1. University of Chicago Press, 1994.

Adams, Brett, Chitra Dorai, and Svetha Venkatesh. "Novel Approach to Determining Tempo and Dramatic Story Sections in Motion Pictures." *2000 International Conference on Image Processing, 2000. Proceedings*. Vol. 2. IEEE, 2000.

Ancuta, Katarzyna. "Spirits in Suburbia: Ghosts, Global Desires and the Rise of Thai Middle-Class Horror." *Horror Studies* 5.2 (2014): 233–247.

Appadurai, Arjun. "Disjuncture and Difference in the Global Cultural Economy." *Theory, Culture & Society* 7.2 (1990): 295–310.

Assmann, Aleida. "Memory, Individual and Collective." *The Oxford Handbook of Contextual Political Analysis* 9 (2006): 210–226.

Bear, Jordan. "From Magician to Metal Brain: The Embodiment of Illusion in Early European Film Theory." *Studies in European Cinema* 5.1 (2008): 17–29.

Beller, Jonathan L. *Desiring the Involuntary: Machinic Assemblage and Transnationalism in Deleuze and Robocop 2*. Rey Chow, Harry Harootunian, and Masao Miyoshi. *Global/local: Cultural Production and the Transnational Imaginary*. Duke University Press, 1996. 193–218.

Bellin, Joshua David. *Framing Monsters: Fantasy Film and Social Alienation*. SIU Press, 2005.

Bergfelder, Tim. "National, Transnational or Supranational Cinema?: Rethinking European Film Studies." *Media, Culture & Society* 27.3 (2005): 315–331.

Bergmann, Martin S., and Milton E. Jucovy. *Generations of the Holocaust*. Columbia University Press, 1982.

Besnier, Niko. "Language and Affect." *Annual Review of Anthropology* 19.1 (1990): 419–451.

Bhabha, Homi K. *Nation and Narration*. Routledge, 1990.

Bradfield, Bruce. "The Dissociation of Lived Experience: A Relational Psychoanalytic Analysis of the Intergenerational Transmission of Trauma." *International Journal of Psychoanalytic Self Psychology* 6.4 (2011): 531–550.

Braga, Luciana Lorens, Marcelo Feijó Mello, and José Paulo Fiks. "Transgenerational Transmission of Trauma and Resilience: A Qualitative Study with Brazilian Offspring of Holocaust Survivors." *BMC Psychiatry* 12.1 (2012): 134.

Branigan, Edward. *Point of View in the Cinema: A Theory of Narration and Subjectivity in Classical Film*. Vol. 66. Walter de Gruyter, 1984.

Buse, Peter, and Andrew Stott. Eds. *Ghosts: Deconstruction, Psychoanalysis, History*. London: Macmillan, 1999.

Chateau, Dominique, and Martin Lefebvre. "Dance and Fetish: Phenomenology and Metz's Epistemological Shift," *October* 148 (2014): 103–132.

Cheah, Pheng. "Spectral Nationality: The Living on of the Postcolonial Nation in Neocolonial Globalization." *Boundary* 2.26 (1999): 225–252.

Crane, Susan A. "Writing the Individual Back into Collective Memory." *The American Historical Review* 102.5 (1997): 1372–1385.

Crofts, Stephen. "Concepts of National Cinema." *The Oxford Guide to Film Studies*, 1998. 1–10.

Davis, Colin. *Haunted Subjects: Deconstruction, Psychoanalysis and the Return of the Dead*. Springer, 2007.

———. "État Présent: Hauntology, Spectres and Phantoms." *The Spectralities Reader Ghosts and Haunting in Contemporary Cultural Theory*. Eds. Del Pilar Blanco and Esther Pereen. Bloomsbury, 2013. 54–50.

Del Pilar Blanco, María, and Esther Peeren. Eds. *The Spectralities Reader: Ghosts and Haunting in Contemporary Cultural Theory*. Bloomsbury Publishing USA, 2013.

Derrida, Jacques. *Margins of Philosophy*. University of Chicago Press, 1982.

Dink, Lusin. *Andre Zvyagintsev: The Return, the Banishment, Elena: How Fathers Exile their Children*. PhD Dissertation. İstanbul Bilgi Üniversitesi, 2014.

Dor, Joël. *Introduction to the Reading of Lacan: The Unconscious Structured Like a Language*. Other Press, 1998.

Durkheim, Emile. *The Rules of Sociological Method and Selected Texts on Sociology and Its Method*. Simon and Schuster, 2014.

Erll, Astrid and Ansgar Nünning. Eds. *Cultural Memory Studies: An International and Interdisciplinary Handbook*. Berlin and New York: de Gruyter, 2008.

Evans-Campbell, Teresa. "Historical Trauma in American Indian/Native Alaska Communities: A Multilevel Framework for Exploring Impacts on Individuals, Families, and Communities." *Journal of Interpersonal Violence* 23.3 (2008): 316–338.

Ezra, Elizabeth, and Terry Rowden. *Transnational Cinema: The Film Reader*. Taylor & Francis, 2006.

———. *George Méliès*. Manchester University Press, 2000.

Felsen, Irit. "Transgenerational Transmission of Effects of the Holocaust." *International Handbook of Multigenerational Legacies of Trauma* (1988): 43–68.

Foakes, Reginald Anthony. *Hamlet Versus Lear: Cultural Politics and Shakespeare's Art*. Cambridge University Press, 2004.

Franotović, Tanja. "Exiles on the Road: The Role of Cinematic Journeys in the Creation of New Structures of Belonging and Cultural Knowledge." *Ars Aeterna* 1.1 (2009): 53–62.

Freud, Sigmund. *Five Lectures on Psychoanalysis*. Norton, 1990.

Halbwachs, Maurice. *On Collective Memory*. University of Chicago Press, 1992.

Hardt, Michael, and Antonio Negri. *Empire*. Harvard University Press, 2000.

Harwood, Sarah. *Family Fictions: Representations of the Family in 1980s Hollywood Cinema*. St. Martin's Press, 1997.

Herzog, James. "World beyond Metaphor: Thoughts on the Transmission of Trauma." Eds. Bergmann, Martin S., and Milton E. Jucovy. *Generations of the Holocaust*, 1982. 103–119.

Higbee, Will, and Song Hwee Lim. "Concepts of Transnational Cinema: Towards a Critical Transnationalism in Film Studies." *Transnational Cinemas* 1.1 (2010): 7–21.

Jucovy, Milton E. "Psychoanalytic Contributions to Holocaust Studies." *The International Journal of Psychoanalysis* 73.2 (1992): 267–282.

Ignatieff, Michael. "Articles of Faith." *Index on Censorship Wounded Nation, Broken Lives—Truth Commissions and War Tribunals* 25:5 (1996): 110–122.

Kansteiner, Wolf. "Finding Meaning in Memory: A Methodological Critique of Collective Memory Studies." *History and Theory* 41.2 (2002): 179–197.

Karenian, Hatsantour, et al. "Collective Trauma Transmission and Traumatic Reactions Among Descendants of Armenian Refugees." *International Journal of Social Psychiatry* 57.4 (2011): 327–337.

Kestenberg, Judith S. "Survivor-Parents and Their Children." Eds. Bergmann, Martin S., and Milton E. Jucovy. *Generations of the Holocaust.* Columbia University Press, 1982. 83–101.

Kilbourn, Russell. *Cinema, Memory, Modernity: The Representation of Memory from the Art Film to Transnational Cinema.* Vol. 6. Routledge, 2013.

Klein, Kerwin Lee. "On the Emergence of Memory in Historical Discourse." *Representations* 69 (2000): 127–150.

Leeder, Murray. "Introduction." *Cinematic Ghosts: Haunting and Spectrality from Silent Cinema to the Digital Era.* Ed. Murray Leeder. Bloomsbury, 2015. 1–14.

Lev–Wiesel, Rachel. "Intergenerational Transmission of Trauma across Three Generations: A Preliminary Study." *Qualitative Social Work* 6.1 (2007): 75–94.

Lim, Bliss Cua. *Translating Time: Cinema, the Fantastic, and Temporal Critique.* Duke University Press, 2009.

Luckhurst, Roger. *The Trauma Question.* Routledge, 2013.

Mehlman, Jeffrey. "The 'Floating Signifier': From Lévi-Strauss to Lacan." *Yale French Studies* 48 (1972): 10–37.

Metz, Christian. *Language and Cinema.* Vol. 26. Walter de Gruyter, 1974.

Michaels, Lloyd. *The Phantom of the Cinema: Character in Modern Film.* SUNY, 1998.

Minow, Martha. *Between Vengeance and Forgiveness: Facing History after Genocide and Mass Violence.* Beacon Press, 1998.

Olick, Jeffrey K., and Joyce Robbins. "Social Memory Studies: From 'Collective Memory' to the Historical Sociology of Mnemonic Practices." *Annual Review of Sociology* 24.1 (1998): 105–140.

———. "Collective Memory: The Two Cultures." *Sociological Theory* 17.3 (1999): 333–348.

———. *The Politics of Regret: On Collective Memory and Historical Responsibility.* Routledge, 2013.

Ortega, Vicente Rodriguez. *Transnational Media Imaginaries: Cinema, Digital Technology and Uneven Globalization.* PhD Dissertation. New York University. 2007.

Pan's Labyrinth (El laberinto de fauno). Dir. Guillermo del Toro. Picturehouse (2006). New Line Home Entertainment (2007).

Powell, Anna. *Deleuze, Altered States and Film*. Edinburgh University Press, 2007.

Radstone, Susan. "Decolonizing Trauma Theory." *Oxford Bibliographies*.

———. "Reconceiving Binaries: The Limits of Memory." *History Workshop Journal* 59.1 (2005): 134–150.

Radstone, Susan, and Bill Schwartz. *Memory: Histories, Theories, Debates*. New York: Fordham University Press, 2010.

———. "Cinema and Memory." *Memory: Histories, Theories, Debates*, 2010. 325–342.

Radstone, Susan, Janet Walker, and Noah Shenker. "Introduction." *Trauma Theory. Oxford Bibliographies*. 2013.

——— "Key Works in Trauma Theory and Film and Media Studies." *Oxford Bibliographies*. 2013.

Rand, Nicholas and Nicolas Abraham. "Family Romance or Family History? Psychoanalysis and Dramatic Invention in Nicolas Abraham's 'The Phantom of Hamlet.'" *Diacritics* (1988): 20–30.

Rand, Nicholas, Nicolas Abraham, and Maria Torok. "The Sandman Looks at 'the Uncanny." *Speculations after Freud: Psychoanalysis, Philosophy, and Culture* (1994): 185–204.

Rashkin, Esther. "Tools for a New Psychoanalytic Literary Criticism: The Work of Abraham and Torok." *Diacritics* (1988): 31–52.

———. *Unspeakable Secrets and the Psychoanalysis of Culture*. SUNY Press, 2008.

———. *Family Secrets and the Psychoanalysis of Narrative*. Princeton University Press, 1992.

Rosenstone, Robert A. Ed. *Revisioning History: Film and the Construction of a New Past*. Princeton University Press, 1995.

———. "A History of What Has Not Yet Happened." *Rethinking History* 4.2 (2000): 183–192.

Sabbadini, Andrea. Ed. *The Couch and the Silver Screen: Psychoanalytic Reflections on European Cinema*. Routledge, 2005.

Shakespeare, William. *Hamlet*. Norton, 1992.

Shaw, Deborah. *The Three Amigos: The Transnational Filmmaking of Guillermo del Toro, Alejandro González Iñárritu, and Alfonso Cuarón*. Oxford, 2016.

———. "Deconstructing and Reconstructing 'Transnational Cinema'." Dennison, Stephanie. Ed. *Contemporary Hispanic Cinema: Interrogating the Transnational in Spanish and Latin American Film*. Tamesis Books, 2013. 47–66.

Shohat, Ella, and Robert Stam. *Unthinking Eurocentrism: Multiculturalism and the Media*. Routledge, 2014.

Stam, Robert. "Film and Language: From Metz to Bakhtin." *Studies in the Literary Imagination* 19.1 (1986): 109–130.

Stoddard, Jeremy D., and Alan S. Marcus. "More Than 'Showing what Happened': Exploring the Potential of Teaching History with Film." *The High School Journal* 93.2 (2010): 83–90.

Szumilak, Monika A. *Reconfiguring Spanish Subjects: Trans/nationality and Technology in Spanish Narrative and Film after 1992*. PhD Dissertation. University of Michigan. 2005.

Tal, Kali. *Words That Hurt: Reading the Literature of Trauma*. Harvard University Press, 1996.

The Others. Dir. Alejandro Amenábar. Miramax Lionsgate (2011). DVD.

The Return (*Vozvrashcheniye*). Dir. Andrey Zvyagintsev. Kino International (2004). Kino International (2004).

Tulving, Endel. "Concepts of Memory." *The Oxford Handbook of Memory* (2000): 33–43.

Turim, Maureen. *Flashbacks in Film: Memory and History*. New York and London: Routledge, 1989.

Turnock, Julie A. *Plastic Reality: Special Effects, Art and Technology in 1970s US Filmmaking*. PhD Dissertation. University of Chicago, 2008.

Virdi, Jyotika. *The Cinematic Imagination [sic]: Indian Popular Films as Social History*. Rutgers University Press, 2003.

Wertsch, James V. *Voices of Collective Remembering: Test*. Cambridge University Press, 2002.

Wilson, Rob, and Wimal Dissanayake., Eds. *Global/Local: Cultural Production and the Transnational Imaginary*. Durham, NC: Duke University Press, 1996.

Wineburg, Sam, et al. "Common Belief and the Cultural Curriculum: An Intergenerational Study of Historical Consciousness." *American Educational Research Journal* 44.1 (2007): 40–76.

Yacavone, Daniel. "Film and the Phenomenology of Art: Reappraising Merleau-Ponty on Cinema as Form, Medium, and Expression." *New Literary History* 47.1 (2016): 159–185.

2 Haunted Inheritance

Fantasy as Phantom in Guillermo del Toro's *Pan's Labyrinth*

> What is a ghost? A tragedy doomed to repeat itself time and again? An instant pain, perhaps. Something dead which still seems to be alive. An emotion suspended in time. Like a blurred photograph. Like an insect trapped in amber. A ghost.
>
> —Doctor Caseres,
> Guillermo del Toro's *The Devil's Backbone*

Guillermo del Toro's *Pan's Labyrinth*,[1] an Oscar-winning masterpiece, established his reputation as a masterful artist who "set a new model for world cinema."[2] The technical brilliance of the film's plotting, shooting, and editing, not to mention the stunning art design complete with sophisticated and subtle digital effects, would have justified the plaudits showered on the director. But it is his ability to use the mise-en-scène to simultaneously represent and comment on a historically haunting era—1944, post-Civil War Spain—that has elicited the most praise and criticism from critics.[3]

The film tells the story of a girl, Ofelia, who, along with her pregnant mother, Carmen, moves to a country mill where her new stepfather—Vidal, a violent Franquist captain—is stationed. Ofelia meets a shadowy faun with ambiguous intentions; he reveals her true identity: She is a princess, the daughter of the king of the underworld, and she must perform three tasks to rejoin him: slay a parasitic frog living in the roots of a dying fig tree; recover a silver dagger hidden in the lair of a rapacious monster; and sacrifice an innocent (her baby half brother) at the center of the film's namesake, the labyrinth. Ofelia does her best to fulfill the missions set before her as her new stepfather seeks to crush the Republican guerillas surrounding the mill.

Del Toro explicitly describes the imagery used to portray Ofelia and the faun's interaction as fairy-tale discourse. The director's signature phantasmagoric vision has drawn considerable attention.[4] Critics have argued about the "realness" of Ofelia's experience with the faun, a question that del Toro does not address.[5] How to reconcile the fairy-tale discourse with the other, realist components of the film has been a particularly vexatious issue. And, indeed, del Toro's world is ambiguous: At times.

the mystical elements in Ofelia's fantasy appear to influence the events of the people living in the captain's mill, but at other times, the symmetry between her experiences and the particular components of her fantasy suggests that she is instead reacting to the trauma she experiences.[6]

Many explanations for the significance of the phantasmagoric discourse focus on the way it balances political tensions in the film by offering two visions; whereas fascism is the way the world is, fantasy is the way the world seems.[7] To some, the intersection of the two worlds challenges narrative expectations and thereby indirectly offers "commentary on war, obedience and gender relations."[8] Others have seen the imagery's implicit reference to "key codes and conventions of children's literature" as a gloss on fascism; the phantasmagoria represents it as images of the "taboos of human nature."[9] Several critics have approached the surrealistic dimension of the story from the psychoanalytical perspective of collective repression; phantasmagoria is seen to challenge the official national memory of the Spanish Civil War.[10]

Del Toro's own explanation for his vision likely accounts for the critical inclination to interpret his use of phantasmagoria in terms of fascism. He spoke of a desire

> to uncover a common thread between the 'real world' and the 'imaginary world,' which I found in one of the seminal bloodlines within fairytales: the bloodline of choice... I thought it would be great to counterpoint an institutional lack of choice, which is fascism, with the chance to choose.[11]

Because fairy tales represent the chance to choose, they are suitable for representing the disorienting effects of fascism on society; they are also appropriate for mediating those horrible dimensions of Spanish fascism that were repressed.[12]

My interpretive position concurs with the reigning view that the phantasmagoric imagery represents a traumatic experience, a rupture of some sort, figured by the realist and phantasmagoric dimensions of the film. However, I invoke Nicolas Abraham and Maria Torok's conceptualization of fantasy to interpret the central ambiguity of the film. If we read the phantasmagoria as a sequence of fantasies defined as a symptom of preservative repression, then they do not simply reflect a need to parry the danger of Vidal or fascism more generally. Rather, we must understand the fantasies as products of a trauma caused by the unconscious obligation to preserve a shameful secret. To uncover the secret, it is first necessary to identify the affective context that triggers Ofelia's fantasy production, Abraham's "reality." This will guide our reading of the film's cinematographic idiom and will reveal how the exquisite and meticulous details of del Toro's phantasmagoric mises-en-scène communicate information that extends beyond its association with renewal myths or children's fairy tales.

The film's cinematographic idiom encourages this approach. The symmetry between Ofelia's daily experience and the texture of her fantasy may be construed as two permutations of her life, one conscious, the other unconscious. Indeed, the filmic juxtaposition of two layers, one subterranean and magical, and the other the earthly plane of the captain's mill, suggests an analogue of a psychic topography. The simultaneous coexistence of reality and the faun's world inside Ofelia indicates that the distinction between both has been eroded. This suggests that if the phantasmagoria embodies an allegorical dimension of the film, it must be understood in terms of a specific pathology afflicting Ofelia as a distinct character. This allows us to shift our view from questions about how the fantasy discourse comments on fascism in order to focus more narrowly on *what caused* her to produce a fantasy in the first place. Once we uncover how the phantasmagoric imagery conjures an embedded family saga, we will be in a better position to (re)situate it within the social and historical context of the film's Franquist setting; we will be able to see how it allegorizes the structure and processes of a collective psyche, of Spain itself.

The Affective Context

As delineated in Chapter 1, phantom films are structured by the temporality of fantasy production. The film's first frames reveal compositional elements pointing backward toward prior significations. We are first shown Ofelia dying, with bloody hands and face, yet almost instantly, the blood dripping from her nose reverses the direction of its flow. While many critics have interpreted this backward gesture as a demarcation of the opening's metanarrative function to "set up a duality" between fascist reality and escapist fantasy,[13] no one has considered the possibility that it is directly linked to the ambiguity of Ofelia's fantasy.

The opening lines of *Pan's Labyrinth* are narrated by a disembodied voice. The narration, which begins just as the blood recedes back into Ofelia's nose, situates us within a graveyard, the "underworld," a place where neither "lies" nor "sadness" exists, where a king awaits the return of his daughter, Princess Moanna, who escaped long ago. The reference to subterranean topography calls attention to the location's status as a screen for the unconscious. The allusions to crypts (an underground palace), and desolation over the loss of a daughter, raise the possibility that the death of Ofelia's father (which lead her mother to remarry) is the "reality" that demands psychic reorganization, that is, the loss of the tailor is a causative agent of Ofelia's fantasies.

More specifically, the discorporate preamble anchors Ofelia's fantasies in a context of inhibited or blocked mourning as the result of a need to preserve an unspeakable secret. This idea is supported by the rhetorical effect of the overdetermined denial of the existence of "lies" in the land of the king, which implies the possibility that the assertion (namely that no lies existed in the land) is false, suggesting it conceals something that cannot be spoken. The denial calls to mind the famous Shakespearean line "The lady doth protest too much, methinks," which is spoken by Hamlet's mother, Gertrude, to him in the drama. Her comment refers to Hamlet's production of a play in which the central character, a queen like Gertrude, declares that she will never remarry if her husband dies.[14] Hamlet's drama within a drama tacitly critiques his mother's decision to marry his uncle, Claudius, when his father died. This chain of thought, which alerts us to the possibility of a link between *Hamlet* and *Pan's Labyrinth*, is not gratuitous: Ofelia's name, not to mention her madness and tragic demise, implicitly connects her to *Hamlet's* Ophelia, and the issue of a mother remarrying is what initiates the development of the film's plot.

The discorporate voice evokes the unseen presence of a secret in the psyche; it establishes a discursive boundary that separates the content of its narration from the ensuing mimesis, signaling its communicative function as a gloss for the latter. Its disappearance mimics how the unconscious excludes a shameful saga from a psyche's (perceptual) awareness. The disembodied narrator also evokes the ghost of Hamlet's father; his injunction that Hamlet take revenge on Claudius is a facade; it is meant to detract Hamlet from his unconscious awareness of the silenced shame. *Pan's Labyrinth*'s disembodied narrator figures a similar type of apparition.

The narrator alleges that Ofelia's departure from the underworld is the source of her royal father's inconsolable grief. His use of the word "escape" to describe her withdrawal from her father may be construed as a cryptic condemnation of her psyche's inclination toward expansion in the wake of his loss; accommodating the loss is a precondition for the gradual, assimilative work of mourning. Ofelia's "escape" renders her father grief-stricken because it points to her unconscious investigation of knowledge about him that is prohibited from awareness. That this implied (psychic) transgression lies at the root of her fantasy production is suggested by the overlap of the disembodied narration with the imagery of her and her mother en route to Vidal's mill.

The mimeses begin by establishing Ofelia's preoccupation with books, *libros*, which tacitly affirms the narrator's implication that she is indeed investigating prohibited knowledge. As in English, the word "book" is used to connote "records," such as "registers," "licenses," and "registrations," as well. Ofelia's insistence on bringing so many books intimates a commitment to an inquiry or inspection. If the narrator condemns Ofelia's "escape," however, Carmen champions it; she speaks of the "free" (fresh) air of the country, *al aire libre*, as a preferable alternative to reading. Indeed, Carmen dismisses the fairy-tale books as objects not worthy of Ofelia's affective attachment, given her age—right at the cusp of adolescence. The context of Carmen's words inverts the priorities and positions presented in the preamble. Her words encourage Ofelia to "move on," to withdraw from the father. This conflict between two different inclinations, one preservative and one expansive, is the "reality" that triggers Ofelia's production of a fantasy.

Directly after Carmen utters these comments, her pregnancy-induced nausea brings a halt to the trip. This break in the flow of the mimesis, which has only just begun, signals the initial stages of Ofelia's psychic disintegration: During this standstill, she has her first vision of the imaginary world that will soon engross her. *Freed* from the car to *explore* the environs while her mother recuperates, Ofelia discovers a Celtic statue that is absent an eye; after replacing its stone eyeball, which is on the ground, Ofelia sees a saga that is prohibited from consciousness. This gesture causes a stick bug to crawl out from the statue's *mouth*, a metonym of language.

The stick bug, a member of an order of insects known as the *Phasmatodea,* or "phantom bug," is redolent with spectral significance. The name, derivative of ancient Greek, is inspired by the insect's capacity for camouflage, which makes it extremely difficult to spot. As a result, its sudden movement appears as an apparition. The causal link between Ofelia's act and the stick bug's emergence more precisely delineates the unconscious processes that operate in fantasy production. If we construe the gaping hole that marks the mouth as the location for assimilative speech, the stick bug's materialization also marks the mouth as the site where lying language is given expression. The stick bug is the imagistic realization of deception, concealment, phantoms, and prohibited psychic assimilation; it is the phantasmagoric representation of the return of a phantom (Figure 2.1).

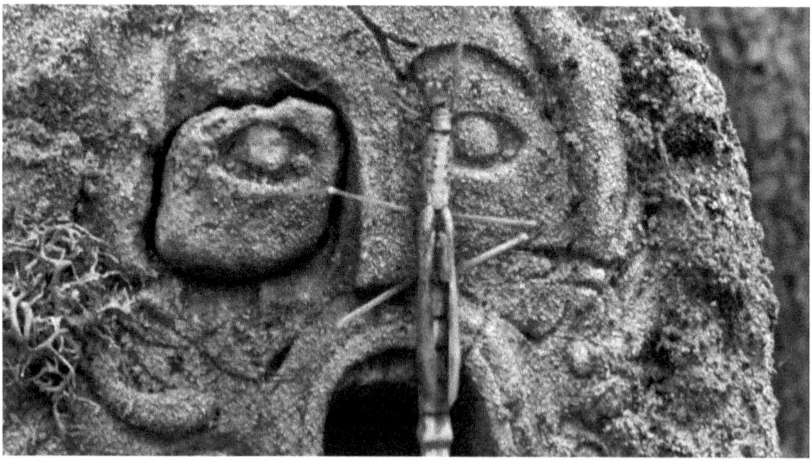

Figure 2.1 Initiation of fantasy: The "phantom bug" emerges from the mouth of the statue after Ofelia has reinserted the left eye.

The causality intrinsic to the sequence of acts—Carmen's prohibitions against reading fairy tales, her subsequent pregnancy-induced nausea, and Ofelia's fantasy production—warrant closer inspection. The film's unambiguous attention to the particles of floating pollen in the scene emphasizes Carmen's fecundity; because her queasiness obstructs the flow of the trip, it implies that something about her pregnancy relates to Ofelia's fantasy production. The film's representation of an interrupted journey bears comparison to obstacles in self-fashionings. It anchors the blockage to Ofelia's self-fashioning in a context of investigations and prohibitions, and to Carmen's fertility. When these associations are reconciled with the reversed shot of blood streaming back into Ofelia's nose, we see in this backward gesture a cryptic reference to a return to one's origin, or more specifically, one's *bloodline*.[15]

Preservative Lexical Strategies

While the manifest content of the preamble refers to Ofelia's origins as a princess, it is significant that although terms such as "your highness," "your majesty," and "princess" dot the dialogue, never once is the Spanish word *real*, "royal," used. This linguistic aspect of the story is noteworthy. The theoretical premise underlying this analysis suggests that this word is hidden because of its connection to some unspeakable drama regarding the nature of Ofelia's royal origins: in fact, the Spanish word *real* is a homophone; another meaning of the word is "real," as in the sense of "true" or "authentic."

I argue that this meaning has undergone an unstated transformation: It has been transmuted in the story into its homonym *real*, "royal," with its set of entirely different associations. In other words, the "royal" conceit of the fantasy enacts a lexical and phonetic encryption that elides the meaning of the word *real* as "true." The faun's insistence that Ofelia return to her royal parentage is now revealed as subterfuge. To take literally the narrator's claim of her true regal origins is to mistake the manifest linguistic meaning for its latent content. The "quest" to return the princess Ofelia to her royal father, the manifest content of the fantasy, must now be read more specifically as related to her need to keep preserved some unspeakable *truth* about her bloodline.[16]

This reading is supported by a network of linguistic subterfuges executed through prohibitions and interdictions throughout the film. Carmen not only voices an interdiction against reading fairy tales, but she also implicitly imposes a prohibition against using the word "father" to speak of the dead man. These two expressions follow the Celtic statue scene and accentuate the sense of censorship that permeates relations between Ofelia, her father, Carmen, and Vidal.

Into this context we must also insert the faun, whom Ofelia meets late at night during her first night at the mill. She is led to a labyrinth by the fairy, who is a disguised emanation of the stick bug. Several critics have seen in the faun a father figure of sorts, one who guides and disciplines; most have read the faun's paternal role as restoring the absent authority of Ofelia's father.[17] When the faun first meets her, he more concretely identifies himself as the horned creature incised in the obelisk at the center of the labyrinth. He also identifies the baby, the *niña*, as Ofelia, which suggests he is a disguised incarnation of the deceased father, the tailor, whose misery Ofelia is tasked to relieve.

The faun's characterization stages the way a phantom works to ensure that the psyche stays on task, resists its own assimilative inclination, and therefore preserves the status quo in the wake of a traumatic loss. The status quo is to forgo freedom and return to the father's crypt. The story of Ofelia's royal lineage, which is the *sole* rationale for undergoing the trials that the faun sets out for her, suggests that it is the false—not *real*—nature of these would-be revelations that motivate them.

The deceptive strategy is meant to trick Ofelia's psyche by substituting a story of her father's loss and therefore deny that she herself has suffered any loss that needs accommodation. Carmen extenuates the emotional impact that the death may have had on Ofelia as well but on another level. Directly after Ofelia has seen the stick bug, when mother and daughter are back in the car moving toward the mill, Carmen insists that Ofelia address Vidal as "father." Ofelia resists. Carmen justifies inserting the word "father" into her daughter's mouth in nebulous terms: He has been "so very good to us, daughter, you can't [even know] know how much."[18] She dismisses the word's referential function, "it's only a word, Ofelia, nothing but a word," to drain it of affective charge.[19]

A similar resistance to acknowledging Ofelia's father is evidenced in ellipses that mark references to him in other parts of the film. Although Carmen mentions him, briefly, at Vidal's dinner table, he quickly ends the discussion, effectively prohibiting her from speaking more about him. The audience learns that he died during the Civil War (the details remain elisions in the script) and that he sewed the captain's men's uniforms; Vidal censors her before she reveals anything substantial. The silence instituted by the captain exposes an uncanny network of thwarted speech at play at his dinner table, where the adult characters convene to eat.

In phantom films, eating scenes virtually always function as metaphors for the obstacle to self-fashioning that befalls the protagonists. We have established how naming presupposes the psyche's cognizance of the assimilation of experiences.[20] Vidal's dinner party scene is nothing if not a portrait of a problematic naming; del Toro's representation reflects an intuitive understanding of a link between blocked or suspended verbalizations and problematic self-fashioning.

Consider the conversation between Carmen and a couple of the wives who attend the dinner. The dialogue is initiated when the doctor's wife questions why Carmen is not eating. Carmen replies that she has no appetite; this leads the mayor's wife to ask Carmen how she came to know the captain. Carmen tells them of how, during the war, Ofelia's father sewed the captain's men's uniforms. A year after the tailor's death, she and the captain "met again," *nos volvimos a encontrar*. The verb *volvimos* (inf. *volver*), "to return, to come back, to start again," elicits discomfort in Vidal, who releases Carmen's hand from his own on the table. The catty women sitting opposite Carmen raise their eyebrows in suspicion. Vidal interjects to excuse his wife's naiveté for believing that such a worldly crowd would find her silly stories of interest. This statement circumscribes Carmen from speaking more about their romance. Because this silencing gesture conclusively denies her the opportunity to speak about a timeline for her and Vidal's romantic history, it raises the possibility that something about the timeline is unspeakable and cannot be shared.[21]

More information is provided in the film's only other reference to their romance, when Ofelia asks her mother why she married Vidal. The scene takes place during their first night at the mill; it directly precedes her first meeting with the faun, discussed earlier. When the scene begins, Carmen and Ofelia are talking about night noises; Carmen explains to a slightly fearful Ofelia that the "house is old, it moans and complains as if it speaks."[22] This account of a house that speaks prompts Ofelia to ask her mother why she "had to get married." Carmen responds that she was "lonely for too long," but this explanation does not sit well with Ofelia. She counters, stating that Carmen was never alone, for she, Ofelia, was always with her. At this juncture, Carmen winces in pain and asks Ofelia to narrate a story to the fetus of her brother in order to soothe his inquietude with her voice. Carmen's pregnancy-induced pain recalls her earlier nausea because it also deflects Ofelia's question about what she meant by being lonely.

Ofelia compliantly narrates a story about a magical rose endowed with power to bestow immortality. The rose grows alone on the top of an enormous mountain of black stone in a desolate and sad country. Because poisonous thorns surround it, it is blocked from bestowing its power on people, who are unable to reach it. The rose wilts as a consequence of this blockage. Ofelia concludes by observing that humans fear pain more than they want immortality. As she narrates the story, images of her fetal brother aglow in warm red and gold colors are interspersed with images of a rose; in addition, images of the mountain, distinguished by its palette of blues and grays, which dominate the scenes of the labyrinth/crypt, also appear.

These latter images displace the image of Ofelia speaking to her mother's protruding belly. The substitution disembodies Ofelia's voice, echoing the sense of otherness that was produced by the film's opening narration. Because that voice bracketed information that related to Ofelia's father's secret, its repetition here suggests that it performs a similar denotative function, that is, Ofelia's narrative and the images should also be construed as bracketed and therefore pertinent to the secret as well.

There is lexical evidence to support this interpretive position. Recognizing how Ofelia's story emerges in the wake of her dissatisfaction with her mother's account of why she married Vidal, we can see how it represents Ofelia's version of what lies behind the silenced affect bound to Carmen's unsatisfying articulation of her reasons. The word for "romance story" in Spanish is composed of the two words "rose," *rosa*, and "novel," *novela*. However, the word "rose," *rosa,* is also used to refer to accounts of salacious romantic engagements, as in the term "tabloids," *prensa rosa*. In this light, Ofelia's story suggests Carmen and Vidal's romance involves something poisonous that harms like a "thorn in the side."

The interpolation of images of the fetus with those depicting the rose, when Ofelia's narration becomes disembodied, intimates a contiguity between the rose and her unborn baby brother. The appearance of the stick bug amid these images, just as she approaches the narrative about the poisonous thorns, links both images to the presence of a phantom. While most critics view the story as a metaphoric account of Carmen's loneliness, the appearance of this rose on Ofelia's clothing when she returns to the crypt at the end of the film suggests, alternatively, that she is, in fact, the (unconscious) referent of her story.

When juxtaposed with Ofelia's previous conversation with her mother about the haunting effects of a house that "speaks" in "groans and complaints," we can hear her story as a disguised articulation about a haunted "house," or "lineage," *casa*. The impotence of the rose refers to the inability of a lineage to thrive beyond the death of its members. Read in tandem with scandalous connotations of a romance and the association between these and circumstances surrounding the marriage between Carmen and Vidal, as well as Ofelia's unborn brother, this invites an interrogation of Ofelia's paternity. Indeed, it suggests that Vidal is not only the father of the unborn son but also the father of Ofelia.[23] A close examination of the elements comprising Ofelia's fantasy will bear this out. Del Toro's phantasmagoria becomes fertile ground for extrapolating this drama as it is inscribed in the film.

The Trials

Before Ofelia sets out on her first task, she dons a dress, sewn by her mother, to wear to a dinner given in honor of the arrival of Vidal's new family. Critics have noted the striking resemblance between the dress and that worn by Alice in Wonderland, with its bold colored dress and white apron, and they interpret it as del Toro's nod to escapism implicit in children's literature.[24] The context in which Carmen reveals the dress to Ofelia, however, yields other interpretive possibilities. First, just before she presents the dress, Carmen has made it very clear that she wants Ofelia to make her father, Vidal, proud of her poise at the dinner. The elegant dress, meant to be an object for Ofelia's coming of age, elicits from Carmen a betrayal of her own disappointed transition to adulthood: "What I wouldn't have done for a dress like that when I was your age."[25] Second, Carmen's turn as a clothier suggests an affinity with the profession of her former husband. This congruence perhaps relates to conditions leading to her marriage with the tailor, and her sense of a less than satisfying coming of age.

Ofelia sheds the dress in order to complete the first task assigned by the faun; her disrobing also signals that the context is no longer one of coming of age but of full-fledged motherhood. Her objective is to retrieve a key from a toad hiding in the roots of a gargantuan and sickly fig tree. Its appearance is uncannily libidinal, visually echoing the floating pollen of the fantasy initiation scene. Moreover, the tree's form (curling, symmetrical branches) suggests a fallopian and ovarian motif, which is also mirrored in the faun's horns. Ofelia climbs through a suggestively vaginal opening at the tree's base; crawls through a narrow, cervical passageway; and approaches the toad in a womb-like chamber under the tree. These gynecological significations represent Ofelia's journey to the toad in the roots of a tree as a journey to her genealogical origins. The fig tree and its fruit are implicated in Western society as tropes related to sexual vulgarity and shame. Adam and Eve covered their sexual organs with fig leaves after transgressing God's prohibition,[26] and "making the fig," *dar una higa*, gesture (with the thumb between the forefinger and middle finger) is recognized in Spain to refer to (unsanctioned) copulation (Figure 2.2).[27]

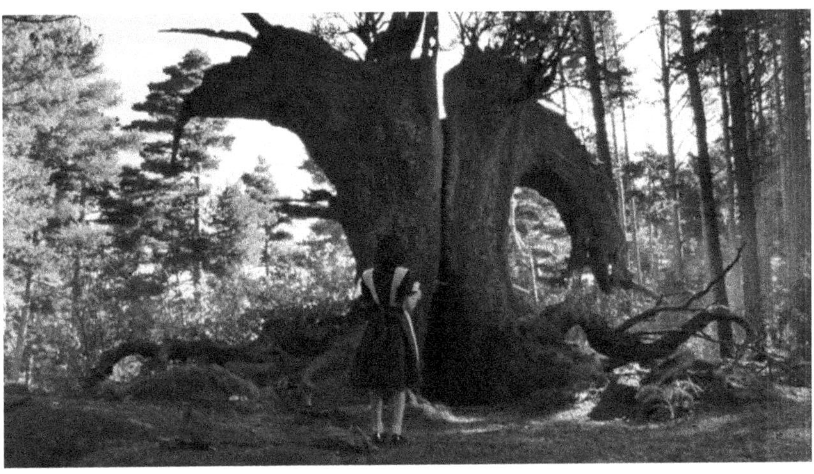

Figure 2.2 Ofelia standing before the dying fig tree.

The salience of the root motif is also heightened by the significance of the mandrake root in the film. Promising it as a cure for Carmen's pregnancy pains and hemorrhaging, the faun hands it to Ofelia with instructions to prepare it in milk and drops of her blood. As she pricks her finger over the mandrake, she sees it animate, tossing and turning in the milk in symmetry with Carmen's tossing in bed. She later awakes feeling rejuvenated and healthy, and Ofelia's magic potion seems to have worked, that is, until Vidal finds it. Ashamed of Ofelia, and of her own susceptibility to the charm of the root, Carmen responds by throwing it in the fireplace, chiding Ofelia for her belief in magic.

The root's ancient and highly overdetermined mythology invites a wide range of interpretations. Most significant for our analysis is its appearance in a transaction between the sisters Leah and Rachel in Genesis 30. Rachel, Jacob's infertile second wife, desires Leah's mandrakes; in exchange, Leah is permitted to sleep in Jacob's bed and subsequently ends her own spell of infertility. The faun's bequest of the root, an object at the center of an interchange of spouses in a Biblical text about family origins, tacitly implicates the tailor in a context of problematic fecundity.

When we read this together with Ofelia's retrieval of a key from the guts of the toad at her biological roots, we find affirmation that the man Ofelia knew as father, the tailor, was not, in fact, her biological father; rather, his place in the roots of her family tree was emptied of his presence and occupied by someone else, much as the enormous toad disrupted the growth of the fig tree. Ofelia's task declares the fact of the tailor's displacement, but the imagery also suggests that he was aware and unavoidably complicit in this deed. The phantasmagoric toad who swallowed the key and blocks expansion is none other than a figure of an unpleasant affective situation that had to be denied assimilation: it declares how the tailor had "to put up with," or "stomach the toad," *tragar sapo*, that is, to swallow and not voice his feelings about something.[28]

The symmetry between the fallopian motif and the faun's horns reinforces the idea that the tailor knew he was not Ofelia's biological father. Although most critics have interpreted the faun's physique in terms of its mythical resonance with the Greek Pan archetype, a goat-god or horned beast, a "god of revelry and fertility,"[29] the "horns," *cuerno*, may also be more concretely construed as marking him as a "cuckold," *cornudo* (Figure 2.3).

The faun is depicted as a giant Billy goat, or *cabrón,* to denote someone who was "cheated by his wife," *engañado por su mujer*. The etymological link between the verb "to cheat," *engañado*, and the word *genesis*, the origin or mode of formation, links cuckolding and conception. This chain of signification is linguistically reinforced by fact that the word for "key," *llaves*, which was buried in the toad's gut and was the source of the tree's demise, is a word commonly used to substitute the taboo word "horns" in speech. The faun incarnates the concept of a cuckold, just as

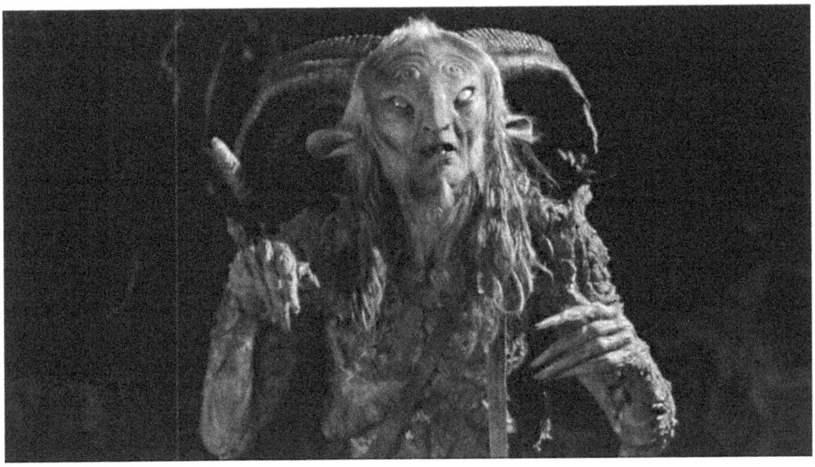

Figure 2.3 The faun's horns.

the frog animates the concept of someone who swallowed an uncomfortable experience related to "keys," that is, "horns." He is the spectral representation of the drama of a husband who has witnessed his wife's deception and was given horns. The father not only knew about his wife's infidelity but also knew that it led to Ofelia's conception. Cuckoldry is the source of Ofelia's origins and the source of the demise of the tailor's family tree.[30]

The physical images of curves and spirals that link concepts of biological genealogy to the faun's cuckolded position also shed light on the symbolism of the labyrinth trope. The labyrinth is an appropriate spatial representation of the cuckold's horns; the word *laberinto* cryptically refers to its unspoken Spanish synonym, *dédalo*, itself a synonym for *lio*, which means a "tangled mess," "fling," or "romantic affair" implicated in scandal. Just as the archetypal labyrinth in Greek mythology was constructed by Daedalus to hide and conceal the offspring of an adulterous affair between Pasiphae and the white bull given to her husband Minos by the god Poseidon, so too does it figure in Ofelia's fantasy as a symbol of a concocted means to hide the unspeakable secret of her adulterous origins.

The Pale Man

The labyrinth figures the psychically excluded or shut-up "reality" of Ofelia's true paternity. Its resemblance to a prison that keeps captive the part-man part-bull progeny of an adulterous relationship brings clarity to the specificity of certain details in what is perhaps the most celebrated phantasmagoric scene of the film, the Pale Man scene. For example, while virtually all critics have seen the Pale Man as a monstrous representation of Vidal and, by extension, fascism, the revelation that Vidal is the biological father of Ofelia brings to the fore explicit aspects of his character that resonate with his symbolic identity. For example, the pallid skin tone of this ghoulish avatar associates him with the white bull that fathered a child with the adulteress Pasiphae. The Pale Man's chalky pallor brings to mind the figurative Spanish expression *pálido como la cal*, "pale as limestone," as well as the expression *a cal y canto*, "to be shut tight, silenced," which evokes the Pale Man's encrypted status. Indeed, the chemical components of limestone, which make it a quality sealant—properties that are the source of the etymological derivation of the verb *callar*, "to silence, hush, keep secret,"—may explain why the faun provides Ofelia with chalk, another form of calcium carbonate, to enter and depart from his crypt. As the bubbling of the chalk trace marks indicate, it is an effective material to ensure that anything within its perimeter will be secure and locked in.

Other details, such as the dinner setting, also point to this symbolic subtext. Every review of the film notes how the setting of the Pale Man scene constructs dinner party symmetrical to the one Vidal hosts at the mill: at both, a man sits at the head of the long table in front of a fireplace (Figure 2.4).

The fact that Ofelia concocts this moment, which eerily resembles an event that she did not observe, further implicates an act of witnessing in the shameful drama that haunts her. Indeed, the pervasive

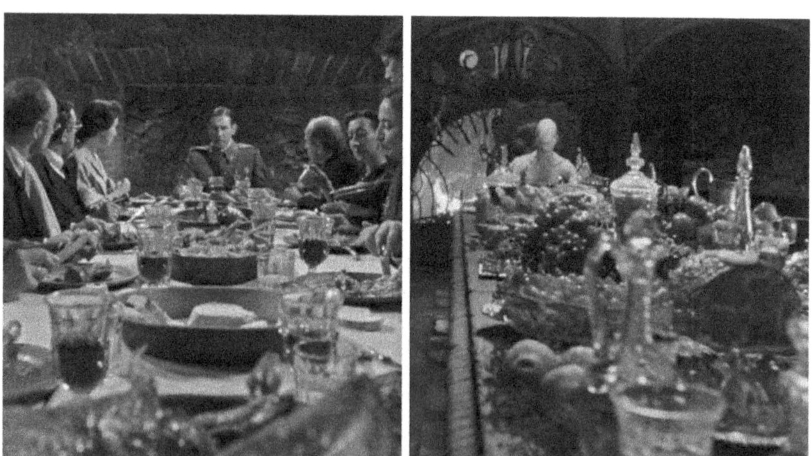

Figure 2.4 The captain and the Pale Man's dinner tables.

presence of eye imagery in the film, from Ofelia's replacement of the eye of the Celtic statue, to the monocle worn by Vidal as he cleans his watch, to the eyes implanted into the palms of the Pale Man, may be read as a veritable ocular poetics born of an unutterable experience of witnessing.[31]

The faun's explicit prohibition against eating any of the delectable food that Ofelia sees on the banquet table makes it clear that what is seen cannot be psychically named. The Pale Man's inability to eat the sumptuous feast before him (the folds of skin and his coloring suggest he was once corpulent but is now malnourished) symbolically stages the repercussions of psychic dyspepsia, a function of his hermetic concealment. Ofelia's physical hunger, a result of her mother's interdiction against eating dinner because she disappointed Vidal, symbolizes her psychic hunger for assimilative expansion. Significantly, the object that Ofelia chooses to consume tacitly enunciates the very drama that is precluded from digestion.

Although several critics have noted that Ofelia selects a fruit to eat, as opposed to the viands or sweets that are loaded on the table, their interpretations of its significance align with the general tendency to read the film as an allegory of resistance against fascism. Thus, Ofelia's consumption of the "forbidden fruit" is viewed as a defiant (often viewed as feminist) gesture against the patriarchal order of fascist rule. There is no doubt that Ofelia's transgression is analyzable in this way, but these persuasive readings fall short of explaining just why Ofelia chose a "grape," *uva*, instead of, say, a strawberry or cherry or persimmon. As my analysis of the fantasy has shown, these details often function as lexical fragments or symbols that cryptically intone a dimension of the concealed unspeakable drama.

Such is the case with the word "grape," which linguistically echoes the film's prominent display of visual motifs related to gynecology. Etymologically related to the Latin term for ovaries, the word *uva* also denotes the vine upon which the fruit grows, *la vid*; thus, it not only resonates with the arboreal motif related to genealogical origins but also aurally calls to mind Vidal's name thus linking him to her roots. The lexical fragments "grape" and "vine" cryptically point to the biological source of Ofelia's lineage, but the fruit, by metonymy, refers as well to the juice it produces, "wine," *vino*. *Vino* is homophonous with the conjugated third-person past-tense form of the verb "to come from," *venir*,[32] which yields another example of how operative linguistic strategies shape her choice of the grape: for Ofelia, eating the grape symptomatically constitutes an attempt to assimilate the source from whence "she came," *Ella vino de su padre—Vidal.*[33]

The evocative semantic resonance between grapes, vines, wine, and biological origins widens when we consider how grapes are featured in medical etymology related to eyes. For example, the vascular layer of the eye, or choroid, which contains the connective tissue of the eye, is named the *uvea*, because it resembles the darkened skin of a grape. The choroid is marked by the dark-colored pigment melanin, which helps limit uncontrolled reflection within the eye, which would potentially result in the perception of confusing images.[34] These two physiognomic characteristics of the choroid, the membranous texture and dark pigment, are given striking prominence in the Pale Man's two eyeballs, which Ofelia is moved to inspect closely.

First, Ofelia's close scrutiny causes her to look away from the grape; the subtle but significant eye gesture registers unconscious awareness of a link between eyes and the grapes. These connected emotional stimuli point to two separate aspects of the drama of Ofelia's conception. When she eats the grape, she is the daughter who wants to digest and name the context of her origins. In thus doing, however, Ofelia threatens to uncover the source of the tailor's shame: he was a husband who was aware of this cuckolded status.[35]

This association between grapes and eyes discloses a logic that makes intelligible the Pale Man's actions consequent to Ofelia's ingestion of the grape, which awakens him. The obvious causality between Ofelia's transgression of the faun's (the tailor) injunction against eating and the animation of the Pale Man brings to the fore his symbolic significance in the fantasy. If the duplication of the Vidal's dinner scene suggests that the Pale Man is a phantasmagoric representation of the former, then his presence in Ofelia's fantasy must be understood as a refracted dimension of the tailor's shame. This is confirmed by the sequence of the Pale Man's actions.

First, he reinserts his eyes into their sockets, which are located in each of his hands. The eyes, resting on a golden platter before him, evoke tropes of witnessing in Catholic rituals,[36] while the holes in his palms evoke the marks corresponding to the crucifixion wounds of Christ, the *stigmata*. As signs that mark a painful (physical and) affective experience, *stigmata* implicitly brand their bearer. The Pale Man's gestures thus connect the act of witnessing with the stigmatization by it.[37] When he raises his hands to his head to align the eyes in the palms with the normative location of eyes in the head, his fingers extend beyond the surface of the face, to resemble the most prominent and protruding feature of the faun's head, namely his "horns." His movements cryptically enact the source of the stigma that enforces psychic censorship on Ofelia: the Pale Man literally "puts horns on the head," *poner los cuernos*; he stages Vidal's role in branding the tailor as a cuckold. The tailor's stigma is symbolized and imprinted by the Pale Man's creation of "horns." (Figure 2.5)[38]

While frightening, the Pale Man's eyeless face nonetheless represents what is necessary for preserving the status quo of his crypt: blindness to the duping experienced by the tailor. Ofelia's effort to accommodate her unconscious knowledge of her parentage threatens the integrity of

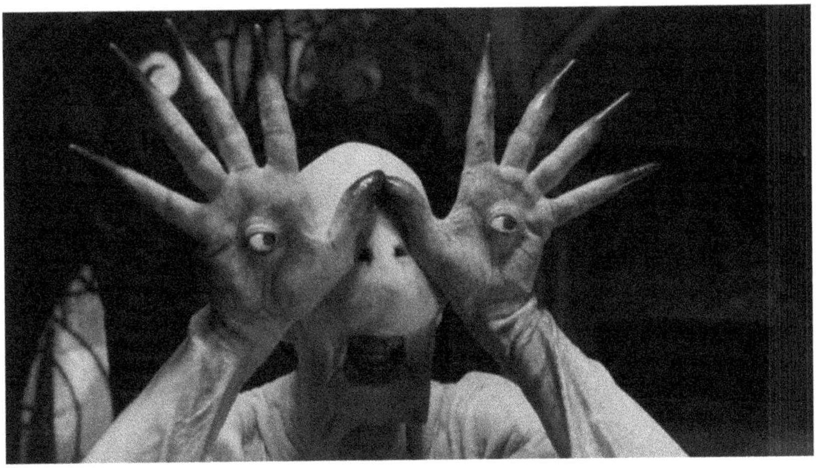

Figure 2.5 The Pale Man "puts horns on the head."

this crypt. The Pale Man's "nakedness" emblematizes the "unraveling," (also, "to be naked,") *desnudar*, of something that had been *binding*, like a "knot," *nudo*. Ofelia's unconstrained ingestion of the grape, a blatant transgression of the rules of the task, is tantamount to severing her filial obligation to preserve the tailor's secret. Ofelia's experience in the Pale Man's crypt reveals the (psychic) stakes of "bearing one's soul and speaking freely," *desnudarse*: it will expose the secret and lead to the unraveling of psychic integrity.

Having ascertained how the symbol of the Pale Man fits in with the larger drama of the tailor's secret, we can appreciate the subtext of del Toro's allusions to bloodthirsty, ruthless destroyers of innocence, which are displayed in murals in the crypt. Many have noted the influence of Spanish painter Francisco Goya (1746–1828) on del Toro's set design, especially *Saturn Devouring His Son*, a tableau belonging to the Black Paintings, which Goya painted on the walls of his dining room.[39] Del Toro substitutes the Pale Man for the Greek god Cronus, who consumed his child because he fears that it will supplant him, as he supplanted his own father; the painting allegorizes how a child's life is devoured by an unconscious obligation to preserve a parent's secret.[40] The alignment of the Pale Man with Cronus, a metaphor for the passage of time, also sheds light on the clockwork nature of a phantom's psychic existence. The mechanized nature of the Pale Man's response to Ofelia's ingestion of the grape and the hourglass that establishes temporal parameters within which she must complete her task both emphasize how the subjective temporality of a haunted descendant is always defined by the traumatic moment of an ancestor's life.

Vidal's Phantom

The assumption that the film is a critique of Fascism grounds most critical interpretations of Vidal's character, which see him as an emblem of the extreme depravity of the political ideology. In light of the foregoing discussion, however, I suggest that preserved silence may also be implicated as a source of Vidal's cinematic subjectivity. Just as the dinner scene, fraught with thwarted speech, yielded encrypted content related to Ofelia's fantasy, so also does it serve as a crucial starting point for an investigation of Vidal's patrimony. After Carmen excuses herself from the table upon Ofelia's return to the mill, the party resumes, and one of the captain's men asks Vidal about the lore surrounding his father. According to legend, the man begins, Vidal's father died in battle in Morocco but not before smashing his watch against the *suelo* (the English subtitles read "a rock," but the word *suelo* means literally "earth, land"), to commemorate the exact moment for his son. Vidal denies the very existence of the watch, thus enveloping the object in unspeakable silence and performing the scene's second prohibition against linguistic expression.

Vidal's refutal, even though the watch is an object of his obsessive interest throughout the film, suggests something about his father must be concealed. The story, which links Vidal's father with the "earth," presents him as a loyal Spanish officer during the Rif War of 1920 (also known as the Second Moroccan War). But the multivalent word *suelo*, which can mean both physical earth and also "soil" in a geopolitical sense, complicates the picture: if understood in its latter sense, Vidal's father's acts tacitly point to a link between Moroccan soil and the site of his *suelo de patria*, or ancestral homeland.[41]

Vidal's disavowal of knowledge about the watch emerges as an ellipsis generated by this implicit connection between Morocco and his father.[42] Since Vidal clearly inherited the watch whose existence he denies, his behavior justifies an investigation of another form of paternal inheritance, namely a secret about an ethnic identity. Vidal's refutation is symptomatic of the psychic obligation to carry a moment in time that is shrouded in silence. Indeed, del Toro's consistent framing of the watch's appearance (often as Vidal wears a loupe and toys with its gears, repairing and reviving it) with visual echoes of the huge gears and wheels in Vidal's study, and in the millwheel attached to the building outside, reveals the mill itself to be crypt-like, holding Vidal who lives *under his father's watch* and *in his father's time*.

Secrets of Tainted Blood

The seemingly incongruous placement of the scene depicting the treatment of gangrene, suffered by the Republican guerilla Frenchie, bolsters this interpretive position. Although the scene occurs outside of both

Ofelia's and Vidal's story lines, and thus does nothing to forward the plot, del Toro's meticulous storytelling process and attention to detail suggests that it serves some thematic purpose. The scene depicts the amputation of Frenchie's infected leg. The surgery justifies why the rebels need the antibiotics, which the doctor and house manager Mercedes smuggle from the mill; it also provides an explanation for Vidal's fury over the fact that they have been stealing it. Upon his discovery of a smuggled package of antibiotics in the woods, the camera closes in on Vidal's face; the juxtaposition of Vidal's face and the vial of antibiotics implicitly present a semantic opposition: Vidal, whose name comes from *vida*, "life," and "antibiotics," *antibiótico*, which means "anti-life." The antibiotics, the object Vidal most wants to control, are precious because they *purify the blood.*

Vidal's obsession with antibiotics is a symbol fragment that permits reconstruction of a secret of his ethnic identity.[43] Having seen how Ofelia's fantasy encrypts her genealogy through arboreal metaphors of branches and roots, it is not surprising to find an echo of this lexical resonance here. These links imbue the amputation scene with much greater symbolic significance than its loose relationship with the unfolding of events might suggest. The *Oxford English Dictionary* records that the word "to amputate," *amputar*, derives from the Latin *amputare*, "to prune around (a tree)." The amputation, literally an excision of *tainted blood*, evokes the idea of pruning a *family tree.*

This sense clearly reverberates with Vidal's obsession with Spain's "clean," "new," *limpia y nueva* race, which he claims his son will represent. His penchant for purity may now be interpreted as a symptom of his own shameful drama of a hidden (ethnic) bloodline. I will illustrate in the following how construing the source of Vidal's behavior as symptomatic of haunting by a shameful secret of ethnic identity explains the distinctive features of his violent streak as something more determined than a representation of the evils of fascism. Rather, Vidal's assertion of his pure line is symptomatic of a phobia-inducing phantom, which "haunt[s] in order to move the haunted persons to expose a concealed and unspoken parental fear."[44]

Vidal's references to a "clean" and "new" Spain, along with his concerns about pruning a family tree, evoke the political mantel of husband-and-wife team of Isabella I of Castile and Ferdinand of Aragon II, who in 1492 completed the so-called Reconquista, or Christian Reconquest of Spain from Muslim rule.[45] Eager to attract papal blessings and, in Isabella's case, gripped by genuine religious fanaticism and belief in the protoracist doctrine of "clean blood," *limpieza de sangre*, Spain's ruling classes endeavored to prove themselves free of Moorish or Jewish "taint."[46] The urgency of this endeavor was shaped by the "confounding presence of the converso," Muslim or Jewish people who had undergone baptism to convert to Catholicism as a means to remain in Spain.[47]

Oftentimes, these converts continued to practice their religion in secret, which marked them as crytpo-Muslims or crypto-Jews; thus, "fear of betrayal or unmasking stimulated by the Inquisition and exacerbated by the great mobility of the *conversos* was foundational to their identity."[48]

Many scholars have noted that the status of the *converso* became, curiously, an *inherited* status, which affected the descendants of families who had converted generations earlier.[49] This was also the case for those *conversos* who left Spain as a result of expulsion edicts. Significantly, a majority of those expelled from Spain went to Morocco, which offers a historical context for the implied reference to this country as Vidal's "fatherland."[50] The fact that Christians categorized Muslims "as a type of infection, disease or pollutant that threatened the health of the Christian population"[51] if they continued to perpetuate their own bloodlines makes sense of Vidal's desire to amputate a family tree. Vidal's interrogation of the housekeeper Mercedes and his murder of the doctor, which reveals a fixation on identifying and eradicating incognito insurrectionists "under [his] nose," may also be interpreted as a symptom of a concealed *converso* identity. His apprehension over enemies in his own home betrays an anxiety over foes hiding in his family lineage.

Converso Phantoms

The Pale Man scene offers clues that point more precisely to the details of Vidal's hidden ethnicity. I submit that while there is no doubt that the tailor's cuckolded shame comprises the central material of the mise-en-scène, it nonetheless also resonates with lexical symbols in the film's idiom that point to a shameful legacy haunting Ofelia's biological father. I suggest that this fold over derives from the fact that the secrets of both the tailor and Vidal were ultimately generated by the same collectively repressed experience—the genealogical purges carried out by the Inquisition tribunals. I will show how the film's characterization of Vidal draws from a symbolic lexicon associated with the Inquisition to represent his cinematic subjectivity as haunted by his father's secret (Moorish) identity; I will then illustrate how the tailor's silencing of his cuckolded status may point to his haunting by a Jewish one.

The architecture of the Pale Man's crypt includes details such as articulated archways, pillars, and tiled mosaics, which evoke Moorish, or Mudéjar, influence. Moorish domination in Spain between 711 and 1492 left Spain with lasting examples of classical Islamic architecture.[52] During the reconquest of the Iberian Peninsula from the Moors in the eleventh to fifteenth centuries, subject Muslims were allowed to retain Islamic laws, customs, and religion and to live in their own quarters in return for owing allegiance and paying tribute to a Christian monarch.[53] Inflected with Mudéjar resonance, the crypt tacitly alludes to Vidal's Andalusian roots.

Vidal's unconscious awareness of a Mudéjar identity is manifested symptomatically as sadism when he tortures Frenchie, whose leg was amputated earlier; this suggests a link between Vidal's cruelty and the context of pruning a family tree. Psychically, the pruning is effected by the exclusion of words that resonate with the shameful secret; this leads to an idiom of expression that is constituted by patterned muteness, such as that experienced by a "stutterer," *tartamudear.* Frenchie suffers from this affliction of speech as well as gangrene. His condition, a result of tainted blood and obstacles to speaking, convokes for Vidal an unconscious awareness that motivates the precise approach he takes to Frenchie's torture.

The phonetic overlap between the word *mudear*, which connotes "the notion of muteness,"[54] and the word Mudéjar (they are phonetically indistinguishable) brings greater clarity to the unconscious source of Vidal's acts. Frenchie is a Republican and thus is perceived as anathema to Vidal's national pure-blood ideals. His offer to *free* the stutterer if he is able to "count to three without s-s-stuttering," *cuentas hasta tres sin t-t-tartamudear*, recalls Ofelia's desire to escape the underworld.[55] It suggests Vidal's unconscious desire to free himself of the condition of imposed muteness. On the other hand, the torturous conditions virtually vitiate any confidence in the possibility of release.

This conflict explains the extremity of Vidal's violence toward Frenchie. If we listen to the word *tatamudear*, we can hear that two words are combined in its phonetic structure: *tata* and *mudear.* John Beusterien explains the verbal merger as a lexical marker of spoken stuttering: The *tata* represents the delivery of word in a stutterer's speech, whereby repeated consonants "are followed by an 'a' sound."[56] Still, the fact that the *word* that is pronounced *tata* connotes *father* or *grandfather* also suggests that the combination might be *heard* as "father's muteness" or even "father [the] Mudéjar." Either way, the speech impediment mutely recapitulates for Vidal an unconscious awareness of Andalusian origins, which was transmitted unwittingly to him as a shameful patrilineal legacy. The "vocal handcuffs" of the stutterer enrage Vidal because they tacitly point to his Mudéjar patrimony.

If Vidal is choked by his ethnic origins, it is because they were deemed shameful and hidden by his paternal ancestors, who likely became *conversos* during the Inquisition. Vidal's torture sequences, which are gruesome in del Toro's unapologetic vision, reenact, with an arsenal of implements, the means used to brutalize and elicit confessions to uproot enemies of the Inquisition tribunals. Earlier, Vidal's brutality toward the father and son farmers was also triggered by an interrogation that is more specific than emblematically fascist. Suspicious of the farmers, Vidal questions them about their activities; it turns deadly once the son claims that his father is "an honest man," *hombre honradao*. The ensuing discussion, with references to "uncovering the truth," *descubrir*, and "no homeland," *ni patria*, culminates in the murder of both father and son. When he discovers two young rabbits among the men's belongings that validate the integrity of their story, he commands Mercedes to prepare them. Although Mercedes claims they are too small to provide much meat, Vidal insists.

Vidal's desire for young blood resonates with the Pale Man's hunger for young blood; his determination to eat recalls Ofelia's when she ate the grape. This resonance links the (biological) father's and daughter's eating motivations and invites us to reexamine the representation of food in the Pale Man scene, the site where the substance of their individual secrets mesh. Recall that the Pale Man, Vidal's monstrous doppelganger, does not touch the abundance of delicacies on his table. The dishes he does not ingest include large platters of blood-red congealed jellies, a huge ham, shellfish, and wine, all of which tacitly reference halal and kosher dietary restrictions. Indeed, the meal evokes the Inquisitorial tradition of gastronomically enforcing Muslim and Jewish converts to prove their religious fealty to Christianity, a practice reflected in *un almuerzo de Cristiano Viejo*, "the meal of old Christians."[57] The Pale Man's refusal of the food suggests an inability to digest some key truth indicting pork, blood, alcohol, and shellfish.

If Vidal's desire for his son to be born in a "clean" Spain constitutes an unconscious attempt to assert non-Muslim identity, his monstrous alter ego's refusal to eat suggests another, gastronomically concealed, oppositional signification of the word "clean": *halal*, or "lawful," food. *Halal* refers to food that is deemed "ritually appropriate," in accordance with religious notions of purity cleanliness.[58] When Vidal prepares to torture Mercedes, his sexual innuendos implicitly equate his body with impure non-halal food. With Mercedes's arms bound, Vidal pulls out the rations she had pilfered for the men she had secretly been aiding; "Chorizo ... *tabaco* ...," he says, rifling through her satchel. "If you had asked for *it*, I would have given *it* to you, Mercedes."[59] The ambiguity of the pronoun "it," *lo*, is curious: The stolen goods would need to be spoken of in the plural, *los*. Read with the sadomasochistic and psychosexual undertones of his behavior as he proceeds (unbuttoning his shirt and lowering his suspenders, things he did not do for the male Republican he tortured earlier), however, it becomes clear that the "it" refers to the *chorizo*, signaling a deeper, religiohistorical context for the matrix of sexual and political oppression that unfolds in the scene: Vidal's symptomatic assertion of his "non-halal" phallus cryptically articulates an anxiety about blood purity.[60]

Mercedes's subsequent actions and words, which suggest a subliminal awareness of the underlying context, support this interpretation. While Vidal's back is turned and he begins fiddling with his torture implements, Mercedes produces her paring knife tucked away in the folds of her apron. She frees herself, stabs him in the back, and slashes at him, finally holding him hostage with the blade inside his cheek. She threatens him: The English subtitles read, "Don't you dare touch the girl [Ofelia].

You won't be the first pig I've gutted!" She rips his mouth open and runs away. The original Spanish dialogue, however, reveals an alternative subtext. Instead of "gutted," Mercedes actually uses the verb *degüelle*, "to slit the throat." Speaking of the non-halal "pig," *cerdo*, in the metaphorical context of slaughter (ritual or otherwise), suggests another, unarticulated word, *marrano*. *Marrano* not only refers to pigs in a zoological or culinary sense but also to dirty swine in a pejorative sense, which aligns with the way Mercedes is speaking of Vidal. Although the word has come to mean "pork" in contemporary Spanish usage, it has a serpentine etymological history: While there is no consensus on its exact origin, some sources locate it in the Arabic *muharram*, "forbidden thing."

The *OED* defines the term as a Spanish word that "was used insultingly of converts to Christianity from Judaism and Islam," especially to those who professed conversion in order to avoid persecution. Although by the sixteenth century its derivatives were "present in this sense in several Romance languages" to refer specifically to Jews, it seems to have been used more generally before the forced conversions of Muslims in the early sixteenth century, who were at the time distinguished from Jews by the term *moriscos*. It became an epithet and means of accusation for Inquisition-era Spaniards who could indict their neighbors before the tribunals. That the term implied a *secret adherence* to *prohibited* religious rituals that were ostensibly practiced in *underground*, sequestered rooms, catacombs, and sub rosa caves, moreover, deepens its connection with the semiotic arrangement of a phantomatic crypt.

Mercedes's use of the verb *degollar* is actually foreshadowed in an earlier scene; here Vidal views his reflection while shaving, which elicits from him a strange and pathological response. He stares into his mirror while his father's watch stares up at him next to the shaving cream. Pausing to look at it ticking beneath him, he turns back to the mirror, draws it toward him, and gestures as if slitting the throat of his mirrored image. The juxtaposition of his fleeting glances (from his reflection, to the watch, and back to his reflection again) implies that Vidal sees his father's image interred within his reflection. The word "to shave," *aeitar*, derives from a fifteenth-century Latinate borrowing of the word *appectare*, "to devote oneself." Vidal's self-decapitating gesture stages his status as a sacrificial victim of his staunch efforts to conceal his father's secret. Living under his father's watch he is caught in a bind that obstructs his ability to swallow the secret truth of his Muslim origins.[61]

Vidal returns to the mirror again after Mercedes mutilates his (and by psychic proxy, his father's) face. Wincing in pain, he stitches back together his cleaved mouth, he becomes a *tailor*.[62] Vidal's assumption of Ofelia's "father's" vocation in this moment reaffirms his identity as Ofelia's birth father, while it also insinuates that both the tailor and Vidal are haunted by a shameful *converso* heritage: The identities of both are the products of tailored genealogies (Figure 2.6).

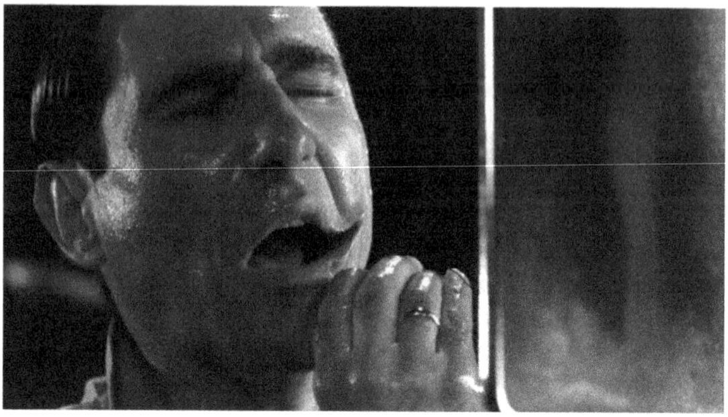

Figure 2.6 Vidal "tailors" his mouth.

Symbols that buttress the idea that the tailor was Jewish abound in the film's idiom. Lexically, the homophone *corte*, which means both "incision" and "[royal] court," connects the concept of laceration to the (false) "royal" context of Ofelia's fantasy. The word "incision" was commonly used in the brilliant and vicious literary wordplay of fifteenth- and sixteenth-century Jewish court jesters to refer to Jews; jokes ostensibly about acts of cutting and tailoring frequently pertained to circumcision, bodily evidence of Jewish identity. The salience of the discourse of fabrics and circumcised foreskins, usually contextualized by references to "hoods," explains why the epithet *ropera*, "clothier," became a word that mocked a *converso's* Jewish heritage or former faith.[63] Jewish tailors represented the negative essence of (Jewish) converts; their "lifelong occupation [was] a pretense unstitched before our eyes: for a tailor *hacer* [to do, sew] means *mentir* [to lie]."[64]

If Ofelia's fantasy is textured by these subtle allusions to Jewish experience, it is not a stretch to assume that the tailor's cuckolding trauma itself may have been informed by a preexisting (unconscious) need to cipher a Jewish identity in his family lineage. For example, a cuckold is often described in terms of "being made a fool," *hacer majer a*, which resonates with the Jewish court jester's ostensible *raison d'être*. In the same vein, "to wear a hood," *capuchin*, with a pointed "top," *pico*, evokes the sharp corners of a cuckold's "horns."[65] We may thus construe his concealment of his knowledge of Carmen's betrayal as symptomatic of his being haunted by a phantom of concealed Jewish identity.[66]

Imagistic evidence in the film further attests to the tailor's concealed Jewish identity. Consider the robe he wears when Ofelia returns to him in all his "royal" glory at the end of the film. Not only does the loose gown evoke that worn by the aforementioned Jewish jesters, but yellow clothing in general came to be associated strongly with Jews in Spain during the Inquisition.[67] The incisions in which the Pale Man places his eyes, which implicated the tailor's branding as a cuckold, can now also be read as an implicit reference to the stigmata of difference experienced by Jewish *conversos*. As the jester literature viscerally demonstrates, even "a lifetime of forced labor in the attempt to adopt Christian piety [was] not enough to redeem [Jews] of stigma."[68] That Jews were likened to (spiritually) blind witnesses of Christ's sacrifice[69] also deepens the context of the tailor's decision to shroud the fact of his cuckoldry in silence.

Finally, the images of the Pale Man's consumption of children and the pile of worn shoes that Ofelia observes in the crypt, both of which evoke the consequences of this stigma, provide further evidence of the tailor's concealed Jewish identity: Whereas the former evokes sensational blood libel cases associated with *conversos* in Spain (which, according to one scholar, directly influenced Queen Isabel's decision to expel the Jews in 1492),[70] the latter replicates gruesome photos of children's shoes piled high at Nazi concentration camps.[71]

The psychoanalytic reading of the film presented thus far reveals the presence of two intricate secrets generated by the Spanish Inquisition. It is now time to delineate how the secrets of the central characters also allegorize a collective psychic scar that is evident in the film's alignment of their pathologies. The visual synergy between the gears and wheels that appear in the mill's architecture and in the captain's watch, as well as the different phases of the moon present in outdoor scenes, evokes a sense of transgenerational rotation, suggesting that the temporal and spatial setting of the Franquist control must too be seen as symptomatic of collective preservative repression.

Historical Extension

The parallels between Inquisition era and Franquist Spain emerge out of the film's idiom and are readable as a return of the repressed. Commentators on the Spanish Civil War have recorded that history was indeed repeating itself in 1939, as it had hundreds of years before; Falangists and Republicans alike chose to deracinate and exterminate their enemies as though they too were Inquisitors, gunning each other down in town centers as examples.[72] The severe dysfunction visible during those years exposed what can only be explained as pathology, the Civil War constituting its most recent symptom. Indeed, the presence of a priest at the captain's dinner table demonstrates the church's participation in the tyranny of the fascists.

The Catholic priest at Vidal's dinner table cites the Church's involvement with the fascists' ruthless methods of suppressing cultural heterogeneity and political pluralism ("God has already saved their souls... What happens to their bodies hardly matters to Him"), recalling the very specific and collaborative relationship between the Church and the monarchy's campaign to homogenize and purify Iberia. Vidal's censorship of Carmen's words, and his later condemnation of Ofelia's fairy-tale books, reverberate with the censorship of linguistic diversity and of the proscription of Jewish and Muslim books, plays, poetry, and other texts which lead to their concealed and proliferation through silent practice. Juxtaposing the Spanish Inquisition beside the Spanish Civil War reveals that Spain's two bloodiest nation-building projects share a modus operandi that resembles a post-traumatic pathology more than it does a coincidence.[73]

The theory of the phantom equips us with a tool to uncover a new form of cultural historiography. It reads the massive trauma of the Inquisition as the genesis of an encrypted collective secret that was transgenerationally transmitted. The film's depiction of the Civil War steeped in so much residue of an earlier, medieval propensity toward social deracinations, implicitly asserts that the work of (collective) assimilation of the collective trauma of the Inquisition was not complete, notwithstanding the projection of ideology as illusory nourishment. In its labyrinthine system of cryptic significations, the film reveals how historical trauma is perpetuated in the lineages that shield it.[74]

The link between genealogies and the legacy of unspeakable collective trauma is strengthened by their coincidence in the symbol of the mandrake in the film. In Genesis, Leah exchanges the root for pregnancy; in *Pan's Labyrinth*, the root is equally efficacious, as the concoction prepared by Ofelia greatly palliated Carmen's physical discomfort. The root's power on both women suggests that knowledge about it belongs to the language surround of Jewish women. Vidal's fury at discovering the mandrake may not just be about childish superstitions but about Jewish traditions that taint his visions for a new and clean Spanish blood. Carmen is shamed by Vidal and throws the root into the fire, it shrieks and writhes in agony. Legend connects the root's maddening shriek to its deracination.[75]

The film's metaphorical substitution of the act of burning for that of uprooting evokes the public method of burning alive *conversos* found guilty of heresy by the Inquisitors. The mandrake's shriek recapitulates in distorted form the screams of those victims who suffered because the policies of the Inquisition had deracinated their genealogical roots. The immolation of the mandrake calls to mind the rituals of public penance of accused heretics, the auto-da-fé, during which countless *conversos* were condemned and burned at the stake.[76] The film's cryptic homage to such victims links the subtext of Vidal and Carmen's reactions to Spain's troubles in 1945; Carmen's immolation of the Jewish root stages a concealed trauma sublimated from the aftermath of witnessing the brutality and social severance of the Inquisition.

In the Spanish imagination, the literary and operatic figure of Carmen emblematizes an essential "Spanishness." This may explain why Vidal viewed his Carmen's womb as a vessel for reproducing a new and clean Spain. Recent research has argued that Carmen's signifying status, however, is more ambiguous; the valorization of Carmen's gypsy features is understood as a "conflation of national, ethnic, and racial identities," that covers up "cultural anxieties."[77] The "symbolic centrality of Gypsies in Spain's collective imaginary (as opposed to their actual marginality in society)" is especially paradoxical in light of how Carmen is repeatedly misidentified in the earlier representations of her as a seductive figure of Spain. In one account, she is mistaken for a Moor and then as a Jew.

Why a woman with illegible origins became a "synecdoche of Spanishness"[78] has been explained in different ways. One cultural critic suggests that character of Carmen is a cipher for the collective memory of "crucial but repressed non-white, non-European, and non-Christian elements that are the legacy of [Spain's] Jewish and Moorish past." Illegibility was reconfigured as an exoticized outcast onto which the repressed legacy can be "*safely* projected."[79] (emphasis mine). Carmen's figuration is a product of a national identity constructed through the literal expulsion of Jewish or Moorish populations;[80] this brings into clearer focus dimensions of Carmen's characterization in *Pan's Labyrinth*.

The affective power of his wife's name is suggested by Vidal's persistent choice of music, which he plays on a wind-up gramophone located in his room at the core of the mill. He repeatedly plays songs that invoke the "Gardens of Granada,"[81] *Casa Carmenes*, which refer to houses in Granada that enclose within them grape vineyards and fruit trees with high walls. The resonance between grape vines, protective walls, and fecund fruit trees with the symbols that communicated the gynecological context of Ofelia's secret suggests that Carmen, whose name derives from the Arabic word *karm*, "vine,"[82] may more literally symbolize with the context of Vidal's birth.

Granada, and its famous *carmenes*, is the legacy of the Islamic Emirate of Granada, which surrendered to Ferdinand II and Isabella I (the Catholic Monarchs) in 1492, an event that completed the "reconquest" of Andalusian Spain from Muslim control.[83] The Monarchs soon after made the celebrated Alhambra Palace, located in Granada, the seat of their rule and the Inquisition.[84] Although the terms of Muslim surrender explicitly permitted the inhabitants of the city to continue religious practice, by 1499, forced Christian baptisms began, creating the *converso* class. The violation of the treaty incited an armed Muslim Revolt, which was quelled but led to the mandate that Granada's Muslims must be expelled or baptized if they stayed.[85] Vidal's affective attraction to the songs that celebrate the "Gardens of Granada" effectively conceal, through the trope of garden fecundity, the site of his unutterable roots.

The figure of Carmen offers a means to repair the shameful injury that afflicted the ancestors of descendants of the Inquisition. Through her reproductive capacity Vidal hopes to transform his ancestor's shame; Carmen is an appropriate vehicle because her very national configuration is constituted by collective repressions of the same sort. But Carmen's birth is problematic. Shocked by the screaming mandrake, Carmen goes into labor and gives birth to a son, only to die of severe hemorrhaging suffered during the labor.

Carmen's outflow of blood evokes the draining of blood from the Spanish social fabric that transpired as a result of the expulsion of Jews and Moors, the very populations her seductive figure is meant to disguise. Although the union of Castille and Aragon with the marriage of Ferdinand and Isabella was used to manufacture the idea of national unity, Carmen's experience points to the hemorrhaged origins of this nation premised on the expulsion of other languages and cultures that had long existed on the Iberian Peninsula. Her death figures Spain's diminished social corporeality; Spanish identity became a pale version, a shell of its former self.

The characters in *Pan's Labyrinth* have been bequeathed a psychic predisposition dating back to the Inquisition. This situational context comes to the foreground when the faun tasks Ofelia to sacrifice the life of her newborn brother so that she may finally return to the king. Ofelia, standing at the center of the labyrinth, refuses to sacrifice the baby. The faun is incredulous; why would Ofelia "deny her ["royal"] lineage," *cuna*; why would she "sacrifice her sacred right," *derecho sagrado*, to protect this baby? The faun's query as to why Ofelia, who has "been humiliated and ignored" by the "snot" *musco*, is curiously incongruous. How could an infant she barely knows cause such indignity? The film's cut to Vidal emerging from the labyrinth just as the faun articulates this question suggests that *he* may in fact be the unstated referent, connected to the baby, his son, by metonymy. This idea is supported by Ofelia's response to the faun that she "repudiates it/him," which would be puzzling if the implied object were her brother since Ofelia has just refused to hand him over.

Ofelia's internal repudiation of Vidal, while she simultaneously refuses to hurt his son, reenacts the tailor's position as one who protected a baby fathered by Vidal and concealed or swallowed the shameful humiliation it brought upon him. Ofelia reveals her willingness to die in order to preserve this secret. This is why she reunites with the King of the Underworld in the scene after Vidal shoots her. Ofelia returns to the "refuge" or "asylum"—other connotations of the word "sacred," *sagrado*—in order to consecrate her ultimate submission to the rules of her father's crypt, where the secret is concealed.

The scene distills the religious and biological symbols that pointed to Ofelia's irresolvable question of origins. It stages a tableau of redemption for the penitent Ofelia; although no one to my knowledge has called attention to this, the scene powerfully evokes the aural and visual spectacle associated with another religious ritual popular in Spain, the *auto sacramental*.[86] The *auto sacramental* was a ceremony at which the Inquisition tribunal "judged and punished prisoners for violations against the Catholic faith. It was a ritual performance, symbolically reenacting the Last Day when all sinners stood before the throne of God,"[87] and was deployed as an instrument to publicly shame sinners accused of disobeying Catholic precepts.

Del Toro's set evokes the setting of these pillories, which were aimed (mostly) toward Jews but any *converso* was a potential target. The high platforms where the king and Carmen sit, for example, replicate the tall structures built for the tribunal officials, those who passed judgment.[88] The height and majesty of these sets enhanced the effect of the ritual on the collective, who were threatened with excommunication if they did not participate and bear witness to the sins of heretics.[89] Del Toro's set replicates the grand and public dimensions of the ritual, but he refracts this "frightful theater of cruelty"[90] to focus on its emotional impact on a family line.

The allegorical implications of this scene, which mimics the bestowal of divine judgment on Ofelia, seem to me more metapsychological than metaphysical. A visual resonance between the architecture and design of the king's and Pale Man's crypts, evidenced in complicated tiling patterns, arches, and ornamental metals, establishes the fact that the royal court and the Pale Man's crypt are different versions of one and the same crypt. The golden hues of the scene, and the king's yellow robes, moreover, locate us in a context of encrypted Jewish identity. The prominence of antler racks adorning the king's throne, visually links the judgment scene to the cuckold's horns.

The *auto sacramantale* dramatized what the final moments of human destiny would be like.[91] Judgment focused on the doctrine of free will, repentance, and grace, and emphasized the inseparability of choices and consequence. These themes are reflected in the king and faun's praise for Ofelia's *choice* to sacrifice her own blood instead of that of the baby's. They reveal that protecting the order and authority of the king's crypt is paramount. The unanimity of their sentiments bespeaks a deeper connection: If the faun is a figure of the cuckolded tailor whose immediate secret haunts Ofelia, the king is the ancestor whose family was shamed and punished as Jewish *conversos*. Ofelia's choice is lauded because it protects the crypt, a domain inhabited by all of the tailor's ancestors, whose lives were shaped by the consequences of their ancestor's (the king's) shame.

Ofelia's penitence shores up the king's royal authority, just as a penitent *converso* bolstered the Inquisition's regulations. The substance of her repentance was manifested in her choice to reject of the truth of her origins.[92] Her refusal to engage in the faun's ultimate "trial," *prueba*, was "proof," *prueba*, that she can remind blind to unconscious awareness of the truth of her paternity, *prueba de paternidad*, which haunts her. Ofelia's return to her father's domain exempts her from punishment for escaping it, thus fulfilling the primary objective of a fantasy, namely, to preserve the status quo. The fantasy also heralds her imminent inclusion into its realm: She will join her Jewish ancestors and all those descendants whose lives were shaped by their need to preserve a secret about an ancestor's problematic Jewish parentage.

The judgment reaffirms the codes and conventions that are necessary for keeping the secret intact. *Pan's Labyrinth* is sensitive to the capacity of a collective to transmit the content and affects of a silenced trauma as "cryptic lexical parcels of unutterable tales."[93] The film's meticulous attention to the transmission of Vidal's son from Vidal to the victorious rebels summarizes the mechanism of Spain's collective psychic haunting, which perpetuates through time just like the labyrinth itself. Mercedes's assured retort to Vidal that his son "won't even know your name" reveals the son, now orphaned, as a symbol of a young Spain haunted by the ellipses of its effaced origins.

The film ends as it begins, with the disembodied narrator, who refers to Ofelia's centuries-long reign, during which she ruled with "justice and kindness," and received public adoration. Below the surface adulation, the narrator intimates that Ofelia's enduring rule, centered around the preservation of a collective secret, is a fundamental element of Spanish history. Commenting that those who care or dare to look may apprehend traces of her reign and her domain, the narrator suggests that Spain continues, via unexamined transmission, to reenact dramas of its shameful exclusionary origins. The synchronization of this comment with the image of the stick bug vivifies the ongoing nature of haunting. Del Toro's historiography of a collective lineage yields a vantage point for viewing the processes by which the Spanish collective engaged in the activity of self-fashioning in the wake of the Inquisition; the film presents Franquist fascism as an index of the unutterable shame of the Inquisition.

Notes

1 *Pan's Labyrinth* (*El laberinto del fauno*), Guillermo del Toro, Sergei Lopez, New Line Home Video (2008), DVD.

2 Paul Julian Smith, "*Pan's Labyrinth* (*El laberinto del fauno*)," *Film Quarterly* 60, no. 4 (2007): 4.

3 Antony Beevor, *The Battle for Spain: The Spanish Civil War 1936–1939* (London: Phoenix, 2007). This historical period has inspired a huge number of Spanish films. Laura Hubner, "*Pan's Labyrinth*, Fear and the Fairy Tale" in *Fear Itself: Reasoning the Unreasonable*, eds. Stephen Hessel and Michele Huppert, vol. 61 (Amsterdam: Rodopi, 2010), 46, citing a study by Barry Jordan and Rikki Morgan-Tamosunas, states that "more than half of the nearly three hundred historical films produced since the 1970s are set during the Second Republic, the Civil War and Francoism."

4 Several critics have examined the similarity between del Toro's vision and that represented in Victor Eric's 1973 drama *The Spirit of the Beehive* (*El espíritu de la colmena*), which is considered a masterpiece of Spanish cinema and the unstated source of inspiration for del Toro's film. See Joanna M. Barros, *Re-membering Identites: Terror, Exile and Rebirth in Hispanic Film and Literature* (PhD Dissertation, Duke University, 2010); and Robert J. Miles, "Reclaiming Revelation: Pan's Labyrinth and the Spirit of the Beehive," *Quarterly Review of Film and Video* 28.3 (2011): 196.

5 This was especially an issue of great interest to fans of the film. I encountered countless fan forum postings and blog entries that contest whether or not Ofelia's magic world was real or imagined. A. O. Scott's *New York Times* review claims "That realm, in which Ofelia is thought to be a long-lost princess, may exist only in her imagination. Or maybe not: its ambiguous status is crucial to the film's coherence." Cf. Jennifer Orme, "Narrative Desire and Disobedience in *Pan's Labyrinth*," *Marvels and Tales* 24.2 (2010): 228. On leaving the question obscure, see the DVD commentary track.

6 A. O. Scott, "In Gloom of War, a Child's Paradise," *New York Times* 9 December 2006, claims that the "ambiguous status is crucial to the film's coherence," Margaret R. Yocom, "*Pan's Labyrinth/El Laberinto del Fauno* (Review)," *Marvels & Tales* 22.2 (2008): 34, and Smith, "Pan's Labyrinth," 8–9, who discusses how the lack of a sense of discontinuity of perspective contributes to this ambiguity. See also Barros, *Re-membering Identities*, 211, who suggests that fantasy remakes reality.

7 Mark Kermode, "Pan's Labyrinth," *Sight & Sound* 16.12 (2006): 22.

8 Yocom, "Pan's Labyrinth," 347. See also Barros, *Re-membering Identities*, 208.

9 Hubner, "Pan's Labyrinth," 55; Roger Clark and Keith McDonald, "A Constant Transit of Finding: Fantasy as Realisation in *Pan's Labyrinth*," *Children's Literature in Education* 41.1 (2010): 52.

10 Kam Tsuei, "The Antifascist Aesthetics of *Pan's Labyrinth*," *Socialism and Democracy* 22.2 (2008): 232. Barros, *Re-membering Identities*, 206–207, 224; Hubner, "Pan's Labyrinth," 46–47; Miles, "Reclaiming Revelation," 195, speaks of the "pact of forgetting." Yocom's discussion of the "state of stories in the aboveground world" also suggests that the film engages with historical repression.

11 "Guardian interview at the National Film Theatre with Director," cited by Kermode, "Pan's Labyrinth," 20–24.

12 Cf. Barros, *Re-membering Identities*, 246:

> In fact, his film rightly suggests that, as not only other writers and artists but numerous trauma theorists and psychologists have been advocating for years, the only way to successfully remember and remake the past—particularly a traumatic one—is through fantasy and retelling.

13 John Perlich, "Rethinking the Monomyth: *Pan's Labyrinth* and the Face of New Hero(ine)" in *Millennial Mythmaking: Essays on the Power of Science Fiction and Fantasy Literature, Films and Games*, eds. John Perlich and David Whitt (Jefferson, NC: Mcfarland, 2010), 107, claims the first two scenes "set up the duality of Ofelia/Moanna (both her death and life) and instigate a compelling storyline." See also Barros, *Re-membering Identities*, 231.

14 Shakespeare, *Hamlet*, Act 3, scene 2.

15 Cf. del Toro's own use of this term to refer to the connection between fairy tales and issues of choice cited earlier.

16 Like Hamlet's ghost, the faun walks with a secret, seeming to reveal one while withholding another: "your father is in the underworld, let there be no secret." But why must Ofelia undergo trials if she is recognized?
17 José Arroyo, "Pan's Labyrinth," *Sight & Sound* 16.12 (2007): 67: "Just as the figure of the father recurs structurally to distort, refract and evoke various versions of patriarchal terror, so Ofelia, the innocent child, also carries multiple meanings."
18 *"Ha sido muy bueno con nosotras, hija, no sabes cuanto."*
19 *"Es una palabra, Ofelia. No es más que una palabra."*
20 Esther Rashkin, *Unspeakable Secrets and the Psychoanalysis of Culture* (Albany: SUNY, 2008), 30.
21 The chronology of Ofelia's origins is unclear. Ofelia tells Mercedes that her father died at the beginning of the war, which was 1936. Since the film is set in 1944, Ofelia is nine years old, and the film takes place in 1944, placing her conception around the time Carmen and Vidal met for the first time, when the tailor sewed uniforms for Vidal's soldiers. Earlier in the film, Ofelia tells Mercedes that her father died at the "beginning of the war," which must have been 1936.
22 *"Aqui las casas son viejas. gruñer—se quejan ... A que parece que hablan."*
23 Del Toro's editing supports this interpretation cinematographically when he shifts his focus from the mountain rose to Vidal's study just as Ofelia says, "forgotten and lost at the top of that cold, dark mountain, forever alone, until the end of time."
24 Hubner, "Pan's Labyrinth," 51, 56.
25 *"Lo que hubiera dado yo de pequeña por tener un vestido así."* Cf. Hubner, "Pan's Labryinth," 57: "There is a certain awe surrounding the female body in the uterine imagery of Ofelia's fantasy world, the infinite circular archways and interiors and the shots of Ofelia's baby brother in the womb."
26 Genesis 3:7.
27 The expression puns on the Spanish word "fig," *higo, and higa*, "female genitals."
28 Cf. Charles Emil Kany, *American-Spanish Euphemisms* (Berkeley: University of California Press, 1960), 187, where he cites the euphemistic use of *sapo* to connote "vulva" and "prostitute," sexual connotations of *sapo*. See too, Calderon de la Barca's famous *Teatro comico breve*, in which a key of honor *(la llave de mi honor)* figures in a story involving a soldier and cuckoldry of a husband who is aware of his position; Ted Lars Lennard Bergman, *The Art of Humour in the Teatro Breve and Comedias of Calderón de la Barca*, vol. 201 (Tamesis Books, 2003), 54.
29 Richard Lindsay, "Menstruation as Heroine's Journey in *Pan's Labyrinth*" in John W. Morehead, ed., *The Supernatural Cinema of Guillermo del Toro: Critical Essays* (Jefferson, NC: McFarland, 2015), 183.
30 Kany, *American-Spanish Eumphemisms*, 192: "In Mexico, *cornudo* is euphemized by *buey* 'ox,' and *llaves* 'keys' may replace *cuernos*." Cf. Ofelia's use of the verb *casarse*, "to marry," derives from *casa*, "house," or lineage.
31 There is an uncanny resonance between this nexus of symbols and those contained in E.T.A. Hoffman's 1817 short story "The Sandman" ("Der Sandmann"), which Abraham and Torok have argued symbolizes "the lasting effects of secrecy in the family." The overlap between both narratives with regard to eyes, specifically the absence of eyes marked by "merely black holes," as well as the theme of fraudulent deception, will be discussed further later. Nicholas Rand and Maria Torok, "The Sandman Looks at 'The Uncanny': The Return of the Repressed or of the Secret; Hoffman's Question to Freud" in *Speculations after Freud: Psychoanalysis, Philosophy, and*

Culture, eds. Sonu Shamdasani and Michael Muenchow (Florence, KY: Taylor and Francis, 1994), 196.

32 I am grateful to my student Tjos Hansen who pointed out this linguistic connection.

33 Cf. Rosario Caballero, "Cutting across the Senses: Imagery in Winespeak and Audiovisual Promotion" in *Multimodal Metaphor*, eds. Charles Forceville and Eduardo Urios-Aparisi (Berlin: Walter de Gruyter, 2009), 78, where she examines Spanish "winespeak" discourse as grounded in a metaphorical frame of organic processes: "The juice extracted from grapes changes considerably along its life inside both oak casks and bottles—a process referred to as breeding or ageing (*crianza*) ... [which] foregrounds the social and kinship dimensions of wine."

34 See *OED*.

35 This chain of associations is linguistically supported: *vid* (grape/vine) → source of Ofelia's paternity → *vid.*, abbreviation of *vide*, Latin imperative singular of *videre*, "to see," which is used in Spanish texts after a term or phrase that should be looked up elsewhere in the document or book.

36 The eyes on the platter evoke gothic imagery of St. Lucy, the patron saint of the blind, whose name Lucia (from the Latin word *lux*, light) was venerated as the protector of sight. See Ante Skrobonja, Amir Muzur, and Tatjana Culina, "The Cult of St. Lucia, Patroness of the Eyes: Some Examples from Croatian Ethnomedical Tradition," *International Ophthalmology* 25.1 (2004): 37–41. I am grateful to my student Christopher Chan for this reference.

37 Cf. the Spanish expression "to know something like the *palm* of one's hand," *conocer algo como la palma de la mano*, which converges with the sense of intimate knowledge obtained through the act of witnessing.

38 Cf. the distinctive wattle or goiter of the Pale Man, which evokes the image of a turkey, and its concomitant semantic association with the expression "to make a fool (out of someone)" as in "You can't fool me," *No soy guecho* in Mexican Spanish. See Kany, *American-Spanish Euphemisms*, 53.

39 In light of the foregoing discussion, the location of the *Black Paintings* in the dining room raises the possibility of viewing the painting as a symbolic attempt by Goya to introject, or *digest* intrapsychically, a trauma he had experienced. Art critics have noted how Goya's *Saturn* reflects a particularly violent, even psychotic, dimension of the god's character. See Jan Jagodzinski, "Is Kronos Eating Our Children? Historical Fathers," *Youth Fantasies: The Perverse Landscape of the Media* (Palgrave Macmillan US, 2004), 69–85.

40 See María Teresa DePaoli, "*Fantasy and Myth* in Pan's Labyrinth: Analysis of Guellermo del Toro's Symbolic Imagery" in *Magic and the Supernatural,* eds. Scott. E. Hendrix, Timothy J. Shannon (Oxford: Inter-Disciplinary Press, 2012). Interface Research and Publications Project (2012), 50, who suggests that the psychopathological condition of the Cronus Complex lies at the center of *Pan's Labyrinth*. While DePaoli, citing Jungian analysts, calls attention to the "destructive ingestive process which hinders the [child's] capacity to exist separately and autonomously from the parent," her focus is on how Cronus "aims to make [the child] a part of himself, to continue living through him," which is quite different than Abraham and Torok's notion of a life whose development is curtailed as a result of the unwitting inheritance of a shameful secret.

41 The defeat at Annual, a Spanish settlement in northeastern Morocco, on July 22, 1921, sparked tremendous political crises, and historians describe it as the Disaster of Annual. The general (recalling that Vidal's father was a general who died in Morocco) commanding the men garrisoned at Annual,

Manuel Fernández Silvestre, is also the subject of much military folklore. He died and his remains were never discovered; some witnesses write that he committed suicide amid the slaughter of 15,000 Spanish men. See José Álvarez-Junco, "The Formation of Spanish Identity and It's Adaptation to the Age of Nations," *History & Memory* 14.1 (2002): 13–36.

42 Ibid., 32–33.

43 The focus on Vidal's eyes echoes the theme of blindness that permeates the Pale Man scene. Vidal, who uses binoculars and a loupe throughout the film to aid his vision, is blind to his own secret identity.

44 Nicolas Abraham and Maria Torok, *The Shell and the Kernel: Renewals of Psychoanalysis*, vol. 1 (Chicago, IL: University of Chicago Press, 1994), 181.

45 The Inquisition was established as a court to "inquire into the heresy of Christians of Jewish origin," in 1478; see Henry Kamen, *The Spanish Inquisition: A Historical Revision* (New Haven, CT: Yale University Press, 2014), 12, 22.

46 Mathew Carr, *Blood and Faith: The Purging of Muslim Spain* (New York: The New Press, 2009).

47 Barbara Weissberger, "Motherhood and Ritual Murder in Medieval Spain and England," *Journal of Medieval and Early Modern Studies* 39.1 (2009): 7–30.

48 Natalia Muchnik, "Being Against, Being with: Marrano Self-Identification in Inquisitorial Spain (Sixteenth-Eighteenth Centuries), An Essay," *Jewish History* 25 (2011): 153.

49 Miriam Bodian, *Hebrews of the Portuguese Nation: Conversos and Community in Early Modern Amsterdam* (Bloomington: Indiana University Press, 1999), 7; italics mine. See also Weissberger, "Motherhood," 8.

50 Bernard Lewis, *Cultures and Conflict: Christians, Muslims, and Jews in the Age of Discovery* (Oxford: Oxford University Press, 1996).

51 Donald Walter Wood, *Speaking through the Prophets: Aljamiado Legends as Spaces of Historical Negotiation* (PhD dissertation, University of Georgia, 2012), 40.

52 See D. Fairchild Ruggles, "The Alcazar of Seville and Mudejar Architecture," *Gesta* 43.2 (2004): 87–98.

53 Ibid., Ruggles delineates the way Mudéjar architecture reflected different monarchical positions with regard to national and religious identity.

54 John Beusterien, "Did Cervantes Stutter?," *Bulletin of the Cervantes Society of America* 29.1 (2009): 213.

55 In the Spanish version of the script, the words "without s-s-tuttering" are italicized, suggesting that they warranted special emphasis.

56 Beusterien, "Did Cervantes Stutter?," 215, explains the orthographic difference between *tata* and *tarta* as a result of "normal linguistic evolution in Spanish."

57 Wlad Godzich, "From the Inquisition to Descartes: The Origins of the Modern Subject," *Surfaces Revue Électronique*, Université de Montréal (1992): 14. See also Carr, *Blood and Faith*, for a description of how Muslims were forced to eat pork or drink alcohol to prove they had converted.

58 Pork, wine, and blood are non-halal; whether shellfish, a non-kosher food, could be eaten is controversial among various denominations of Muslims—namely, fish and seafood. See J. M. Regenstein, M. M. Chaudry, and C. E. Regenstein, "The Kosher and Halal Food Laws," *Comprehensive Reviews in Food Science and Food Safety* 2 (2003): 111–127.

59 "*Si me lo hubiera pedido... se lo hubiera dado, Mercedes.*"

60 This analysis benefited from critical discussions with my perspicacious student, Christopher Chan.

61 The slitting of his throat may also be read as the slitting of his father's throat, evoking the patricidal anxieties in Goya's *Saturn Devouring his Sons.*
62 Carmen says instead, "*El padre de Ofelia le confeccionaba los uniformes,*" or, "*Ofelia's father made [the captain's] uniforms.*"
63 *Moriscos* were also vilified for the practice of circumcision, which identified them as others through physical features, but literary trends reveal a prevalence of references to Jewish tailors in this regard. This may be due to the brilliant self-lacerating poetry of the *ropero* Anton de Montoro, who was a *court* jester in the court of Juan II of Castile (r. 1406–1454). Cf. Francisco Márquez Villanueva, "Jewish Fools of the Spanish Fifteenth Century," *Hispanic Review* 50.4 (1982), 404, who states that Montoro "brought to the fore ... what it felt like to be a *converso*. ... His case helps us to understand why "virtually all Spanish court jesters were and had to be Jews."
64 George A. Shipley, "Vidriera's Blather," *Revista Cervantes* 22.2 (2002): 91.
65 See Kany, *American-Spanish Euphemisms*, 193.
66 Muchnik, "Being Against," investigates the process of identity construction of crypto-Jews.
67 For fools' gowns, see Villanueva, "Jewish Fools"; for Jews and yellow clothing, see Pamela Anne Patton, *Art of Estrangement: Redefining Jews in Reconquest Spain* (University Park: Penn State Press, 2012), 23.
68 Villanueva, "Jewish Fools," 404.
69 Pamela Anne Patton, *Art of Estrangement*, 76. The fact that the tailor is also "crowned," *coronar*, in this image reflects, again, on his cuckolded status, see Kany, *American-Spanish Euphemisms*, 193.
70 Weissberger, "Motherhood," 192, states that "Ritual Murder recounted by Damian de Vegas played a decisive role in the royal deliberations on the fate of the Spanish Jews in the two years prior to the issuance of the Edict of Expulsion."
71 Clark and McDonald, "A Constant Transit of Finding," also note this implicit reference.
72 Paloma Aguilar Fernández, *Memory and Amnesia: The Role of the Spanish Civil War in the Transition to Democracy*, trans. Mark Oakley (New York: Berghahn Books, 2002), 39:

> Franco devised the idea that his government, although essential new, had re-established the tradition of other supposedly glorious periods in the history of Spain. He also claimed to link up with eras in which order, unity and Catholic values had reigned through the country, in which respect he resuscitated the myth of El Cid and the memory of the reign of the Catholic Monarchs ... as the executor of the Catholic and Spanish imperial tradition in accordance with traditional legitimacy.

73 Carr, *Blood and Faith*, claims that *morisco* expulsions have more modern resonances in the official language of security concerns about alien populations who might have allegiances beyond the state in which they live that could result in treachery.
74 Recent studies on the genetic signatures of people in Spain and Portugal provide evidence of the mass conversions of Sephardic Jews and Muslims to Catholicism in the fifteenth and sixteenth centuries after Christian armies wrested Spain back from Muslim control. See Susan M. Adams et al., "The Genetic Legacy of Religious Diversity and Intolerance: Paternal Lineages of Christians, Jews, and Muslims in the Iberian Peninsula," *The American Journal of Human Genetics* 83.6 (2008): 725–736.
75 Shakespeare, *Romeo and Juliet* Act 4, Scene 3: "Shrieks like mandrakes' torn out of the earth."

76 Simon Whitechapel, *Flesh Inferno: Atrocities of Torquemada and the Spanish Inquisition* (Creation Book, 2003).
77 José F. Colmeiro, "Exorcising Exoticism: 'Carmen' and the Construction of Oriental Spain," *Comparative Literature* 54.2 (2002): 126–128. Colmeiro says that "a recent poll in the European Union revealed that, after Don Quixote and Don Juan, Carmen was the fictional character most identified with Spain." The essentialization of Carmen derives from two sources: the 1845 novella by Prosper Mérimée and its later development in the 1875 French opera by George Bizet.
78 Ibid., 137.
79 Ibid., 130. Colmeiro suggests that "Spaniards themselves had helped create this confusion of identities as a nationalist act of resistance against foreign influences. The Spanish aristocracy reacted against the French and Italian models imported by the Bourbon monarchy during the Enlightenment because of the perceived threat to national identity. Thus the Spanish elite started identifying with and imitating the customs in music, clothing, speech, and entertainment of Madrid's lower classes, considered more Spanish and authentic (the 'majos' and 'majas' portrayed by Goya)." See also Ella Shohat and Robert Stam, *Unthinking Eurocentrism: Multiculturalism and the Media* (New York: Routledge, 2014), 45, where they discuss repressed Sephardic Jewish traditions that remain alive in Roman Catholic Mexican American families in New Mexico and Texas.
80 Ibid., 129.
81 Smith, "Pan's Labyrinth."
82 Ibid.
83 Leonard Patrick Harvey, *Islamic Spain, 1250 to 1500* (Chicago, IL: University of Chicago Press, 2014) x, *et passim.*
84 Ibid., 337.
85 Ibid., 150 *et passim.*
86 For a detailed illumination of the visual aesthetics of the ritual, see Errol L. King, *Production of Meaning: Spectacle as Visual Rhetoric in the Auto Sacramental* (PhD dissertation, University of Arizona, 2012).
87 Maureen Flynn, "Mimesis of the Last Judgment: The Spanish Auto de fe," *The Sixteenth Century Journal* 22.2 (1991): 281.
88 Ibid., 287, 296.
89 Francisco Bethencourt, "The Auto da fe: Ritual and Imagery," *Journal of the Warburg and Courtauld Institutes* 55 (1992): 155.
90 Ibid., 161.
91 Frederick E. Danker, "Emblematic Technique in the Auto Sacramental: Calderon's No hay mas fortuna que Dios," *Comparative Drama* 6.1 (1972): 42, cited by King, *Production of Meaning*, 17.
92 Conversos's repentance consisted of the "wholesome abhorrence of heresy." Ibid., 149 *et passim.* Cf. del Toro's emphasis on how the fairy-tale form enabled him to explore questions of "choice."
93 Esther Rashkin, *Family Secrets and the Psychoanalysis of Narrative* (Princeton, NJ: Princeton University Press, 1994), 46.

Bibliography

Abraham, Nicolas, and Maria Torok. *The Wolf Man's Magic Word: A Cryptonymy.* Vol. 37. University of Minnesota Press, 2005.

Abraham, Nicolas, Maria Torok. Trans. Nicholas T. Rand. *The Shell and the Kernel: Renewals of Psychoanalysis.* Vol. 1. University of Chicago Press, 1994.

Adams, Susan M., et al. "The Genetic Legacy of Religious Diversity and Intolerance: Paternal Lineages of Christians, Jews, and Muslims in the Iberian Peninsula." *The American Journal of Human Genetics* 83.6 (2008): 725–736.

Álvarez-Junco, José. "The Formation of Spanish Identity and Its Adaptation to the Age of Nations." *History & Memory* 14.1 (2002): 13–36.

Arryo, José. "Review of *Pan's Labyrinth*." *Sight & Sound* 16.12 (2006): 66–68.

Barros, Joanna M. *Re-membering Identities: Terror, Exile and Rebirth in Hispanic Film and Literature*. PhD Dissertation. Duke University, 2010.

Beevor, Antony. *The Battle for Spain: The Spanish Civil War 1936–1939*. Hachette UK, 2012.

Bergman, Ted Lars Lennard. *The Art of Humour in the Teatro Breve and Comedias of Calderón de la Barca*. Vol. 201. Tamesis Books, 2003.

Bethencourt, Francisco. "The Auto da fe: Ritual and Imagery." *Journal of the Warburg and Courtauld Institutes* 55 (1992): 155–168.

Beusterien, John. "Did Cervantes Stutter?" *Cervantes: Bulletin of the Cervantes Society of America* 29.1 (2009): 209–221.

Bodian, Miriam. *Hebrews of the Portuguese Nation: Conversos and Community in Early Modern Amsterdam*. Indiana University Press, 1999.

Caballero, Rosario. "Cutting Across the Senses: Imagery in Winespeak and Audiovisual Promotion." *Multimodal Metaphor*. Eds. Charles Forceville and Eduardo Urios-Aparisi. Walter de Gruyter, 2009. 73–94.

Carr, Matthew. *Blood and Faith: The Purging of Muslim Spain*. The New Press, 2009.

Clark, Roger, and Keith McDonald. ""A Constant Transit of Finding": Fantasy as Realisation in *Pan's Labyrinth*." *Children's Literature in Education* 41.1 (2010): 52–63.

Colmeiro, José F. "Exorcising Exoticism: "Carmen" and the Construction of Oriental Spain." *Comparative Literature* 54.2 (2002): 127–144.

Davies, Ann, Deborah Shaw, and Dolores Tierney. Eds. *The Transnational Fantasies of Guillermo del Toro*. Springer, 2014.

DePaoli, María Teresa. "Fantasy and Myth in *Pan's Labyrinth*: Analysis of Guillermo del Toro's Symbolic Imagery." *Magic and the Supernatural*. Eds. Scott E. Hendrix and Timothy J. Shannon. Inter-Disciplinary Press, 2012. 49–54.

Fernández, Paloma Aguilar. *Memory and Amnesia: The Role of the Spanish Civil War in the Transition to Democracy*. Berghahn Books, 2002.

Flynn, Maureen. "Mimesis of the Last Judgment: The Spanish Auto de fe." *The Sixteenth Century Journal* 22.2 (1991): 281–297.

Godzich, Wlad. "From the Inquisition to Descartes: The Origins of the Modern Subject." *Surfaces* 2 (1992).

Harvey, Leonard Patrick. *Islamic Spain, 1250 to 1500*. University of Chicago Press, 2014.

Hei Tsuei, Kam. "The Antifascist Aesthetics of *Pan's Labyrinth*." *Socialism and Democracy* 22.2 (2008): 225–244.

Hendrix, Scott E., and Timothy J. Shannon. Eds. *Magic and the Supernatural*. Interface Research, 2012.

Hessel, Stephen, and Michèle Huppert. Eds. *Fear Itself: Reasoning the Unreasonable*. Vol. 61. Rodopi, 2010.

Hubner, Laura. "*Pan's Labyrinth*, Fear and the Fairy Tale." *Fear Itself. Reasoning the Unreasonable*. Eds. Stephen Hessel and Michèle Huppert. Rodopi, 2010. 45–62.

Jackson, Rosemary. *Fantasy*. Routledge, 2013.

Jagodzinski, Jan. "Is Kronos Eating Our Children? Historical Fathers." *Youth Fantasies: The Perverse Landscape of the Media*. Palgrave Macmillan US, 2004. 69–85.

Kamen, Henry. *The Spanish Inquisition: A Historical Revision*. Yale University Press, 2014.

Kany, Charles Emil. *American-Spanish Euphemisms*. University of California Press, 1960.

Kermode, Mark. "*Pan's Labyrinth*." *Sight and Sound* 16.12 (2006): 20–24.

Kinder, Marsha. *Blood Cinema: The Reconstruction of National Identity in Spain*. University of California Press, 1993.

King, Errol LeRoy. *Production of Meaning: Spectacle as Visual Rhetoric in the Auto Sacremental*. PhD Dissertation. University of Arizona, 2012.

Lewis, Bernard. *Cultures in Conflict: Christians, Muslims, and Jews in the Age of Discovery*. Oxford University Press, 1996.

Lindsay, Richard. "Menstruation as Heroine's Journey in *Pan's Labyrinth*." *The Supernatural Cinema of Guillermo del Toro: Critical Essays*. Ed. John W. Morehead. Jefferson, NC: McFarland, 2015. 182–200.

Miles, Robert J. "Reclaiming Revelation: *Pan's Labyrinth* and the Spirit of the Beehive." *Quarterly Review of Film and Video* 28.3 (2011): 195–203.

Muchnik, Natalia. "Being Against, Being with: Marrano Self-Identification in Inquisitorial Spain (Sixteenth–Eighteenth Centuries). An Essay." *Jewish History* 25.2 (2011): 153–174.

Newitz, Annalee. "Pan's Labyrinth—Can Fantasies Rescue Us from Fascism?" *Wired*. CNMN Collection, 7 February 2007.

Orme, Jennifer. "Narrative Desire and Disobedience in *Pan's Labyrinth*." *Marvels & Tales* 24.2 (2010): 219–234.

Pan's Labyrinth (*El laberinto del fauno*), Guillermo del Toro, Sergei Lopez, New Line Home Video (2008), DVD.

Patton, Pamela Anne. *Art of Estrangement: Redefining Jews in Reconquest Spain*. Penn State Press, 2012.

Perlich, John and David Whitt. Eds. *Millennial Mythmaking: Essays on the Power of Science Fiction and Fantasy Literature, Films and Games*. McFarland, 2010.

———. "Rethinking the Monomyth: *Pan's Labyrinth* and the Face of a New Hero (ine)." *Millennial Mythmaking: Essays on the Power of Science Fiction and Fantasy Literature, Films and Games*. Eds. John Perlich and David Whitt. McFarland, 2010. 100–28.

Rand, Nicholas, and Maria Torok. "The Sandman Looks at 'The Uncanny': The Return of the Repressed or of the Secret; Hoffman's Question to Freud." *Speculations after Freud: Psychoanalysis, Philosophy, and Culture*. Eds. Sonu Shamdasani and Michael Muenchow. Florence, KY: Taylor and Francis, 1994.

Rashkin, Esther. *Family Secrets and the Psychoanalysis of Narrative*. Princeton University Press, 1992.

———. *Unspeakable Secrets and the Psychoanalysis of Culture*. SUNY Press, 2008.

Regenstein, J. M., M. M. Chaudry, and C. E. Regenstein. "The Kosher and Halal Food Laws." *Comprehensive Reviews in Food Science and Food Safety* 2.3 (2003): 111–127.

Ruggles, D. Fairchild. "The Alcazar of Seville and Mudejar Architecture." *Gesta* 43.2 (2004): 87–98.

Scott, A. O. "In Gloom of War, a Child's Paradise. Palgrave MacMillan," *New York Times* 9 December 2006.

Shipley, George. "Vidriera's Blather." *Cervantes: Bulletin of the Cervantes Society of America* 22.2 (2002): 49–125.

Shohat, Ella, and Robert Stam. *Unthinking Eurocentrism: Multiculturalism and the Media*. Routledge, 2014.

Skrobonja, Ante, Amir Muzur, and Tatjana Culina. "The Cult of St. Lucia, Patroness of the Eyes: Some Examples from Croatian Ethnomedical Tradition." *International Ophthalmology* 25.1 (2004): 37–41.

Smith, Paul Julian. "*Pan's Labyrinth* (*El laberinto del fauno*)." *Film Quarterly* 60.4 (2007): 4–9.

Thormann, Janet. "Other Pasts: Family Romances of *Pan's Labyrinth*." *Psychoanalysis, Culture & Society* 13.2 (2008): 175–187.

Tierney, Deloros. "Transnational Political Horror in Cronos (1993), *El espinazo del diablo* (2001), and *El labertino del fauno* (2006)." Eds. Ann Davies, Deborah Shaw and Doloros Tierney. *The Transnational Fantasies of Guillermo del Toro*. Palgrave Macmillan, 2014. 161–182.

Villanueva, Francisco Márquez. "Jewish Fools of the Spanish Fifteenth Century." *Hispanic Review* 50.4 (1982): 385–409.

Weissberger, Barbara F. "Motherhood and Ritual Murder in Medieval Spain and England." *Journal of Medieval and Early Modern Studies* 39.1 (2009): 7–30.

Whitechapel, Simon. *Flesh Inferno: Atrocities of Torquemada and the Spanish Inquisition*. Vol. 3. Creation Books, 2003.

Wood, Donald Walter. *Speaking through the Prophets*. PhD Dissertation. University of Georgia, 2012.

Yocom, Margaret R. "Pan's Labyrinth/El Laberinto del Fauno (Review)." *Marvels & Tales* 22.2 (2008): 345–348.

Zipes, Jack. "*Pan's Labyrinth* (*El Laberinto del Fauno*) (Review)." *Journal of American Folklore* 121.480 (2008): 236–240.

3 Uncanny Reunions, Filial Obligations, and the Trope of Haunting in Andrey Zvyagintsev's *The Return*

INDIEWIRE: Nevertheless, if you had to give a brief description of your film.
ZVYAGINTSEV: I would say that it's about the metaphysical incarnation of the soul's movement from the Mother to the Father.[1]

Praised for its elegant and eloquent understatement, Andrey Zvyagintsev's *The Return* portrays a journey to an uninhabited island undertaken by two teenage brothers, Ivan and Andrei, with their taciturn and demanding father, who has returned home after a twelve-year absence. Because the film raises many questions about character motivation—such as the reason behind the father's absence as well as the underlying objective for traveling to the remote island—yet leaves them unanswered, and because its stunning imagery foregrounds the ineffable silent power of Nature, critics ascribe to it a "mystical" or hermetic quality, which itself is almost universally attributed to the influence of Andrei Tarkovsky's brilliant oeuvre and metaphysical aesthetics. This is a valid observation, for Tarkovsky's creative legacy is indeed evident;[2] Zvyagintsev's film shares Tarkovsky's interest in "dreamtime" as well as the camera techniques he uses to signify distinctions among states of consciousness.[3]

But Tarkovsky's aesthetic sensibility alone does not illuminate the enigmas that permeate the film, which centers on a tense drama between father and sons. For example, quite a few critics have seen Ivan's suspicion of and resistance against his father as an Oedipal struggle;[4] others see it as an implicit social commentary on the problem of absent fathers in Russian society.[5] The consensus, however, is that initiation into manhood is the central theme of the film.[6] I accept this interpretation. But I construe more narrowly what the transmission of masculine knowledge means. If the film is about the father's transmission of important information to Ivan as he enters adolescence, it is also about a family secret and the unconscious obligation to conceal it.

Compositional Structure

I base this on the supposition that the events of the father's return and the fishing trip are components of a fantasy created by Ivan in response to a traumatic experience. I will delineate how the film's opening mise-en-scène is demarcated as a distinct informational domain with clear temporal and spatial boundaries, and I will show how the information contained within that domain represents this traumatic experience. Zvyagintsev's unambiguous partitioning off of this material allows us to see the journey that follows as a fantasy produced by Ivan to resist the psychic reorganization required to assimilate the trauma.

Some critics have raised questions about the status of the father's return. Understanding that the father is an Abrahamian symbol in Ivan's fantasy is a definitive response to these concerns; indeed, the third narrative segment in the film confirms this interpretation of the central narrative and indirectly of the introductory scenes. The final segment assumes a photo-journal idiom that "offers a competing version of [the] events" that took place on the journey;[7] most critics concur that this segment presents the most intractable enigma of the film. Its idiom is sharply distinct from that of the journey, which precedes it. As in the transition between the first and the second segments, this distinction implicitly communicates that boundaries have shifted and that a different information domain is being defined. Furthermore, the father's image is absent from the photos.[8] Philip Cavendish notes that the photo-journal component operates as a "film within a film" and a "text within a text" to guide viewers' interpretation of its central narrative component.[9] This makes sense. The third segment is a rereading of the journey, in the same way that the journey itself rereads, in the form of a fantasy, Ivan's affective experience.

The photos themselves call attention to cinematographic techniques used elsewhere in the film. One example is the film's frequent deployment of backward gazes (such as the repetition of shots that zero in on the car's rearview and side mirrors), which capture the complex crosscurrents between Ivan and his father at particularly fraught moments. The use of regressive perspectives is another visual trope: Ivan watching his father with binoculars, for instance, which evokes Ivan's status as a double, or witness, of his father's actions.

The Opening as Prologue

Prologues are important in Russian literature. Russian literary scholars Peter Steiner and Sergej Davydov point out that prologues and epilogues bracket the main events of a plot and link them to their larger context—an important aspect of any work's literary effect.[10] Other Russian scholars call attention to practices of "ensembling," that is, the binding of "texts of different styles and genres"[11] into specific forms of communication to which the prologue serves as a guide. The opening scenes of *The Return* (the ones that occur on Sunday on the watchtower)[12] fulfill both the contextualizing and the interpretive functions of a literary prologue and are more helpfully seen in that light than as part of the film's main narrative. Specifically, these scenes introduce us to the communicative patterns that inform—that *are*—the plot, that is, an unspoken secret between mother and son. In its focus on this theme and its language, the prologue illuminates everything that follows, in particular, the relationship between fathers and sons as displayed on the fishing trip. The introductory scene on the tower is a crucial visual and linguistic gloss upon the rest of the film.[13]

Like *Pan's Labyrinth, The Return* opens with disembodied sounds: in this case, the slap of splashing water. The juxtaposition of the splash with underwater images hints at a subterranean world like that of Ofelia's fantasy—this too is a concealed realm in which the splashing sound may be resonating with an awareness as yet unconscious. By the end of the film, the viewer will understand that the prolonged underwater shot of a sunken boat foreshadows a watery grave; even before that, the camera's trajectory from the stern of the boat to the bow visually hints at the recontextualization to come and supports an interpretive strategy of retrospection (Figure 3.1).

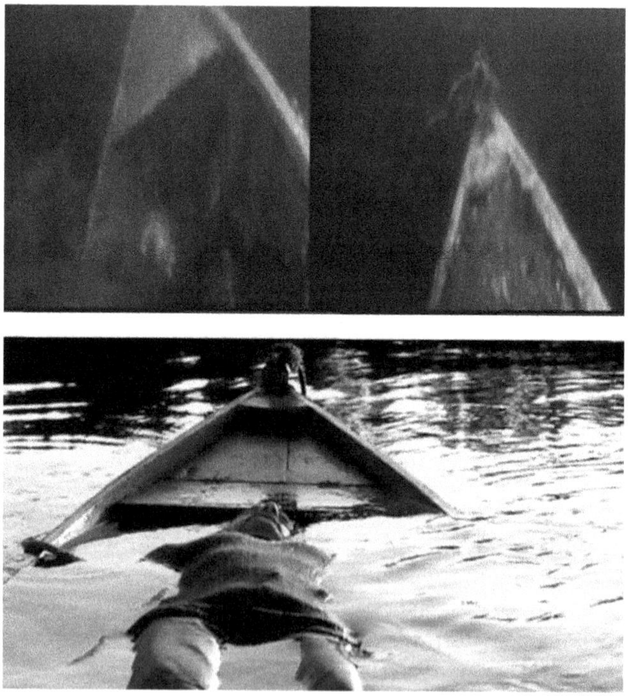

Figure 3.1 Three distinct shots of boats' "noses."

This backward gesture at once suggests (from the very outset) the concept of "return" and hints at the central enigma of the film—the truth that lies inaccessibly sunken beneath the surface level of signification.

So too does the slow focus on the bow of the boat. The Russian word for this, *nos*, also refers less metaphorically to the nose proper and, as in English, is implicated in numerous connotations of concealment—"to hide something under someone's nose," "to stick one's nose into someone else's business," or "to lead someone by the nose, i.e., deceive them." In Russian, you can also "leave someone with his nose" or "make a fool of him," *ostavit' s nosom*. The single word *nos* thus summons up concealment, trickery, and snooping, all at the same time.

This is not just an idiosyncratic interpretation on my part. The nose is important in Russian literature. Vladimir Nabokov concludes that in Russian folklore, it conveys "connotations of deception, delusion and inquisitiveness,"[14] and Magdalena Vintrova suggests that it calls attention to the "permeable boundary between reality and fantasy." Nikolai Gogol's famous story about the search for a missing nose, for example, is understood by many critics as a classic example of the ambiguous nature of that organ, and Vintrova points out that Gogol "relies on the power of a lexical pun to drive home his focus on the porousness of this [reality/fantasy] border: reading the Russian word *nos* backwards spells *son*, or 'dream.'"[15] Furthermore, Vintroya observes, images of the nose operate in Gogol's story "as diagnostic tools sniffing out the status of the protagonists' minds and of the social climate they inhabit."[16]

For all these reasons, the image of the submerged boat's *nos* is a tacit hint to expect more than one level of meaning and to anticipate the fluid oscillation between reality and fantasy that characterizes phantomatic haunting. More particularly, the spectrum of meaning attached to the word and concept of *nos* invokes the unconscious as an implicit gloss on the drama that follows it. The first line of spoken dialogue in the film supports this view. Like those first splashing sounds, the dialogue is disembodied: "*Prygajte, kak dogovarivalis'! Kto spustitsja po lestnice, tot trus i kozel*!" ("Jump as agreed. He who descends [by] the ladder is a coward and a goat.") This injunction, together with the suggestive composition of the film's opening, focuses us narrowly on the unconscious causative source of Ivan's fear. Most critics read it as an adolescent challenge to Ivan's masculinity;[17] they view his traumatized state when his mother finds him, hours later, still atop the tower, as the consequence of his fear of heights. Towards the end of the movie, this is how his brother Andrei describes Ivan's refusal to follow him and the father up the ladder to the platform: "*On vysoty boitsja.*" ("He is afraid of heights.") I argue, rather, that the very issue that traumatizes Ivan isn't his fear of heights but the fact of something submerged in his unconscious.

The disembodied allusion to a prior "agreement" suggests that Ivan is terrified by a pact which, in the context of the opening underwater imagery, evokes simultaneously an unconscious pact and an unconscious binding—in this case to conceal a secret on behalf of an unknown other. It further suggests that it is not the narcissistic vulnerability of young males that is the power behind this pact. In literary contexts, the word Ivan invokes to describe his fear, *strashnaia*, conjures the sense of an uncanny presence or even possession; his use of it to denote physical and emotional paralysis approaches the possibility of psychic haunting.[18]

Once we consider that the disembodied words "as agreed" may also reference an unconscious contract—to past unconscious one to cooperate with an unknowable ancestor to conceal a secret—we can analyze the language of the statement to unveil hidden lexical relationships between the words "goat," "coward," and the verb "descend," which provide more information about the silenced drama. First, the nouns "goat," "coward," and the verb "descend" are all included in the threat contained in the injunction.[19] The threat establishes that "descent," *spusk*, is an infringement of the agreement. While the immediate context makes clear that the literal reference is to "descending" by ladder, the intensity of the fear it elicits in Ivan suggests that a less literal reference is in play as well, concealed by the more obvious one. That is, to focus on one denotation of "descent" (the sense of going down ladders) is to displace other connotations of the word, such as *semeinyi spusk* and its synonym, *proiskhozhdenie*, "family descent or origins," and *padenie*, "fall" or "downfall."

This cluster of words, in the context of the earlier ominous "coward" and "goat," begins to define for us how Ivan actually heard that introductory injunction. Note first that the threat implicates the linguistic process of *naming* as the source of shame. The word "goat," *kozel*, connotes not only the animal but also, as we saw in *Pan's Labyrinth*, a "cuckold."[20] The hint of illicit sexual encounter is strengthened in the phonetic overlap connecting *trus*, "coward," and *trusy*, "bed linens, underpants." These associations suggest that it is not acrophobia that is responsible for Ivan's irrational fear but the resonance between two distinct types of descents. The boys' conscious agreement about the ladder evokes the unconscious agreement that haunts Ivan about another kind of descent and a clandestine sexual affair.

It is worth noting that "goat" in its meaning of cuckold derives from an obscene dialect of Russian called *mat*.[21] The "term *mat* itself derives from the Russian word for 'mother,' a component of the key phrase *yob tvoyu mat*' ('fuck your mother')," which is the basis of an "oral lexicon comprising thousands of phrases, exclamations, interjections, and idiomatic expressions, all enveloped in a nimbus of transparent synonyms and coded euphemisms."[22] It is a "set of refined and complex linguistic structures which, to some extent, function as a 'shadow language' of standard Russian."[23] One linguist has suggested that *mat* generates an aesthetic of transcendence over the limits of polite discourse, where accusatory words and those that describe sexual acts are excluded.[24] Its poetics are governed by substitutions based on phonetic similarities and thereby engage in acts of hiding within language. In the film, the *mat* word *kozel* points to an experience that cannot, for reasons yet to be determined, be named. Because the experience is hidden behind a *mat* word, it is implicitly linked to a sexual act.

Furthermore, the prologue's command that we "read backwards" suggests that what Ivan fears is not something in the future (the jump from the tower or the climb down the ladder) but something that has happened already (his descent into a forbidden secret). The dialogue between Ivan and his mother, later, on the same tower, links his fear and the concealment of his "descent." He tells her that he would have died of fear had she had not come, and she is perplexed by his apparent surprise at her presence. "Darling, what are you talking about? I'm here with you."[25] The fact that she has to assure him of this implies that on some level, he is somewhere else. Yet he has not moved from the tower. How, then, to explain his absence? One explanation is that he has had a dissociation. The film visually marks the gap between the time the other boys leave the tower and the time when Ivan's mother arrives, with the image of a sky blazing in the pinks and oranges of a setting sun. The mother's discarnate voice, which accompanies the searing image of Ivan paralyzed atop the tower, also fosters the sense of distance between Ivan and his mother's physical world (Figure 3.2).

The fetal curl of Ivan in his terror atop the tower evokes childbirth, another clue to his state of "elsewhereness." And here too, a disembodied voice, this time the mother's, intimates the presence of a menacing secret, echoing what transpired on the tower before she arrived. If the first scene cryptically identifies the precipitant of Ivan's dissociation as a shameful secret about illicit romance, cuckoldry, and illegitimate descent, then the

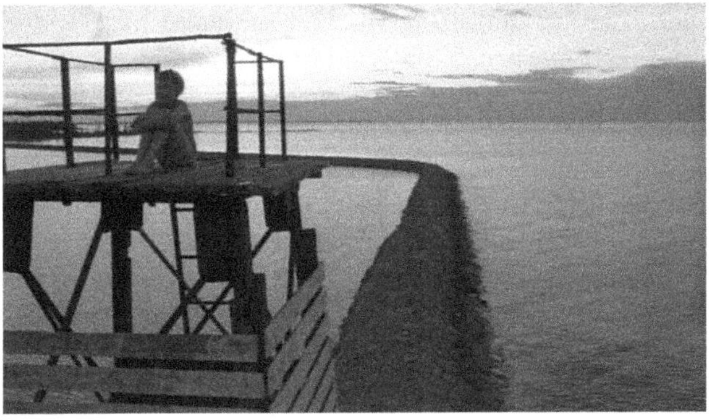

Figure 3.2 Ivan in a fetal position on the tower.

second scene's reiteration must be understood as occurring *in the wake of* his psychic disintegration. In other words, the scene in which Ivan and his mother establish a partnership to conceal a secret (about his "shameful" descent by ladder) parallels another partnership that has undone him—which preserves a secret about an illicit liaison and its illegitimate issue.

Let me be clear. Ivan's pact to conceal the fact of his descent does not refer to his own illegitimacy. Since the secret he asks his mother to keep is *his own*, we must reject an analytic position that interprets his acts and words as referring to an unsettling disruption in her psychic life. Indeed, the film's representation of the mother as an empathic conduit for psychic expansion in the wake of traumatizing adolescent experience makes it clear that if the inherited demand that Ivan "not descend" into the world of the unspoken imprisons him in a pathological relationship, the mother-son bond he enacts is not that shared with his own mother.

Rather, the verbal stirrings of the secreted word "goat" points to the survival of a memory trace derived from the father's experience. In contrast to the mother's commitment to Ivan's self-fashioning, such as suggesting that he can "jump another time," the father's censorial disposition throughout the film, not to mention the ellipses that mark his language, reveals him as the stranger within Ivan's psyche. The father's tight grip on what Ivan can say and do (especially, as we shall see, what he can physically ingest) evokes the way a phantom takes over a subject's mind and informs actions related to self-fashioning. Ivan's pact with his mother, then, must be seen as a symptomatic attempt to exorcise the effect of his father's "phantomogenic words": "coward," "goat," and "descend." To use Nicolas Abraham and Maria Torok's terminology, Ivan "stages" sharing a secret with his mother to "relieve his unconscious by placing the effects of the phantom in the social realm."[26]

Ivan's performance stages his haunting by the secret pact between the father and *his* mother, Ivan's paternal grandmother, who figures as a silent but important component of the fantasy. [27] While the film provides no overt information indicating whether the Babushka, who lives with the boys and their mother, is maternal or paternal, historians have noted that the general pattern of Russian domestic life had, as a strong rule, the understanding that a woman left her family at marriage and joined the household of her husband.[28] This interpretive position suggests a psychoanalytic corollary to Zvyagintsev's perplexing metaphysical explication of "what his film is about," which I cite in this chapter's epigraph. While the director leaves unclear the particular referent of the familial term "Mother" when he states that his film concerns "the metaphysical incarnation of the soul's movement from the Mother to the Father," the foregoing analysis offers a more precise optic for understanding: The film is about the "incarnation" of a (secret's) movement from the Mother (Babushka) to her son, the Father.

The tower scenes thus teach us to view the father's return as a figuration of the phantom, that is, as a fantasy. Like the faun in *Pan's Labyrinth*, the father is a vision triggered by a child's attempt to exempt himself from the awareness that he has infringed upon an agreement to conceal a secret and the psychic reorganization that must result from this awareness. Also like the faun, the father has a deceptive purpose—to resuppress the child's awareness of the secret, all the while subjecting him to trials that test the extent of his unconscious commitment to resist self-fashioning. Keeping in mind the phantom's objectives proves enormously helpful when it comes to decrypting the father's sparse but affectively powerful communications.

The Fantasy of the Father's Return

The words that trigger Ivan's breakdown and the resulting "trip" reappear in the first scene after the prologue, in the narrative proper, where we see his struggle with self-knowledge begin. He finds his brother and the other boys in a subterranean space splattered with muddy puddles. The setting visually echoes the film's watery first frames and is another evocation of the unconscious. When Andrei sides with the boys who called Ivan a "coward" and a "goat," a physical fight and reciprocal *name-calling* ensue. This war over words reiterates the role of language in catalyzing the psychic crisis that Ivan, in his fantasy, seeks to resolve.

The rash of accusations reinforces the importance of name-calling and also reiterates the link between cowardice, cuckoldry, and bed linens already established in the prologue. For example, Ivan, having all but asked the other boys to name his shame ("What did you say, who is a goat?" *Chto ty skazal? Kto kozel*), identifies Andrei as a goat as well because the latter has torn his shirt. Both brothers are now convicted goats. The verb "tore," *porval*, adds another telling dimension to the linguistic framework that conceals and reveals the boys' secret. Its object, "shirt," *rubashka*, is a word closely linked to the "bed linens" semantic chain, which includes words related to bridal trousseaus. At the same time, as in English, the word is applied to such situational contexts as relational breakups, such as, for example, "our relationship was torn apart by..." The verb "busted," or "riven apart," *razbil* (as in Andrei's lip), has the same semantic range of application, such as "we broke off our engagement." This linguistic subtext implies more than normal fraternal rivalry. Does it point to a rivalry somewhere in the censored scene? Andrei's explicit denunciation of Ivan as "liar," to their mother at the very moment that they learn of their father's return, supports this possibility.

When the boys get home, their mother shushes them twice. These injunctions against speaking, which precede her announcement of the father's return, recall the injunction with which the film begins. It is a prohibition very different in tone from her facilitative actions on the tower; the same difference is reflected in a diffidence with the boys that contrasts with the warmth she displayed earlier. Reading this narrative now as Ivan's fantasy, his mother has become a cipher. She is now a stand-in for another mother, his father's mother when she was young. Reading backwards again, we see her standing in for Babushka on the tower, when Ivan assumes the identity of his father as a young boy. The distant, removed disposition of Ivan's mother evokes Babushka's idiom of care for her son.

This scene is followed by a visual segue that moves us directly from the mother to Babushka and so reinforces the idea that Ivan's mother is an encoded representation of his grandmother. From the image of the mother's back—another suggestion that we too must go backwards to understand her role in the fantasy—the film cuts to an exceptionally long and narrowly focused shot of an unmoving Babushka, whom the brothers pass on their way to look for their father. The camera follows them as they search, taking in the visual and aural dimensions of the scene in their brief glimpse; finding no father, they move on to look for him elsewhere in the house. The camera does not go with them, however. It remains with Babushka, emphasizing her status as an integral component of the fantasy.

In this scene, Zvyagintsev makes ingenious use of the rhetoric of portraiture to establish a framework for later relational connections.[29] Babushka's stillness throughout the shot's thirteen-second duration recalls Ivan's paralysis, suggesting that his elsewhereness and her silence are connected. Although absent of dialogue, the scene is not absent of sound: The *Benedictus* from the Mozart *Requiem*, sung by a chorus and a quartet of soloists, accompanies the visual portrait. The use here of the mass for the dead adds the dimension of loss to the context by which we are slowly defining the silenced drama. It points us to another quartet defined by loss, this one comprised of Babushka, her son, and the two brothers. (The mother is excluded for she is "outside" the family line; this position is reinforced by her literal location outside the house when she tells the boys that their father has returned.)

As the chorus and quartet express mourning in voice, the camera expresses it in Babushka's melancholic demeanor. And it makes clear that pain is the object of its focus as it pans, seemingly incongruously, from her face to the burning embers in a *pech'*, a stove, making an imagistic pun on the word *pechal'*, or "grief." This is another example of the linguistic and the visual reinforcing one another. The information presented in this shot, in other words, must be "heard" to be appreciated. Furthermore, if we translate the image of burning wood into a word, we hear *topit'*, one of whose meanings is "to stoke up," "to warm," "to be heated," "to burn." But, recalling how an unutterable word and its affect may be concealed through a word whose phonetic structure has more than one meaning, we cannot ignore how the word also means "to sink"

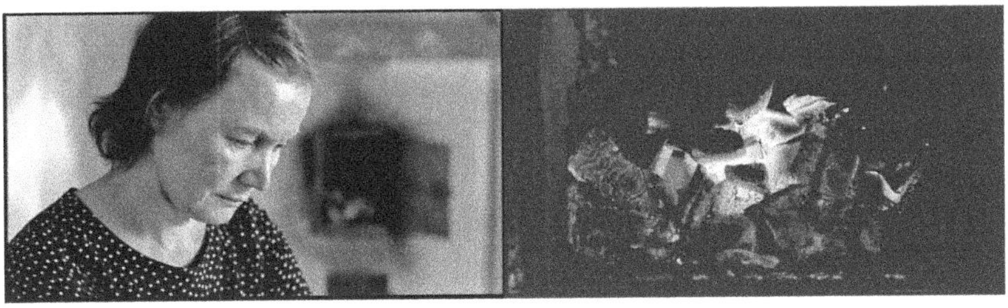

Figure 3.3 Close-up of Babushka's grief-stricken face juxtaposed with the image of the wood-burning stove.

in the senses of "to drown" and "to ruin." The linguistic properties of the word evoked by the image recapitulate and contain the simultaneity of two irreconcilable states of being (Figure 3.3).[30]

Further lexical relationships connect the word *topit'* to a semantic chain of other words evoking the concept of inflamed affectivity—words such as "passion," *teplot*, and "inflame," *gorjachít*, that intimate a drama of inflamed passion may account for Babushká's mournful affect. In the context of the earlier fight between Ivan and Andrei, with its veiled references to conjugal sex, breakups, and cuckoldry, this cinematographic portrait conjures an embedded saga of a tragic love triangle involving two brothers and the wife of one of them.

More details may be derived from the lexical information offered in the image of the fire itself, which features not only the blaze but also the resulting charred and burnt wood. The Russian word for "fire," *ogon'*, is obviously connected to a chain of words whose meaning devolves on acts of burning, including singeing, scorching, and smudging. Less obviously, one of its synonyms, *koster*, or "bonfire," is also a synonym of the word "smudge," *gryaznoye pjatno*. It belongs to a lexical inventory of words, such as "spot," *pjatno*, and its synonyms, "blight," "stain," and "mark."

The imagistically underrepresented connotation of the word *topit'* in its meaning "to sink" evokes the same affective experience of dishonor compressed within the words "fire" and "smudge." Synonyms include words referring to disastrous turns of events, such as "failure," "collapse," and "to go under." While the sense of "drown" appears to anticipate what happens to the father toward the end of Ivan's fantasy, we should by now be wary of taking much in the film at surface value. In light of the complex net of linguistic information communicated by the stove image, we do better to interpret the father's aqueous descent as the symbolic expression of successful repression: the return to unconsciousness of the secret blot that haunts this family.

As I will elucidate in more detail later, the submerging of the father coincides with Ivan's (first unsolicited) utterance of the word that names him—"papa." Many critics have understood this as Ivan's cathartic triumph over a conflict that consumed him. I think this is warranted; the new capacity to use a contaminated word implies its psychic digestion and the resumption of self-fashioning. But we are reading the journey as a fantasy, and that is the context in which Ivan's triumph takes place. The successful repression symbolized by the father's submersion is *a fantasy* of successful repression. It satisfies Ivan's need *to persuade himself* that the conflict has been resolved—that he has regained his accustomed psychic blindness, repudiated all knowledge of the shameful secret, and thereby preserved the status quo. This catharsis is his painstaking but illusory proof, not that all obstacles to self-fashioning have been overcome but that *there were no obstacles to self-fashioning to begin with.*

The image of the father's sinking body also delineates the linguistic process of repression—the uncoupling of words from contaminating affects. The father's sinking—papa's drowning—denotes not only death by water but also the sense of "flushing" or "washing away." It is the shame of this "papa," and the secrecy around him, that has convulsed Ivan and overwhelmed his capacity to name and absorb it. The phantom's return, therefore, has done its work; it has transmitted to Ivan, via its haunting, the psychic tools and linguistic strategies necessary for preservative repression.

The word *topit'* thus emerges as a keyword, a cryptonym concealing within a singular phonetic structure the passionate underpinnings of a family's shame and the means by which the shame may be flushed away and kept sunken (repressed) and at bay.[31] Further lexical networks between the word "to drown" and others that mean "to cover," "to conceal," "to silence," "to muffle," and "to black out" further outline the missing piece that preservative repression conceals.

This is in the future, however, as Ivan's fantasy of the journey develops. In the meantime, the Babushka portrait provides a visual and linguistic key to the scene that immediately follows it—the first visual perception of the father. Zvyagintsev directly quotes Andrea Mantegna's (1431–1506) famous painting, *The Lamentation of Christ.* Virtually all critics have noted this reference, and many rely on the liturgical literature to explore its religious implications.[32] However, because this image is quickly followed by another one representing Abraham's sacrifice of Isaac, we must not be too quick to assign religious symbolism to the image.[33] Given that the Old Testament story has traditionally been read by New Testament theologians as a prefiguring of Christ's sacrifice, it is likely that Zvyagintsev is less interested in theology per se than in representations of sons sacrificed by their fathers.[34] We will have more to say about this presently (Figure 3.4).

Jesus's mother Mary is the primary lamenter in Mantegna's painting. Zvyagintsev's staging excludes her from his reproduction, but the visual absence of one mother's grief recalls the silenced grief of another,

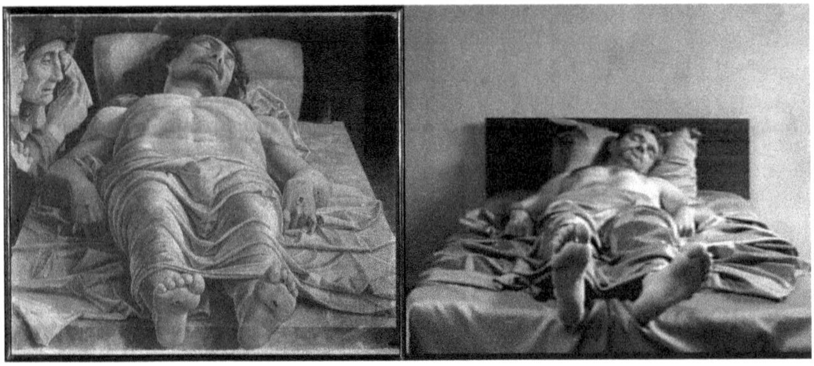

Figure 3.4 Andrea Mantegna's "The Lamentation of Christ"; courtesy of Erich Lessing/Art Resources, NY; juxtaposed with Zvyagintsev's replication of the scene.

Babushka, whose portrait immediately precedes Zvyagintsev's replica.[35] Moreover, the striking resemblance between actress Galina Popova and Mantegna's Mary—the angle of their faces, their grief-stricken eyes, their mournful mouths—visually links Mary and Babushka.

Zvyagintsev's elision of Mary suggests that something about Babushka needs to be removed or hidden. Linens and undergarments are central to Mantegna's painting and are reproduced exquisitely in Zvyagintsev's reconstruction. They reevoke the earlier linguistic network of sex and beds and marriage and adultery that came up first in the prologue and then in the fight between the brothers. The triangular linens that frame the father's genitals in the center of this image mirror the triangular shape of the undergarments that Ivan wore atop the tower.[36] Art historians have noted that Mantegna's intent was to call attention to Christ's humanity (as opposed to his divinity),[37] but Zvyagintsev's recontextualization of the scene in the setting of a bedroom takes this a step further and yields a new vantage point from which to interpret his use of Mantegna's painting.[38]

For example, his substitution of a sea-blue silk sheet in place of the white one of Mantegna's painting hints both at sensuality and at the father's shameful origins. The white sheet conceals Christ's genitalia (even as the folds accentuate them), but the blue sheet imports to the father the stigma of cuckoldry. This symbolism comes from a Bruegel painting (*The Blue Cloak*), in which "an adulterous wife hides her infidelities from her cuckold husband by covering him with a large blue cloak... She hangs a blue cloak, the symbol of lies, around her husband."[39] A blue cloak in Renaissance art was subsequently understood to symbolize lying and deception. Sexual deception is also suggested by the word "silky," *shelkovisty*, which translates a feature of the linen's texture. To

call someone "silky" is to focus on an insincere or "smarmy," *vkradchivy*, aspect of his or her personality.

In Mantegna's painting, the relationship between the marble slab upon which Christ lies and the burial "crypt," or "tomb," that lies beyond it (on the upper right side of the painting) anchors the scene within the period between his mortal death and burial, and his subsequent "resurrection" or "return," *voskresénie*.[40] Zvyagintsev's reproduction extends the implications of this interstitial moment to suggest that what is anticipated by the boys as they rush past their grandmother, the father's return, relates to a shameful saga that was experienced by a mother and then transmitted, silently, to her son. Indeed, the director's substitution of the wood-burning stove for the opening to the crypt in the upper right side of his portrait of Babushka objectifies the saga as something that is both encrypted and related in some way to a "return" or "resurrection." Furthermore, the fact that the fire image ultimately resolves into the door that Ivan and Andrei push open for their first glimpse of their returned father implicitly suggests the shaping of their apperception of him by Babushka's silenced drama. The scene establishes that the father's return is a response to Babushka's entombed secret.[41]

Filial Sacrifice

Our backward-reading strategy is embraced and exemplified by Ivan, who dashes away, within six seconds of seeing his father, to an attic in which is stored a worn trunk.[42] Ivan rummages through it; he pulls out a dusty book of Bible stories with folio etchings, and just as Andrei joins him, he locates, hidden among the pages, a family photo from their early childhood. That the photo was "concealed among the sheets," that is, the pages of the book, implicates it too as a symbol of the family's shame. The close-up of Ivan rifling through the various sheets of the book visually recalls the blue sheet that covered the father, and indeed, both senses are connoted by the word "sheet," *list*, which also signifies the nouns "leaf," "plate," and "paddle." This lexical contiguity is crucial for deciphering a submerged level of discourse that is communicated between the father and his sons on their journey, especially because it intersects with the "blot" and "stain" lexical relationships uncovered earlier.

The family photo confirms that the man the boys just saw is indeed their father. The composition of the picture, in which the father is literally handling a toddler-aged Ivan, is an example of the prolific mentions of "hands," *ruka*, and by extension acts of "handling, handing off, transmitting" in the film. The superimposition of the picture on a photo-plate of a wood engraving by Julius Schnorr von Carolsfeld (1794–1872) of an iconic biblical image—Isaac's binding by Abraham—guides us to view Ivan's family and Isaac's family as similar (Figure 3.5).[43]

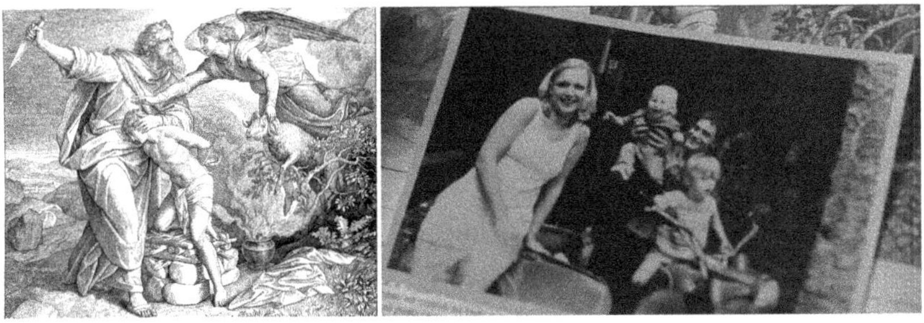

Figure 3.5 Julius Schnorr von Carolsfeld, "The Sacrifice of Isaac"; courtesy of Alfredo Dagli Orti/Art Resources, NY; juxtaposed with screenshot of family photo wedged within it.

Abraham's binding of Isaac as he prepares to sacrifice him as God has instructed refers to an event narrated in Genesis 22. Religion scholars who plumb folklore for preserved collective memories consider this material, called "The Binding" or the *Aqedah*, significant in the spread of both Christianity and Islam. For example, Russian vernacular religious practices, such as rites and festivals, include details that "can be explained as allusions to the *Aqedah*." Most prevalent are the "baking oven as altar" and "the collection or deployment of chopped wood, and knives."[44] These associations reverberate with Zvyagintsev's interest in the image of the wood-burning stove, not to mention his concerted attention to fire management over the course of the fishing trip. One other detail of ritual practices that is related to the *Aqedah* is the frequency with which a "triangle of parents" figures as a catalyst for the plots that shape them.[45] I am postulating that such a triangulation is the core of the secret that haunts Ivan and that the tense shifting alliances among the boys and the father may be seen as symptomatic reenactments of the repressed scenario.

The father's enigmatic character echoes the enigmas of Genesis 22: Nothing is said there of God's motivation for testing Abraham as he does; Abraham says nothing of his intent to Sarah, his wife and the mother of Isaac; and, last but not least, Isaac's father offers him no explanation for his acts.[46] Some scholars have argued that these biblical silences tacitly point to questions surrounding Isaac's paternity; this view aligns with the conclusions I draw from the patterns of silences and lexical displacements in the film.[47]

The "trunk," *grob*, is filled with bed linens, which summons again the now-familiar lexical network of relationships between "bed linens" and "cuckoldry." The phonetic resonance between "trunk" and "tomb," *grobica*, links the concept of memory, metaphorically rendered as a container for memorabilia, to the concept of "crypt," whose image in Mantegna's *Lamentation of Christ* demarcates the place where Christ will be entombed and from which he will emerge in resurrection. The father's endless search for crypt-like containers, his consistent backward glances, his obfuscation of information pertaining to "where he came from," and his fury at Ivan's suspicious demeanor all expose how his identity is shaped by secrets.

The Dinner Scene

The departure of the brothers and father on their fishing trip removes us from Babushka's saga per se and toward how its preservative repression has impacted Ivan's self-fashioning process. This shift in focus is communicated in the dinner that follows the boys' retrieval of the photograph. The plan for the journey emerges during this theatrically staged scene, and so do more details about the drama whose concealment is the source of the journey fantasy in the first place. Critics who focus on the wine and the father's extended disassembling of a chicken (likened to Jesus's distribution of food) have frequently compared the dinner scene to Leonardo da Vinci's *The Last Supper.*[48] Given that visual art is clearly a source of inspiration for Zvyagintsev, this is a persuasive position. However, his spatial setup is simpler and reflects another venerated table scene. This one, *Troiska* painted by Andrei Rublev (1360–1430), is celebrated for its organization of space.[49] Both Rublev and Zvyagintsev, who had a deep appreciation for the former's artistry,[50] rely on triangular structures to represent unseen presences. Although five people attend the table in the film instead of Rublev's three, the virtual silence of the mothers in this scene excludes them from the spatial configuration established by the dialogue among the father and his two sons.

The biblical source of Rublev's painting 'The Hospitality of Abraham" gives strength to this interpretation. This story is recounted in Genesis 18:1–33 and tells of "three strangers fed by Abraham who prophecy Sara's pregnancy."[51] Rublev's elision of Abraham and Sara in his composition of the story emphasizes the harmony among the three guests, who represent God as a trinity, that is, as a shared existence between Father, Son, and the (resurrected) Holy Spirit. The emphasis on the three guests brings into focus the idea of a God whose activating and guiding force takes up residence in the body of a believer in Jesus Christ. Zvyagintsev's "spatial orchestration," premised on an implicit exclusion of the silent mothers, anticipates the metaphoric role of the father in the film. Just as God resides as an inner, activating spirit or principle of his believers' existence, so too does the father function in the lives of his sons (Figure 3.6).

Eating scenes in phantom films point to obstacles to self-fashioning; there is a good example of this in the dinner scene of *The Return*,

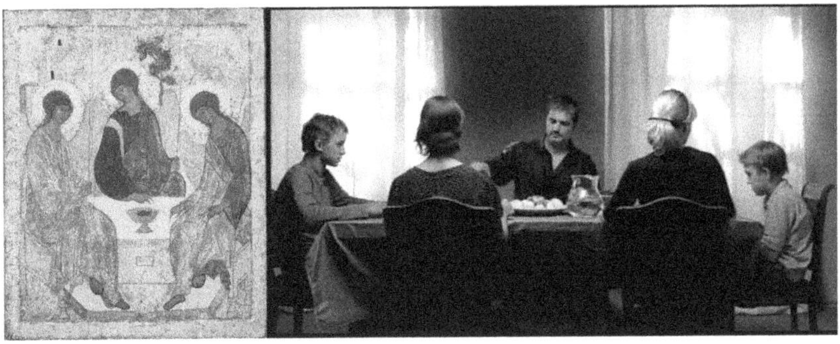

Figure 3.6 Andrei Rublev's Icon of the Old Testament Trinity; courtesy of Scala/ Art Resources, NY; juxtaposed with screenshot of dinner scene.

where an important gloss is provided before the father arrives. Ivan, Ofelia-like, sneakily ingests a cherry before everyone is seated. On his second attempt, he is thwarted by his mother and forced to return the piece of fruit to the bowl. Her silent injunction against ingesting is reminiscent of the doomed fruit in Anton Chekhov's (1860–1904) *The Cherry Orchard* (*Vishnevyj sad*).[52] This play dramatizes the story of a woman who, psychically stymied by the drowning of her son, is unable to save her house and her lineage. Chekhov made an "oft-quoted comment" to the effect that "[p]eople can be having dinner, just having dinner, and at the same time, their happiness is being secured, or their lives are being destroyed."[53] There is another resonance between the film and this play in that the final scene of *The Cherry Orchard* involves the metaphorical encryption of a man, Firs, who articulates confused memories of a murder, inside the ill-fated house/ family lineage.

Following Chekhov's observation, we can look to the way information that pertains to the life trajectories of the diners is embedded within their words and gestures. Once everyone has gathered around the table, there is an extended silence—almost a minute, or a third of the duration of the entire scene—that is finally broken by the father's first utterance. The silence foregrounds and animates the silences and concealment that surround him; at the same time, his power to end the silence demonstrates the objective of his return—to transmit the idiom of concealment through strict control over what passes through the mouth, be it food, drink, or words.

In this case, the father's first words are a command to the boys' mother: "Pour them some wine," *Nalej im vino*. The "them" refers to Andrei and Ivan; the father has already poured wine for the mother and

Babushka and so made them irrelevant to the rest of the scene. Here too those three laconic words communicate a second level of meaning: The word *vino*, "wine," is connected to the concept of "guilt," *tvorit*, in a common Russian proverb: *vino vinu tvori*, "wine causes guilt." In its intransitive form, the verb "to pour," *nalit'*, means "to fill up" as in "to be filled with shame," *napolnjat'sja styda*. If we include in this constellation of associations the lexical networks connecting the words "blame," "stain," "blot," and "smear," the father's command would seem to suggest that drinking wine is tantamount to psychically acknowledging the shameful saga.

But is this really what the father means? Keep in mind that phantoms return to test a descendant's commitment to concealing a secret, not to aid its absorption and psychic assimilation. We must entertain the possibility, therefore, that the father's first command is a trial, like that posed to Ofelia by the faun, or God's command to Abraham to prepare his son for sacrifice. This sense of a trial as "tests" given to young novices in order to assess their progress toward mastery of a skill best captures the father's intentions. The father's instruction that wine be poured for the boys reads superficially as an invitation to assimilate the family stain but more powerfully as the covert beginning of their initiation into the family practice of concealment.

The four phantom films that I analyze all use eating scenes to tell us about the saga that blocks the protagonists' self-fashioning. They are sufficiently frequent in *The Return*, however, to warrant deeper exploration. My view is that Ivan's hunger reflects (and disguises) the thwarting of his self-fashioning processes and is therefore a crucial motivator of the journey's unfolding. The vicissitudes of Ivan's appetite mimic the vicissitudes of his battle with his father, and Zvyagintsev's intense focus on this dynamic is revealing. The father's control over what Ivan eats, and when he eats, is unacceptable to Ivan; for the father, however, the digestive processes of self-fashioning must be organized so as to preserve intact the secret and the family lineage, not to assimilate them.

The dinner scene is an exposition of the father's organizational regimen. The mothers dilute the "wine-blame" that they pour in the boys' glasses, and the father acquiesces silently to this act; this suggests that "watering it down," *razzhizhat'*, is an important principle. "Watering down" or "thinning" the wine diffuses the stain and its affect, as if to "cleanse," "obliterate," "rub away," or "efface," *stirat'* it. This lexical network communicates a strategy for ensuring the preservation of the silenced drama: Diluting and thinning makes the water and wine "digestible" while keeping it thin and transparent enough to allow for the invisible submersion of preservative repression. Effective repression is equivalent to decontamination; once a wine or a word is diluted enough that it can no longer stain—once it is sufficiently "deterged"—self-fashioning can proceed.

If they adhere to this rule in their self-fashioning, the boys can be trusted to fulfill their unconscious family obligations. Note that there is no ingestion in the scene except for the wine, even after the father goes to great lengths to break a roasted chicken up into edible portions. The film represents the chicken as the main ingredient of the meal by placing it in a central position on the table and surrounding it by the family; yet it is not eaten. This may be construed as a tacit comment on the suitability of ingesting "chicken," *kuritsa*. (The word "chicken" is a synonym of the Russian word *trus*, "coward," which we have seen rhymes with "bed linens.") The camera's lingering attention on the father after he handles the chicken bolsters this. He persistently "wipes" his hands, ostensibly to rid them of the grease but more likely to "cleanse," "rub out," and "remove" contamination of his hands by the *word* "chicken." The gestural wiping demonstrates what must be done on the lexical level to effectively "wipe out the memory," *unichtózhit' vospominánie*, of the shameful stain.

Once we see how words, or acts that can be translated into words, can decontaminate lexical fragments stained by the family shame, we can better appreciate the prominence in the film of such watery entities as "downpours," "rain," "puddle," and "sludge, soil."[54] If we extend this list to include elements in the plot where Ivan and Andrei get "drenched" and "soaked," and the escalation of tension over a broken promise to go to a "waterfall," we can see how these disguised references to the word "downfall" evoke the saturating presence of the stain in the boys' lives.

At the same time, the father repeatedly exposes his sons to such muddy and smeary messes; those are the conditions best suited for teaching them the ropes, as it were, of filial binding. Even the opening sound of this remarkable film—that disembodied splash, *plesk*, whose semantic scope encompasses meanings ranging from "stain" to "cleanse or wash"—is an acoustic conveyance of the same network of implications.

The brothers' exposure to this first trial yields mixed results. They do follow their father's order to drink. But Andrei's wish for more is thwarted by the father, as it breaks the rule against uncensored or uninhibited ingestion/digestion, i.e., self-fashioning. And this, of course, is the primary source of tension between the father and Ivan, whose distaste for the wine discloses resistance to his father's rules and to the saga they preserve at the expense of his desire for unthwarted expansion.

The father's control over Ivan's hunger and its satiation is an initiation into the rules of what (including language) may and may not pass through his mouth.[55] The inaugural scene of the road trip portrays another trial, this one in the form of a conversation between Ivan and his father in the car. Again, Zvyagintsev uses visuals—the mise-en-scène itself and the character portraits established within it—to call attention to linguistic and imagistic proscriptions that underlie their conflicts.

The scene that immediately follows the car conversation depicts Ivan awakening, thus suggesting that the conversation was a dream. Moreover, the oneiric dimension of this conversation echoes the dissociative tenor of Ivan's earlier conversation with his mother, when Ivan assumed the identity of his father as a young boy. But if Ivan's mother on the tower represented Babushka, Ivan's father in the car represents Babushka's husband, the cuckold, the man who raised him as a son. This is a conversation between a boy and the man whom the boy was not allowed to love as a father lest he reveal the shameful truth of his paternity.

The father's speech in this scene is tinged with the formality of a previous generation—the generation of the man who raised him. His invocation of the unusually formal word "father," *ottsom*, when he instructs Ivan on how to address him, is an example. Furthermore, we see the entire conversation through the rearview mirror, another backward-looking metaphor that relates its relevance to the unspoken family history. The father supposes that Ivan does not call him "Papa" because he is ashamed of him, and he implies that Ivan has lied about this; both of these charges vividly conjure up the wounded anger of a man who has been rejected by the boy he raised. In this scene, we see how their very compliance with the injunction to keep their secret both binds them and gives rise to endless tension between them. The enigmatic acts by which the father renders himself (and his origins) illegible agitate Ivan, who echoes the affective experience of the man who raised the father with the obsessive suspicion and fear of a presumptive cuckold.

Ivan and his mother talk about the act of concealing his descent; father and son, however, maintain that nothing is concealed at all. Ivan denies that he is lying about being embarrassed by the father, and the father is complicit in the lie; the faces of father and son as we see them in the rearview mirror reveal that Ivan's compliance is insincere and *that they both know it.* And yet, Ivan seals a verbal oath of honesty with "Papa," and the father praises Ivan for his linguistic adherence, "well done," and includes the designatum, "son."[56] The kinship words imply affective attachments that neither possesses at that moment, and they both know this; to deploy them in speech is a collaborative act of concealment, the essence of preservative repression.

Ivan's dream is fantasy-like in its "magical" resolution of the conflict over whose words should be in his mouth, but once he has woken up, he is no longer so complicit. His hunger upon waking is a desire for both psychic and physical assimilation, and he grows increasingly anxious when they are thwarted. He acknowledges this when he complains to Andrei of the imperious power of what "Dad said," "*papa skazal.*"

The father subjects him to a long wait while Andrei is off looking for a restaurant, and Ivan's misery increases. He watches his father's voyeurism from the back of the car, as Zvyagintsev, with extraordinarily deft cutting, tracks a complex sequence of alternating visual images that reflect the lines of vision of both father and son.

First, the father's eyes focus on of the *triangular folds* of the *skirt* of an approaching woman with a very provocative walk. Ivan watches him track her in the *rearview* mirror, a *hand* visible right next to her seductive *behind*. The father's line of sight, therefore, recapitulates the lexical networks that we have seen delineating the secret conditions of his illegitimate birth: the textiles, the folds, the triangles, the hands that point to the "seat" of an illicit sexual affair. It is too much for Ivan to bear, and when the possibility of food finally arrives, he impulsively declares that he has changed his mind, that he has "crossed sides," *perehotel*, and is no longer hungry.

This vision of the seductive woman sets the stage for the next trial in the boys' initiation. Immediately following her passing, Andrei, for whom they have been waiting, is found. The father berates him for his laggardliness and requires of him an agreement to swear off certain acts, such as "looking around, taking in the view." Andrei accepts the father's words into his own mouth, an act of compliance for which the father praises him as he had praised Ivan for his earlier parroting. Moments later, in a restaurant, Andrei hungrily eats his lunch, thus confirming that he has accepted the father's terms; he has digested the command to circumscribe his self-fashioning. Ivan, however, will not eat; he does not accept the father's terms and will not ingest or digest them.

But of course, Ivan must eat if he is to survive; he will have to find tolerable ways to "eat" his father's words. Furthermore, the father recognizes the implications of Ivan's resistance and escalates the intensity of the trial of compliance. He places his watch on the table and announces that Ivan's plate must "be cleaned" within "two minutes," *cherez dve minuty dolzhna byt' chistoj*. The "need" or "necessity," *dolzhna*, that the father invokes is linked by Ivan later in the film to his father's tormenting, when Ivan asks his father what he "needs" from his sons in order to stop tormenting them. What the father needs, his statement cryptically conveys, is for Ivan to comply with the father's strictures, in this case by ensuring that the plate is cleaned. As the photo-plates in the Bible linked the word "plate" with its synonyms "sheets" and "bed linens," we can see in this command the need to deterge ("clean," "wash," or "purify," *chistoj*) the word "plate" of its shameful affect and to demonstrate this purification by eating. This the same logic established in the consumption of watered-down wine.

This is not the end of the struggle, however. A piece of bread falls to the ground (after Ivan insolently tosses it towards his mouth and misses), and he refuses to eat it, claiming that it is "dirty, sordid," *gryaznit'*. He is comfortable leaving the dirty evidence for others to "remove," "let out," as in "to let something out of sight," *vykinem*. In this, however, he unwittingly exposes his weakness as concealer of sordid and dirty secrets, and in response, the father commands twice that Ivan eat the "soup and bread."

This repetition demonstrates the lexical strategy of permitting ingestion of "sordid" objects *while also* preserving the psychic status quo. The camera reveals the bread to be the "dark," *chernyj*, common variety; the word "dark" is synonymous with "smut" and "soil." The extended shot of the soup offers further information. We see it to be a "pottage," *pokhlebka*, (as opposed to the "broths," or "bouillons," *bul'on*, often implied by the general term "soup"). The detergent power of "pottage" derives from its orthography: The word *pokhlebka* literally hides or encrypts the word "bread," *hleb*, within it.[57] The image makes clear that conversion of the word "soup" to its synonym, "pottage," neutralizes the negative charge of the sordid bread and render it (and other stained foods) edible—a task that Ivan must learn to accomplish if he is to survive.

Similar lexical rules are articulated throughout the journey. For example, when a downpour traps the car in a muddy mess, the father communicates to his sons, along with instructions about freeing the car, information about preserving a secret even while transmitting it. For example, he emphasizes the order in which objects must be "handled" and placed. After instructing the boys to cut "branches," *vetok*, a word that also connotes "lineage," he makes clear that they need to be placed *under* the "wheel" or "roller," not "before or in front" of it. This is a cryptic communication that the shameful (lineage) branch must be put under, and thereby concealed, by the wheel. Then, with the branch securely concealed, the secret is transmitted down the lineage, from back to front, from ancestors to descendent. Andrei's turn at the "steering wheel," *rul*, synonymous with "helm," and "rudder," calls attention to his growing mastery of the rules the father has returned to impart.

The father subjects the boys to another intense trial in another downpour; this time, he has the boys raise their "oars," "paddles," also synonyms in Russian of the word "sheet." Rowing in tandem makes the boys "rowers," "pullers," "paddlers," *grebtsy*, words that are lexically connected to the nouns "strippers," "removers," and "lifters" of stains." When the father directs Ivan to "keep the boat's bow in the wave," *derzhi lodku nosom k volne*, during the stormy crossing to the island, he is also imploring Ivan to diffuse his curiosity, to "wash," or "splash" the "nose." Frequent instructions to "change," or "hang wet clothes to dry," while commonsensical, also intimate a more charged proscriptive sensibility.

Another scene focuses on the father's mouth and what will or not pass through it. Ivan is curious about why two fish that the boys had caught were not cooked for dinner and asks what to do with them. Andrei muses that the fish can probably be cooked and asks his father if he knows how, using the verb *umet'*, "to know, understand" "to be able to." The father affirms that he does, with the postscript that he does "not eat fish (now)," because he once "gorged." This is the only personal detail that the father shares with his sons throughout the journey. The father's antipathy toward fish correlates with his growing antagonism toward Ivan's obsession with fishing (lit. "catch fish," *rybu lovit'*). If Ivan's hunger is a metaphor for self-fashioning, fishing, the desire to "catch," "trap," "snare," and "hook," is a metaphor for his inclination to uncover the unconscious knowledge that haunts him. The father's response to Andrei's question communicates a lesson about the consequences of too much inquisition.

Immediately thereupon, the father rises to retire and commands his sons to extinguish the bonfire and bind more tightly the loose assembly of their "tent." The father's warnings about fishing, and his subsequent declaration of the family rules, are understood by Ivan to carry homicidal intentions; indeed, his paranoia about his father's motives transforms him into Isaac during the *Aqedah.* He links the father's words to murderous designs to decapitate him: He views the words in his father's "mouth," *rot,* as the executing agent against his "neck," *rot.* Decapitation refers to Ivan's feeling of being choked and strangled by the father's words. Ivan himself identifies the father's mouth as the source of confusion and fear. Countering Andrei's defense that the father's adult status makes it difficult to not engage in "papa this, papa that" behavior, Ivan claims that one must "peer into the mouth," *v rot zagliadyvat',* of someone [in order to fully assess their trustworthiness]. The pervasive allusions to the *Aqedah*, such as a journey into the deep woods with a father who is silent about his objectives, not to mention the knife trope that stimulates Ivan's murder fantasy, tacitly reprise Zvyagintsev's earlier equation of the *Aqedah* and other kinds of binding filial obligations that can destroy a life.[58]

The conflict between Ivan and his father reaches its zenith on Friday, in an angry explosion after a fishing expedition. We have seen how the father's use of time limits both marks the trials he imposes on his sons and adds to their stringency. This time he actually gives his timepiece to Andrei as the boys are leaving, implicitly placing Ivan under Andrei's "watch." But the boys return hours late, and although it is Ivan whose obsession with fishing is the source of the delay, the father's anger is directed at Andrei. This suggests that it is the elder brother who was being tested here, on his ability to rein in Ivan and ensure that the younger boy will toe the family line and fulfill his binding filial obligations.

The need for this test is intimated in a conversation between Ivan and his father on the shore of the lake. The father tells Ivan to wash his dirty "bowl" (a synonym of "plate," and by extension, "sheet,") after a meal. Ivan, fed up with being commanded, looks around to make sure there are no witnesses and then throws his father's bowl into the lake. When the father joins him and asks where his bowl is, Ivan tells him that it "sunk," *utonula*, in the lake, concealing both his agency and the anger that led him to deliberately dispose of the dish. Meant to pique, Ivan's response surprisingly elicits praise from the father, whose judgment of his son is premised exclusively on how well he conceals the shameful family saga. Ivan's lie denies his instrumentality in the detergent act of sinking the dish and therefore confirms to the father that Ivan is absorbing the rules of preservative repression. Ivan's way of expressing his rage at his father, sinking the dish—is intrinsically decontaminative.

This makes Ivan appear to be a model initiate. Indeed, the father's offer to teach him how to carve a "dish out of birch" communicates appreciation for Ivan's growing competence at (unconscious) deception and the fact that he will expect further such feats of competence in the future. The words "dish" and "carve out" are stigmatized already, and "birch" is tainted by its synonymic relationship to "branch" with its associations of lineage. Ivan's response to his father's ideation of a next phase in his initiation is to cry out that he is incapable of this, that he has "failed," "gone wrong," "strayed," or "gone to seed," *u menja ne poluchitsja*.[59]

Ivan's anguish reveals that he has not yet fully acquiesced to living a life dedicated to the protection of the family secret, but in drowning the bowl, his self-fashioning processes have unwittingly aligned with his father's intentions, and his self-accusation speaks to this realization. In this conversation on the lake shore, the father makes clear that Ivan's life's role is to guard; Ivan's resistance to this life sentence is what induces the father to enlist Andrei and deputize him to accompany Ivan on his fishing expedition.

That the father is correct in assuming that Ivan resists the obligations of guardianship in favor of "fishing" and other acts of unconscious investigation is borne out in the next scene, where Ivan twice declares to Andrei that they "need worms, the native fish will not go for the bread."[60] This observation is a reflection of his obsession with catching what he is fishing for, and the second time it is synchronized with an image of the father emerging from the forest to the beach. The father's knowledge of the island marks him as indigenous; *he* is the "native fish" that Ivan wants to catch. Andrei likens his father to a fish when he later idiomatically refers to the father's willingness to let them go fishing before they leave the island as having been duped by the boys: The father, Andrei claims, "fetched" or "brought" in the "pancake," *blin nravit'sia*, of their fishing gambit. Finally, the duplication of the verb "go to," *poiti*, used first by the father to announce he will "go for a walk," and then by Ivan immediately after when he states that the fish "won't go for," *ne pojdet*, bread, implicitly equates the father's actions with those of the fish.

The father "goes for" his walk, and the boys "go for" their earthworms; the parallel editing of the two excursions shows that their destinations are the same and implies that their objectives are, too. The father goes to the island's sole house, where he digs a deep hole in the center of the foundation and retrieves a trunk. In this is concealed another box that cannot be opened without a key. The correlation between "holes," "female genitalia," and "black boxes" or "cases" in the Russian *mat* offers compelling evidence that the father's excursion is a metaphorical return to the source of his haunting. We have seen how the word "goat" means "cuckold" in Russian *mat* and how its coincidence with the word "descend" triggered Ivan's dissociation on the tower because of its unspoken reference to the father's fallen, sunken, concealed identity. In this way, the father's acts may be construed as a return to his mother's womb, or in the cant of Russian *mat*, his mother's "cunt," the origins of the lowlife father. The boys' excursion, which takes them to the very place where the father dug up the trunk, likewise, is a return to the roots of Ivan's possession by suspicion: his father's illegitimacy. Earthworms are creatures whose natural habitat is the smeary mess of mud and rain; their movements resemble those of a "screw," *chervjak*, replete as those are with sexual connotations, and they are known in Russian as "lowly ghosts," *nizkaya dusha*—fitting symbols of the haunting conditions of the father's birth.

The boys arrive at this same house after the father has left; peering into the windows, they see the dugout pit of moist dirt, the perfect place to collect worms. The spectral resonance of the pit is echoed by Andrei's ghostly hoot as he looks through its windows. The house's windows frame information related to the haunting; they call attention to the boys' status as witnesses who "see through someone," *vid'et naskvoz*, a connection that is repeated when the boys find an abandoned ship whose windows, too, are emphasized by the camera's slow pan. The huge fish that the boys hook there, a metaphor for their father, reinforces the idea that they have found out his truth, something that Andrei unwittingly confirms when he claims that Ivan's explanation for their tardiness stated "the truth," *pravda*.

The father, already angry, becomes enraged by Andrei's affirmation that his failure (to contain Ivan) was a consequence of a "truth" about what they "hooked": His secret has been exposed. The barrage of insults that Andrei hurls at his father when his father hits him in response—such as "riffraff," *svoloch'*, "lowly sod," *gad*, as well as "bitch," *suka*, a pervasive lexical item in Russian *mat*, which connotes both a sense of "betrayal" as well as "bastard," tacitly identifies him as the son of a cuckold. In a self-sacrificial gesture, Andrei exhorts his father to kill him to lessen his anger. The father crouches on the ground where Andrei lies and grabs for the axe that had been used to chop wood for the fires throughout the trip, which is lying in the sand nearby. Significantly, it is Andrei who puts the word "kill," *ubej*, into his father's mouth. These associations between self-sacrifice, wood chopping, and axes evoke the drama of the *Aqedah:* Andrei metaphorically assumes the submissive position of Isaac in relation to Abraham.

But whereas Andrei utters the word "kill" as an injunction, the father repeats it as a question, "Kill you?" suggesting some confusion over the proper object of the verb. Who is it that should be the object of sacrifice? Andrei, for his failure to guard Ivan? Or the father himself, for the fact that he let them discover his secret? This ambiguity is emphasized by a close-up of the father crouched against Andrei with the axe wedged between them.

A resolution to this enigma is suggested when Ivan himself appropriates the word "kill" from the mouths of his brother and father, which compels us to understand each family member as defined by his correlatedness and self-surrender to each other. When Ivan commands that his father stop his actions toward Andre while simultaneously raising the knife he has hidden against his father, he becomes Abraham to his father's Isaac. He states,

> Stop. Don't approach. Don't approach, stop. Stop, don't approach. I would have been able to love you if you were another, but I hate you. Don't you dare torment us. You are nothing, a nobody. Understand? You are a nobody.

It is not the knife he wields that makes Ivan's deranged threat to kill so dangerous, however. It is his revelation of the nothingness at the core of his father's identity that is the true lethal weapon, and indeed this has an immediate effect on the father, who negates it. While the father's denial is frequently interpreted as referring to his biological paternity and cuckoldry, it is hard to reconcile this interpretation with the obvious inversion of the *Aqedah* scene.[61] If the father is reassuring Ivan of his (Ivan's) legitimacy, what do we do with Ivan's assumption of Abrahamic stature in the scene and the father's transformation into Isaac? The only way to make sense of this, and of the climactic scene that succeeds it atop the tower, is to listen, or, as Ivan repeatedly urges his father to do, "to hear" *slyshat'*, what is encapsulated within.

Ivan's use of the derogatory term "nobody," a synonym of the word "worm," to name his father, implies that the secret has destroyed any relational links between them. This context resonates with theories that attempt to explain the mystery of why Abraham would sacrifice Isaac, his long-awaited son: The binding represents an attempt to rectify a broken relationship. Refusing to accept the father's denial, Ivan drops the knife and runs away, with the father and Andrei in pursuit. Ivan's destination, a tower similar to the one in the prologue, tacitly announces that we have come full circle.

Critics have seen the father's interaction with Ivan on the tower as an effort, too little too late, to mitigate the effects of his brutal treatment of his sons. But in Ivan's unnerved scrutiny of the father's hands, soiled by the ladder's grime, which disrupts his ascent, the film suggests another subtext. Indeed, the particularity of the tower setting marks the conflict as connected to Ivan's dissociation on the other tower, which Ivan claims would have killed him had his mother not arrived. Both scenes depict Ivan in a colloquy with a parent over a secret they share.

The father implores Ivan to let him onto the tower platform—specifically to "let me," *pusti menja*, not "let me in," *vypusti menja*, as translated in the subtitles; this leaves open the question of just what the father wants Ivan to let him do. Given that Ivan has just locked a latch that blocks him, it may be that the verb commands Ivan to "release" the lock. Linguists have shown that the perfective aspect of the verb *pustit'* is associated with specific situations "[which] favor interpretations in terms of individual capacity."[62] The father's tacit reference to Ivan's capacity to release the lock is echoed in Ivan's repeated assertion of his (newfound) abilities to "jump," off the tower; Ivan frequently uses the verb "be able to," *moch'*, to assess his competence, or, more accurately, lack thereof, to transcend the trials put before him by his father. In this light, the father's entreaty, buttressed by a chorus of "sons," may now be heard as code to signal that his exchange with Ivan comprises a concealed negotiation over filial obligations.

Ivan's rebuff to his father's plea tacitly acknowledges that he can't handle them, and he beseeches his father to tell him what the father "needs" from him. To shore up his authority to invalidate the father's plea, and to impose his own conditions on the negotiation, Ivan invokes the conditional marker "if," *esli*. Ivan snarls,

IVAN: If you don't leave I'll jump. Hear?! I'll jump. Understand?
FATHER: Never mind, it's ok. Don't move. Wait.
IVAN: Understand me? I jump. Hear? I can. Everything, I can, I caaaannnn....

Because the father responds to this threat to jump with a repeated entreaty to Ivan to "let me, release me," the possibility arises that the father and Ivan's discussion about jumping in fact is a disguised articulation of a threat to "release," "spring," "well forth," or "divulge" the secret. We can also read the father's reply as a disguised plea to be released from the secret too. Read with this linguistic correlation in mind, we can decipher the conversation:

IVAN: If you don't leave, I'll jump (spring → well forth → bubble over *bit'' kliuchom* → beat the keys → reveal the secret). Hear? I jump → reveal. Understand?
FATHER: Never mind. [It's ok, refrain, don't well forth about my secret origins.] Don't move. Wait. [As if this were a trial].[63]
IVAN (INCENSED): Understand me? I jump. Hear? I am able [to spring forth the "key" *kliuch*]. Everything, I can, I caaaannnn....

Critical consensus accepts on face value Ivan's threat to jump, but I am not sure how literally we should understand his bravado. The abject fear on his face as he articulates his defiance, coupled with the terrible vulnerability of the repeated refrain "I can't," in the aftermath when Andrei commands him to help move the father's body, suggests otherwise. What is at stake in this drama is not masculine prowess or physical courage but psychic integrity in the face of an irresolvable conflict between normal adolescent expansion and the suffocating bind of filial obligations.

Ivan's benumbed, catatonic reaction to his father's fall, his easy submission to Andrei's directions, and their reprisal of skills that they acquired along the trip, such as placing branches under the object that needs to be transported through muddy, messy conditions,[64] not to mention the reiteration of instructions such as "use your little hands" to guide Ivan's participation in the activity of dragging their father back to the shore, point to Andrei's assumption of his father's authority and cadence. Andrei's acts have been construed by critics to reflect on the cyclical nature of the transmission of masculine skills that are also metaphorically likened to tools for navigating gendered social expectations in contemporary society. I am persuaded by this interpretive position, but again, as my close reading has hopefully reflected, the film's phantom structure invites us to look even more specifically at the film's final words on the matter.

Once Andrei and Ivan have dragged their father's body back to the beach, very little is said between them beyond the necessary back-and-forth of preparing a boat to launch. The camera tracks many manual transactions between the brothers as they hand items to each other, putting them into the boat or taking them out, which calls attention to the film's ubiquitous subtext of transmission. Andrei, having absorbed all of the father's strictures, is now the authority obliging Ivan, despite his failure before. Such is the impression provoked by the shot of Andrei recoiling the rope attached to the boat's bow; it is Andrei now who is charge of teaching Ivan "the ropes."[65]

Now Ivan is ready to toe the line; this is revealed when his father descends into the water. We have already noted how "descent" figures the return of the phantom to its crypt in Ivan's psyche and successful preservation of the status quo. Now submersion washes out the family stain, and with its return to invisibility, Ivan is finally able to call his father "papa," which he had not been able to do before, even when the father fell off the tower. His psyche has now become fluent with the linguistic rules for preserving secrets.

The magical concurrence of affect and language in the word "papa" shows how fantasy reassures in the face of painful psychic reality. In the fantasy's final scene, the boys find, hidden behind the passenger seat visor, a family photo strikingly similar to the one they had found in the Bible. But in this picture the father is not present; the picture has

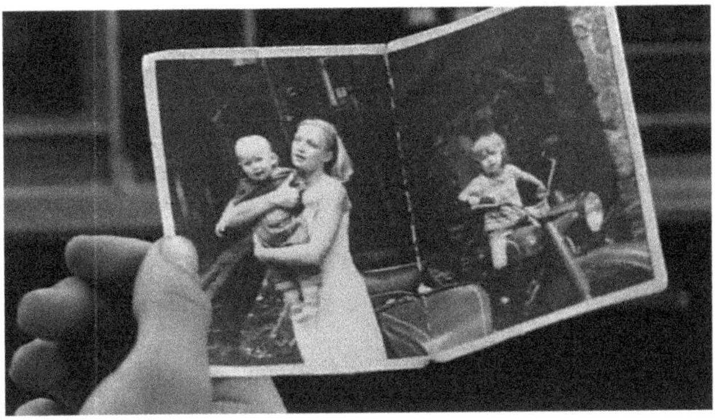

Figure 3.7 The family photo without the father.

been doubled or folded, leaving a jagged edge and nothing more. His absence brings to the foreground the components of the love triangle between a woman and two brothers that was intimated by the fight between Andrei and Ivan in the early segments of the fantasy. Andrei, with paternal gravitas, commands Ivan to "conceal" *spriach'*, the photo, and Ivan hides it. He then comments, "my feet are drenched," *u menia nogi promokli*, which underscores the now-established paradigm of concealment. With its evocation of penetrating stains, the imperfect verb "to get soaked," *promokát'*, and its perfective form, meaning "to blot," Ivan cryptically articulates an unconscious awareness of his new status as a descendent with a secret. Andrei's response—"Take your shoes off" *razuisia*—reaffirms the paradigm: remove, deterge, the contaminated object. The father is gone, but the boys are now joined in the secret communion he returned to enforce. Andrei is now driving the car, as their new partnership becomes the vehicle for preserving repression into the future (Figure 3.7).[66]

Historical Extension

The Return is unique among these four films in an almost complete absence of reference to historical time. In the other films, sociohistorical and cultural contexts emerge from the lexical networks of secreted words. *The Return*, however, consistent with its mystical style, appears to disavow precise historical contextualization. The film was undertaken twelve years after the fall of Soviet rule (2001–2002; the release date was 2003) and some critics have made persuasive arguments about its engagement with post-Soviet experience. Those who are interested in *The Return* as social criticism see this engagement as an introspective examination of the emasculating conditions of post-Soviet reality; insofar as cuckolding is a symbol of emasculation, this is an interpretation that aligns with the reading I have advanced.[67] Critics disagree about whether the father's return is cause for optimism or pessimism. But none of these analytical positions reconcile the historical contexts they propose with the film's extraordinary specificity. If the film invites analogies about post-Soviet society, we must be able to locate it more precisely within the broader cultural realm from which it emerged.

I begin that effort with (what I see as) as Zvyagintsev's overdetermined erasure of history. In Guillermo del Toro's film, *Pan's Labyrinth*, the symbols, represented as phantasmagoria, point to their absent historical context. But *The Return* offers virtually no identifiable historical referents and so requires a different strategy. If the secret embedded in a phantom film is ultimately a piece of an unutterable collective past, then our historical inquiry must note and account for this film's apparent blindness to history. We must ask: What historical context has to be concealed from view?[68]

As we have seen, Zvyagintsev uses hearing frequently and effectively to signal *The Return's* symbolic meaning. It should not surprise us, therefore, that the film's sole temporal marker comes in acoustic form: namely, in twelve lines of a traditional Nekrasov Cossack folk song, *Ne iz sadu* ("It was not from the garden"), buried in the film's last segment.[69] The brevity of this quotation obscures both its importance to the film and its historical significance. It belongs to a cycle of songs memorializing the Cossack Ignat Nekrasov,[70] and with him a crucial moment in Russian history. It was under Tsar Ivan IV (Ivan Vasil'evich, Ivan the Terrible, Ivan *Groznyi*, r. 1553–1584) that "the Cossack energy, their hatred of the Tartars and their habit of living at the expense of pillage"[71] was channeled into empire building. Ivan turned the Cossacks, once a force of chaotic destruction, into guards who protected the borderlands against the Tartars[72] and a central contingent of Ivan's personal army. Nekrasov, the early eighteenth-century founding father of a clan of Cossacks, was the heir to this tradition and to its identity, language, and songs.

It may be startling to read into this fragment of music a historic pointer to the sixteenth century in general and the reign of Ivan IV in particular. But the song communicates a wide range of themes that reverberate strongly with Zvyagintsev's portrait of his young Ivan's problematic self-fashioning. These include ancestor summoning, vigilant defense, and collective identity formation during Russia's own self-fashioning as a nation. They are parallels that establish a link between the generational psychology haunting Ivan and the Russian collective experience at large. There is an affective and aesthetic resonance between the song and *The Return* as well. *Ne iz sadu* recounts the sad tale of two warrior brothers trying to cross the Danube River. The younger one falls into the freezing water; at the point of death, he asks to be remembered to his wife and family.[73] The constellation of brothers; wife; and a dangerous, muddy, and watery mess is as relevant to this film as is the melancholic cadence of the music.

The child Ivan is a boy obsessed with suspicion; Ivan IV was a ruler obsessed with betrayal and with the brutal strategies he employed to protect and guard his political legitimacy.[74] Scholars agree, to varying degrees, that his reign can be understood only with reference to his paranoia.[75] I have neither the linguistic skills nor the space to engage deeply with the formidable scholarship on Ivan the Terrible; as one scholar puts it, "controversies surround almost every aspect of Ivan's reign, from the authenticity and reliability of individual sources to the assessment of the significance of particular events."[76] I will limit myself here to demonstrating how his "symptomatic" behavior points to possession by an unutterable family secret—making this musical reference another gloss by Zvyagintsev on the unconscious rules for family self-fashioning in the presence of a shameful secret about legitimacy.

Ivan IV's Phantom

Historian Edward Keenan details the "grammar" of political tenets that underlay Ivan IV's rule, which is necessary, in his view, to understand it.[77] Keenan claims that dynastic succession was all important in sixteenth-century Russian politics. He notes that the princely house of Moscow adopted the rule of primogeniture after its victory over its rivals (and relatives) in the civil wars of the mid-fifteenth century. The eldest son and a network of interconnected marriages distributed power throughout the clan through systematic inheritance. But "the most important marriage in each generation [was] that of the rulers."[78]

Thus, Ivan IV was born into a society ruled by marriage politics and the relationship between kinship and dynastic status.[79] Indeed, Keenan's example of the surpassing importance of primogeniture is the 1526 marriage of Ivan's father, Vasily III (r. 1505–1533), to Elena Glinsky (1508–1538). Vasily's previous marriage of twenty years had been dissolved for lack of issue. Keenan points out that this dissolution, which undid not only a religious bond but also a stable marriage-related political alliance, was a wrenching prospect to the Russian church as well as to the state. Nevertheless, both acquiesced[80] because "the alternative—the termination of the grand-princely line and a resultant political free-for-all—was a more dismal prospect. They bit their lips, made the necessary arrangements and realigned themselves around the newly-arrived" Elena.[81]

In other words, it was *the ruler's responsibility* to propagate his clan;[82] to seed other than his own was not acceptable. It must therefore have been disconcerting for everyone when it took Elena more than four years to conceive after her marriage to the much older Vasily III.[83] During this long anxious period, Elena made frequent pilgrimages to monasteries to beseech the Mother of God for assistance in conceiving[84] (as her predecessor had without success). Russian hagiographers hailed her long-awaited pregnancy as miraculous, and so was her ultimate delivery of a son in 1530.[85]

The point here is that after almost two hundred years (1240–1480) of subjugation by the outsider Mongols, the Muscovite clan managed to reclaim and maintain sovereignty on the basis of patrilineal transmission of dynastic authority.[86] The resulting stability was new in Russian tribal history and very much in the interest of the Orthodox Church. Some doctrinal issues arose in this new partnership; the princely house was strongly associated with old pagan traditions about the Russian motherland, the *Land Rus'*; and the church put pressure on the princely house to distance itself from these in favor of its newer male-centered doctrine.[87] But it was never possible to suppress completely the older and more familiar model of family authority, in which the womb is the vessel of dynastic continuance, and genealogy and geography are conflated. Thus, the notion of "Russians *dvoeverie* ('dual-religion,' i.e., the retention and mixture of pagan motifs with the newer Christian religion)" was ultimately "raised to the level of ideology. Just as the Russian princes were sacred both as clan ancestors and Christian saints, so the Russian Land was a 'holy land' in both pagan and Christian belief."[88]

The concept of *Rus' zemlia*, Russian land, for example, derived from the belief that the ultimate source of the Muscovite clan's political authority was "moist mother earth," *mat' syra zemlia.*[89] Even the distinctive Russian conception of the Virgin Mary is construed by some scholars as a disguised surrogate for older earth and fertility goddesses.[90] In any case, to the extent that Mother of God worship endured alongside the new patriarchal trends, it affirmed the "connection between royal mother and divine blessing"; Elena Glinsky's "miraculous" conception was a manifestation of this "grace," *milost'*, within the "blessed womb of the *tsaritsa.*"[91] This ambivalent claim represents an attempt to bolster the grand prince's dynastic claims.

In short, although Church and state did their best to translate the popular view of Russia from a pagan motherland into a patrilineal principality, the older vision endured, not least in the divine intercession to which Ivan IV's conception was attributed. The new patrilineal code was further undermined by the long pause between Elena's marriage and her son's conception, which raised suspicions that Ivan was not the child of Vasily III.[92] Historians have noted these in passing, but no one to my knowledge has considered them seriously. The power struggles among the Muscovite princes in the years between Ivan's parents' deaths, and his majority implies that there were questions about Ivan's paternity, but, again, no one has yet drawn a direct line between this scenario and Ivan's ruling grammar. I want to make it clear that I am not arguing that Ivan was in fact illegitimate; I claim only that Ivan's ruling style reflects an (unconscious) awareness of those questions.

Vasily III died in 1533, when Ivan was three years old. His death unleashed complex rivalries among the princes of rivaling clans.[93] These contestations also involved the gentry, known as boyars; boyars ranked below the princes and they were charged with the business of administering the state. The Muscovite political equilibrium depended on a strong central figure, but Ivan's youth unbalanced it. The result was an intensely competitive contest for power among princely Muscovite families and their allies.[94] This struggle has been interpreted primarily as an inherent weakness of the system, which could not sustain itself in the absence of a functioning ruler; as long as Ivan was a minor, there were struggles over who would hold the regency and other coveted distinctions of power and prestige. The conflict was a debilitating obstacle to governance.

Vasily III had established a Regency Council shortly before his death, intending it to protect Elena and Ivan.[95] He appointed Elena's uncle, the renowned and respected statesman Mikhail Glinsky, to the council. Because Glinsky had both a deep attachment to his niece and no personal claim to the throne, Vassily thought he would be able to help Elena navigate through the contentious claims for power.[96] His foresight came to naught, however, when Elena appointed Count Ivan Telepnev-Oblensky, who was believed to be her lover, to the Regency Council. Furthermore, Telepnev-Oblensk's sister, Agrippina Fedorovna Chelyadnin, was Ivan's nurse.[97] Glinsky vigorously opposed these choices, and Elena jailed him. He died of starvation.[98] None of this endeared Elena to the princes or to the gentry; although she was able to take control of the Regency and held it until her death (perhaps from poisoning). But the arrest of her lover Telepnev-Oblensky, along with his governess sister, amidst eight-year-old Ivan's wails, ended, for all intents and purposes, the Glinsky control of Ivan and the Regency.[99]

This drama makes clear that Elena's relationship with Telepnev-Oblensky was viewed askance by many, even her closest relations; the suspicions extended to the conception of her son. They were sufficiently widespread that they were likely a subtext of the discourse to which Ivan was exposed as a young child. Close reading of several examples of Ivan's own speech, as preserved in a set of extraordinary letters, supports this position. The letters[100] were written between Ivan and Prince Andrei Kurbsky, who was active in Ivan's military service and who seems to have been a member of Ivan's immediate circle, until 1562, when Ivan blamed him for a military loss.[101] Kurbsky defected to Lithuania in 1564, thereby earning the enmity of Ivan, who now saw him as a traitor. In a *cri de coeur*, Kurbsky began a correspondence with Ivan, in which he condemned the Tsar's unceasing brutality and the destructiveness of his rule.[102] Ivan's responses are a full-throated defense of his actions, backed up with references to the traumatic aftermath of Elena's death and the catastrophic fire that destroyed Moscow (and parts of the royal palace) several months after his coronation. His language in the letters suggests that these memories were shaped by suspicions about his legitimacy.

Kurbsky himself derides Ivan's epistolary style as unsophisticated, boorish, and an affront to royal decorum; he calls Ivan's prose "noisy," and notes the "messiness" of his shifts from lofty biblical reference to personal memory and from there to crude refutation.[103] Furthermore, he says, Ivan's letters are full of details regarding "beds and body-warmers and countless other things in truth, as if it were the tales of crazy women."[104]

This is a striking comparison. It reminds us that Ivan was brought up by nannies: common women in his mother's service who took care of him. The implicit target of Kurbsky's censure is the residue of the common women's vernacular that he detects in Ivan's speech. In his *History of the Grand Prince of Moscow* (written about nine years after his first epistle to Ivan), Kurbsky insinuates that he must silence discussion about how Russia happened to arrive at its contemporary condition, though he makes an "undisguised reference to Elena Glinsky." Kurbsky's statement is significant in how it represents the linguistic surround, where suspicions about his genealogical origins abound. Kurbsky attributes the cause of Ivan's torturous idiom to Elena's "evil habits,"[105] and it is likely that the nannies' discourse was subject to the same repression. Ivan's nannies lived among the complex currents of a royal household; surely, they must have been highly alert to the "rules" that governed their environment which, though unwritten, still have the power to organize colloquial expression. Furthermore, for five years, Ivan's governess was Elena's putative lover's sister. It was she who managed the nannies, their relationships, and what they did and didn't talk about, all in a highly contested situation in which her self-interest was deeply invested. It is hard to imagine that the simultaneous awareness and suppression of the rumors about Ivan's parentage did not shape the nannies' discourse and therefore Ivan's idiom first as a subject and then as a ruler. The concealed premises and sly metaphors of palace nursemaids gossiping among themselves as they clean, feed, and babysit their royal charge are precisely the kind of linguistic usages that are likely to shape the child's own language.

For example, recall that Ivan's conception was widely cast by historiographers as a miraculous birth, due to the intercession of the Mother of God. Elena's womb was a blessed vessel that bore him, its treasure, to his royal position. Different sources record that when Ivan was especially anxious, he often brought up the topic of treasures, gold, and royal coffers. It is not hard to imagine that he was unconsciously comforting himself with cryptic references to his great value to the realm.

Yet the words also represent a source of agitation, especially in the context of its transmission. For example, Ivan's obsession with the royal treasure and its disposition can be seen in his response to Kurbsky's first accusatory letter. Ivan bitterly recalls the transfer of Elena's treasure to Prince Ivan Shuysky, who had vied with Elena for power before she took firm control of the Regency and who returned at her death to assume the power of Regent. Ivan recounts that the royal treasure was "made into gold and silver vessels," upon which were incised "the names of [Shuysky's] parents, as if they had been their inheritance." Here Ivan is openly lamenting the usurpation of his own inheritance in the context of the absent Vassily; is he also unconsciously defending himself against the whispers that his own patrimony does not in fact belong to him? Later in the letter, Ivan denigrates a sartorial favorite of Shuysky's, which everyone "during the rule of our mother," knew about. The shabbiness of the garment betrays poverty and lack of sophistication. This is proof, Ivan implies, of the Shuysky family hubris.[106]

In this argument, Ivan is defending himself against Kurbsky's accusation that he is a malevolent ruler—*he* does not torment; he is the tormented one. But he is also implicating Shuysky's family in the manufacture of a false genealogy. Furthermore, lexical strategies that connect the words "vessel," *sudy*, and "bed warmer," *grelka*, point to another more intimate context for the treasure discourse,[107] and perhaps implicate Elena (the matriarch of her family) in a similar scheme.

Six months after Ivan's coronation, on June 21, 1547, a catastrophic fire swept through Moscow.[108] Fires were not unusual in that city of many wooden buildings, but this one was the most devastating of a series, and it did not auger well for Ivan's brand-new reign. By now, Elena's mother and two brothers had restored themselves to his good graces, which had altered in the wake of Elena's death, and were wielding a new power at court.[109] But after the fire, a council of boyars and Church clergy argued to Ivan that the Glinskys must be eradicated from his domain for the sake of the dynasty and of public safety. In a letter, Ivan focuses on the terrifying memory of the crowds who followed him in his escape during the fire to the suburbs demanding that he turn over his uncles and grandmother (whom he was suspected of *concealing*).

The Glinskys were accused of deploying sorcery to perpetuate family control over Ivan's rule. The particular spell allegedly used by them entailed the "extraction of human hearts." The verb "to extract," *vynimat'*, is linked etymologically to words meaning "to take out," "to bear," *vynesti*, and "to incubate," bring forth" *vynashivat'*; these lexical indices suggest that the Glinskys were suspect for their role in Elena Glinsky's reproductive process and that their real crime was the one that led to the birth of Ivan.[110]

Similar insinuations about the context of Ivan's conception are found in another letter written by Ivan to the King Sigismund Augustus of Poland-Lithuania (r. 1548–1572).[111] Ivan defensively compares himself in his victimhood to the biblical Adam at the point of his exile from the Garden of Eden (Genesis 2:4-4:24). Tellingly, in his paraphrase of Adam's shame, he uses the word "furs," *shkura*, to designate Adam's concealment of his sexual transgression, instead of the biblical "fig leaves," *smokovnye list'ia'ya.*[112] This locution gives his account a vernacular inflection, both in its affective subtext and in its reference to the intimate everyday objects that nursemaids and their charges talk about.

The treasure passage disguises Ivan's concerns about manufactured genealogies. Here, the use of "fur," and its link to a semantic chain of words associated with "bed-warmer," seems to reference the sexual encounter that might have enabled one. Elena's "vessel" did indeed become the receptacle of royal power. But even while the treasure story articulates concerns about Ivan's conception from the new patrilinear point of view, both of these passages also reflect aspects of the old fertility worship of "moist mother earth," in its pagan form and as conflated with the Christian Mother of God. The "bed-warmer" discourse in particular embeds within it prohibited sexual words associated with the old pagan values and the Russian lexicon of obscenity and imprecation known as *mat.*[113]

Lexical Fragments of *Mat* in Ivan's Memories

John Fennel, the eminent translator of Ivan IV's epistles, identifies *mat* (*The Return*'s "mother's tongue,") as a characteristic feature of the Tsar's language.[114] In Fennel's view, *mat* is the source of the "pure vulgarisms, common abuse, swear-words, which *bespatter* so many of [Ivan's] angrier passages" (my emphasis).[115] This is the ancient vocabulary that was once associated with pagan fertility ritual. In its original context, it appears to have been a lexicon used to conceal clan (that is, genealogical) secrets from outsiders. It is not hard to imagine that in the palace nursery its use helped to identify those who knew of "the secret" of Ivan's conception and exclude the rest of society from this knowledge.

Ivan's *mat*-inflected discourse consistently links the transfer of Elena's treasury to her act of copulation, and I suggest that this raunchy and evocative imagery derives from whispers about his mother's possible sexual transgression that he heard but did not completely understand, which made him fear their implications. For example, a cryptic reference to Elena is included in Ivan's description of the Shuyskys's pretensions to royal authority. Recall his outraged memory of the impoverished outerwear of Shuysky during the rule of "our matriarch." Fennell found this reference odd and the description of the coat convoluted beyond measure. Literally, Ivan states: [the coat was] "green mohair on the marten fur, and the skins were shabby" *shuba byla mukhoiar zelen na kunitsakh, da ke vetkhii;* Fennell understands this to be an awkward depiction of "a shabby marten fur coat lined with green mohair."[116]

If we listen to the words, however, we *hear* another dimension: the word "Elena," is formed by the words "green," *zelen*, and "on," *na*. I submit that Ivan's description unconsciously restates something he had previously "heard": ("our mother") "Elena was on the marten-fur," *kunicah*, or, more likely, "Elena was on the *cavalry*" *konnica* (from *kon*, "horse"), a perfect homonym. The image of a threadbare coat uncomfortably evokes the idea of an exposed body; the affective charge of this description as applied to Elena must have been both unutterable and unbearable to her son. Thus, the worn-out coat, which Ivan attributes consciously to a family of pretenders, refers unconsciously to his own mother's naked body. Encrypted in the description of the coat is an image of coitus that Ivan as a young boy unwittingly absorbed.

A similar sexual connotation shadows Ivan's account of the transfer of Elena's royal treasure. He describes a "furious kicking and stabbing with sharp implements," *nogami pihajushhee osny koljushhe*, as simultaneous with Elena's transmission of the (gold) vessels.[117] This locution too conjures an animated image of coitus: Sharp implements are a common metaphor in Russian *mat* for the phallus and kicking legs for sexual intercourse.[118]

Ivan's account of Prince Shuysky's treatment of him and his younger brother after their mother's death is another example of unconscious awareness. He is enraged at Shuysky's demeanor, which conveyed neither parental concern for the children nor the deference due to a royal master. Kurbsky comments that Ivan's rage seems extreme, yet Ivan is very clear about why and how Shuysky made him so angry.[119]

Here is Ivan's description: Prince Shuysky is "sitting on a bench, leaning his elbow on the bed of our father, [i.e., the late Tsar, father to all Russian people] and putting his foot on a stool." Translating Prince Shuysky's gestures into language, we can see how this vision communicates the *exposure* of Elena's secret. The verb *sidet'*, which means "to sit down," also means "to set out," as in "to display" or "expose." Another meaning of the word "bench," *lavke*, is the location where a shop displays its wares. Shuysky's bent arm signifies both the reliance on the Tsar's bed—the site of conjugal relations—for genealogical legitimacy and the implication of a bent or "branched" lineage issuing from it. The action of Shuysky's leg in placing (sets out, again) his foot on the stool reverberates with "furious kicking (and poking)" that coincided with the transfer of Elena's treasure—and with its sexual subtext. In addition, the word "stool" in Old Church Slavonic, *stolŭ*, referred to the seat of royalty, the throne. Ivan reads Shuysky's gestures as communicating: "I expose the illegitimate branch that grows from the throne." His offense at what he consciously took as Shuysky's disrespectful countenance reflects an unconscious response to suspicions about his paternity and explains why he named Shuysky's acts as the source of his torment.[120]

Ivan's Reign

The encounter with Shuysky suggests that his actions may be translated into language that helps us understand Ivan's political behavior. Here is another example.

"The Taking of Kazan" is a Russian folk song, a fragment of the collective memory of Ivan's reign. It recounts the "gunpowder episode," an anecdote about Ivan dating from 1552. Ivan wants to invade and conquer Kazan, but a wall prevents him from realizing this wish. He has charged his ignition engineer with blowing it up, yet the wall still stands. In his frustration, Ivan lashes out against the engineer, accusing him of treachery and commanding that he be killed on the spot.[121] One brave soldier takes it upon himself to explain the slow combustion habit of fuses. This intercession stays Ivan's fury long enough that the powder has time to explode. Victory is achieved, and the life of the engineer is saved.

According to folklorist Norman Ingham, this song

> serves a purpose: the glorification of the common soldier or cossack who dares to speak back to the tsar. That much is widely recognized. What I want to call attention to is the prerequisite, [Ivan] Groznyi's temper and the imagery with which it is conveyed. Tension is created on two levels at once: the gunpowder that is about to go off, and Ivan's temper, which is on a shorter fuse. This is not so much a song about Kazan' as about the 'Wrath of Ivan Groznyi.'[122]

Ingham analyzes the lexical overlaps between fuses and Ivan's explosive behavior. He claims that the "fixed epithet, *groznyi tsar'*," transmits by its very existence complex information about Ivan's rule. He deconstructs this sobriquet to delineate the broad semantic range of the word *groza,* which, in Ivan *Groznyi,* signified several different aspects of Ivan's behavior.[123] It connoted the fear and awe that Ivan's actions evoked in foreign enemies, but it also conveyed his severity with his own quick and merciless punishments.[124] Ingham notes that for the most part Ivan's *groza* "takes the personal form of hotheadedness, sudden ire," which leads him to punish what he perceives as disobedience.

Some variants of "The Taking of Kazan" include another detail that tells us more about the conditions that trigger Ivan's wrath. According to Ingham, "Ivan Groznyi becomes aggravated by the 'sordidness' *grubiianstvo*, of the enemy Kazanis, who taunt him from the city walls just as he is impatiently waiting for the black powder to go off." In some variants, the taunting "women of Kazan add insult by 'mooning' him!"[125] Ingham is right that the "ribald humor of this affront to the authority figure gave the version entertainment appeal,"[126] but we can note too that the word "sordidness" is the same one used by Zvyagintsev's

Ivan to describe the tainted bread he refuses to eat. In Ivan IV's violent reaction, is he also protecting a sordid secret? Ingham claims that the Kazan' mooning gestures were part of a "rain dance meant to help mire the Russian forces in the bogs,"[127] a scenario that summons the same metaphor of muddy mess that signifies sexual shame in *The Return*; the Kazanis' *exposure* of their buttocks or *backsides* may be construed as a silent reference to Ivan IV's perhaps "backsided" (that is, illegitimate) claim to imperial authority. Even the soldier's calming explanation about the slowness of fuses rests on the fact that they are *underground* and *buried*—not *exposed* (like the derriéres of the taunting enemy).

Thus, Ingham uncovers lexical rules that make sense of Ivan's sudden reversals of behavior, the source of his fiery reputation; here, I will extend his reading to demonstrate a grammar and lexicon of preservative repression (which can also be seen in the soldier's calming explanation) that reverberates with the grammar and vocabulary so carefully delineated in Zvyagintsev's film.

The most compelling link between Ivan's idiom and *The Return* is the film's setting on a remote island, devoid of ties to larger social circulation. Recall that the fantasy of the trip to the island was produced as a way to obscure Ivan's psyche's need to accommodate the tower experience and thereby preserve the status quo. Recall too, how preservation of the status quo requires (unconscious) adherence to a strict regimen of lexical rules to decontaminate words stained by their shameful associations. The film's constellation of geographical isolation, strict regimentation, and preservation of the status quo evokes a similar constellation in Russian history, namely Ivan IV's 1564 institution of *oprichnina*, the name of which derives from a root meaning "separate" or "apart."

I suggest that *oprichnina* served for Ivan IV the same psychic purpose that the island serves in *The Return*; both are sites where preservative repression may be actualized. As I will show, the institution of *oprichnina* created a balance in which Ivan could simultaneously instantiate his secret *and* decontaminate it. The preservative structure of Ivan IV's institution bears a striking resemblance to the fantasy of the young modern Ivan, in that both were triggered by the need to resist psychic reorganization. This being so, we can understand it by identifying the grammatical rules that support it. This is the same perspective embodied in *The Return*.

Oprichnina is a challenge to historians because, as Charles Halperin has shown, contemporary "perceptions of the *oprichnina* were not homogenous."[128] They ranged from diplomatic denials that the *oprichnina* even existed to seemingly banal bureaucratic references to landholding and personnel issues. Halperin notes that this discourse tended to treat the *oprichnina* as "'a fact of life,' too well known to require definition."[129] To some extent that neutrality of tone may have been a function of its administrative context; nonetheless, Halperin suggests, the perception of the *oprichnina* as "normal" is noteworthy precisely because the institution was anything but that. It was a two-tiered structure of administration, founded on two parallel systems of power, an irregularity that is all but denied. The historical sources are enigmatic enough that the *oprichnina* remains the subject of scholarly debate over "specific, factual issues" as well as "broader analytical and conceptual" ones.[130]

Furthermore, the *oprichnina* seems to have been in part a result of Ivan's own need for secrecy, which adds another layer of mystery to its provenance. Most scholars acknowledge that it came about after a series of traumatic losses in Ivan's life. His wife, for whom he had had genuine affection, died in 1560, and her loss is seen as a turning point in Ivan's behavior, "the end of the happy days for Ivan and for Russia; for he lost not only his wife, but his better nature [dobrodetel']."[131] A year later Ivan had ostensibly recovered enough to marry again, but crushing military defeats, which lead to the defection of Prince Kurbsky and his furious first letter, deeply disquieted Ivan. Then, in December 1564, "without explanation, [he]... left Moscow with his wife, sons, treasury, and the religious treasures of the city for an undisclosed location." From there he sent letters that apprised the boyars and the population that he had abdicated the throne.[132] He accused both boyars and clergy of treason and embezzlement.

The boyar response to this was frantic. With Ivan in Aleksandrova Sloboda, a hunting palace that would soon become the site of his *oprichnina* court, the boyars were unable to rule in his absence; but they feared that any faltering of the administration would catalyze unrest among the citizens of Moscow. So, an envoy was sent to entreat Ivan to return to Moscow and the throne.[133] Ivan agreed to rescind his abdication in word; but his conditions demanded the establishment of *oprichnina*, which would give him free reign to seize land and to hound those he deemed as traitors.[134] Desperate to ensure continuity of the court bureaucracy, the envoy submitted to his demands.

Thus, Russia was effectively split into two parts: the "Land," or *zemlischina,* which continued to be governed by the boyar court with Ivan as its dynastic head, and the *oprichnina*, which was ruled by Ivan himself on his terms alone. The result was a state-within-a-state, a fortified island in the middle of the Russian empire. Each domain had "its own government, its own capital, its own treasury and its own army."[135] In addition, while the boyars served as his legatees at his court in Moscow, Ivan established his own *oprichnina* court, which operated along the lines of a monastic system, where the courtiers formed a specific brotherhood devoted to protecting Ivan from betrayers. These people were known as the *oprhichniki.*

These events resonate with preoccupations and patterns that we have already seen as characteristic of Ivan's idiom. First, the accusations of treason and embezzlement, and the very fact that he carried the royal treasure with him, bring to mind the "gold vessels" discourse. Second, there is the peculiarity of the entire abdication crisis. Halperin claims that this threat was "phony" and staged,[136] implying a conscious disingenuousness. Yet the secrecy, the drama, and the threat may be accounted for in another way as well. His threat to reject the throne—to cut off the head of the dynasty, as it were—"stages" the intrapsychic conflict driving his actions, namely the need to separate himself from unconscious knowledge about his royal legitimacy.

I understand this unconscious scenario to be the reality that catalyzed Ivan's production of *oprichnina* (an actualized fantasy). (His unconscious enactment uncannily anticipates the filmic Ivan's dramatization of his possession by his father's secret on the tower, before he sets out for the island.) The *oprichnina* is born out of Ivan's need to exempt himself from an obstacle to self-fashioning generated by his suspicions about his own parentage; it became a tool for the preservation of his psychic status quo. Heeding Charles Halperin's insistence that historians discern "the existence of the *oprichnina* by its symbols,"[137] and building on his work, I will elaborate here on two specific symbols to make my point: amputated dog heads mounted on horses,[138] which emblematized successful raids to seize lands and persecute noble lineages;[139] and the two-fingered Sign of the Cross, which was associated explicitly with the monastic order that Ivan founded, and which was imbued with cleansing and salvific significance.

Priscilla Hunt also interprets Ivan's *oprichnina* idiom as a symbolic system, which she concludes was "compensatory to his extreme anxiety resulting from his sense of betrayal by his people."[140] She argues that *oprichnina* was organized around a personal mythology built on "official ideology of sacred kingship" promulgated in 1547, when Ivan was crowned Tsar. This theology endowed the "'abstraction' of the state and the grand prince's newly assumed rank of tsar with symbolic 'flesh and blood' by associating them with the body of Christ."[141]

Mythology allowed Ivan to resolve the conflict because it allowed him to present

> himself as a heightened form of the organic unity of the state, as a part equal to and condensing the energy of the whole. In so doing, he proved himself a master mythmaker, defining his own sacredness by analogy to the higher paradigms of Christian myth

and in this way brought balance and coherence to "a world made threatening and unmanageable by paranoid delusions of betrayal"; Ivan could "portray himself as a unity where opposites mirrored one another"[142] and effect a balance unavailable to him before *oprichnina* was established.

Hunt reasons that even if it is impossible to prove that Ivan had "access to the sophisticated and elaborate set of assumptions which I believe informed his personal mythology," she is nonetheless still able to discern how they "provided Ivan with a language which encompassed his dual nature in Christ."[143] Her argument anticipates my focus on the linguistic surround that shaped Ivan's identity formation; whereas she zeroes in on the religiopolitical structures of meaning that shaped his identity, I pay attention to what was pressed in between the lines of his language environment as a child. While I am persuaded by Hunt's conclusion that Ivan's *oprichnina* "created a wholeness of self by resolving the conflict between his inherited Christian morality, his pagan blasphemies and his inner [paranoid] impulses,"[144] I locate the source of his symbolic system in his possession by an unconscious knowledge that he is inclined to investigate all the while having to deny its very existence.

Ivan's bipolar actions are likely the source of his legacy in collective memory, which preserves an image of a "split personality."[145] This collective memory may derive from Ivan's undulating behavioral shifts while *oprichnina* was in operation. This would correlate with Halperin's discovery that the only contemporary sources that reflect the *affective experience* of *oprichnina* presence are peasant reports, which recount brutal treatment at the hands of the *oprichniki*. The *oprichniki* disrupted villages that lay in the path of their raids for land, which Ivan claimed to incorporate into *oprichnina* territory. The salience of "splitting," in the memory of Ivan's *oprichnina*, with regard to the Russian royal domain, or in the collective memory of Ivan's bipolar disposition, implores us to see it as a defining grammatical rule of Ivan's idiom. The homographic relationship between "*kroju* from *kryt'*, 'to cover,' [conceal] and *kroju* from *kroit'* 'to cut, sever'"[146] encourages this line of inquiry.

This hypothesis can only be advanced on the basis of lexical links between the secret about Elena's suspected adultery and Ivan's *oprichnina* idiom. Keenan's linguistic analysis of the word *oprichnina* provides persuasive evidence. He argues that the particular legal connotations of this word shed light on Ivan's motivations, yet have been disregarded by historians. The word *oprichnina*, literally "the widow's mite,"[147] was a legal term during Ivan's reign; it referred to a parcel of property belonging to a deceased cavalryman that was kept apart and passed on to his widow, while "the rest of the estate was taken back and redistributed to some other warrior."[148]

Keenan claims that in order to understand the link between the institution and its name,

> we must take Ivan at his word, and consider his term and his actions in the context that we have established, in which his personal life history and family history were both crucial to the system that depended upon them and were at the same time the fetters of his inherited [royal] bondage.[149]

Keenan reads Ivan's use of the word as "paradoxical: he was not a widow, and, since all of Muscovy was in a sense his property, the notion of his taking a small share of it as private was doing something quite outrageous."[150] Keenan sees this as an ironic subtext, a metaphor for Ivan's assault on "centrally dynamic features" of the patrilineal system.

However, it also seems reasonable to read this in terms of Ivan's secret knowledge. In his first response to Kurbsky, Ivan evokes an image of Elena Glinsky "left in miserable widowhood." The Russian word rendered by John Fennell as "miserable" implies poverty, and Ivan details pious Elena as miserabl[y dressed in] "calico cotton," *sitsevkyh*, upon the death of Vassily III.[151] Like the other reference we have seen to threadbare outerwear, this one too engages the semantic network related to "bed linens" and coitus that is so resonant in *The Return*. Ivan's description of Elena's "pious" state of (un)dress evokes an incongruous juxtaposition of religious piety and devotions of a more carnal kind. At the same time, the precarious condition of widowhood, suggested by the evocative Russian description of a widow as a "hanging on by thread," *vdova, visiashchaia na voloske*, hints at the weakness of her connection to Muscovite patrimonial legitimacy. In this way, Ivan's "widow's mite" actualizes the construction of a domain in which Ivan's vigilant guardianship of the widow Elena's mite—the secret of her weakness—can protect both of them from its consequences.[152]

Institutionalizing *oprichnina* meant that Ivan would not have to carry out his vigilance alone. He established a retinue of *oprichnikis,* who swore oaths[153] to sniff out betrayers and protect the domain; in return they were included in the court, a "pseudomonastic" brotherhood, for which Ivan served as abbot.[154] "Pseudo" here reflects Charles Halperin's ironic take that there was very little that was monastic about it beyond being a kind of secret police.[155] Nonetheless, the twofoldness of their united commitment to protect Ivan('s effort to protect his secret) emerges as an important grammatical rule of Ivan's *oprichnina* idiom. The symbolic use to which amputated dogs' heads are mounted on mares yields more information.

The composite symbol, whose meaning derives from the juxtaposition of two components, reifies the significance of amalgamation for Ivan. Halperin has demonstrated how significantly dogs figure in Ivan's idiom, both in his speech (he constantly curses enemies and betrayers as "dogs") and in the use of their amputated heads as an emblem of triumph.

Halperin explains the connection between dogs' heads and successful raids in terms of dogs' talents for hunting and guarding; Hunt links the dogs' heads to the "symbol of Justice: they confronted sinners who had judged the tsar in wrath 'like dogs,' with emblems of their own pollution"; yet another historian sees in the dog symbolism an allusion to the Dominican coat of arms.[156] But there is another possible, and telling, link between the word "dog," *sobaka*, and the Russian *mat*. The "basic oath" of *mat*, Stephen Smith tells us, is "fuck your mother." This imprecation is a "*fragment* (italics mine) of an old Slavic formula *pyos yob tvoyu mat'*, "a dog fucked your mother,"[157] and implies a debased sexual act with a canine. This appears to be another instance where a reminder of sexual transgression is encrypted in the "mother tongue," this time with the word "dog" as a pointer to the putative absent biological father, the intruder into the Muscovite princely bloodline. We can translate Ivan's enigmatic mounting of dog heads on horses as the idea that the *head* of the Muscovite line is a *dog* or perhaps as another disguised articulation of his mother "on the cavalry." The mounting of dogs' heads on horses after a victorious intrusion symbolically stages the unutterable union that, whisperers suggested, brought Ivan to the throne.

Dogs and horses are important in Ivan's idiom because they simultaneously stage yet conceal the secret of his parentage. His particular uses of them suggest preservative rules requiring that the roles of *both* his parents (intruder and his mother as cavalry rider) be dramatized in distorted ways. It is a macabre reminder, both of his great triumphs and of his greatest vulnerability. The combination allows Ivan to transform the nagging suspicion of his mother's shameful union into an emblem of successful intrusions into noble lineages. Halperin has noted the prevalence of brooms in historical accounts of the dog head-and-horse combination and suggested that they represent the "sweeping out" of pernicious threats to the dynasty.[158] I suggest that the target for decontamination might more specifically be the very union that this combination stages. Furthermore, the techniques of torture that Ivan implemented during these raids may also be understood as distorted articulations of the secret whose existence they enact.[159] Forcing victims to ride a mare naked;[160] burning betrayers with "bed warmers";[161] not to mention kicking his victims and poking them with sticks, all recall images of coitus unwittingly described by Ivan himself.

Ivan was apparently indifferent to class or hereditary background when it came to membership in his brotherhood; he created a context in which people of mixed backgrounds were unified in the protection of his authority.[162] Here too, the *oprichnina* enacts both the secret dynastic transgression of his parents' union and Ivan's obligation to protect it. Away from court, the *oprichnikis* were villainous brigands, the source of extraordinary suffering. At court, they were a "monastic brotherhood created to protect the unity of the nation and the purity of the faith."[163] "Unity of the nation and purity of the faith" may have been commonplace epithets in Russian politicoreligious discourse, but the words had a specific charge for Ivan. If his violent raids (energetically carried out while *oprichnina* was in operation) are translatable as distorted enactments of his mother's unutterable sexual communion, then his creation of a dominion that was governed by religious symbols of salvation may be understood as a decontaminating complement of the raids, necessary for the preservation of his psychological status quo. The monastic order of *oprichnina*, excluded from the dictates of dynastic rule, functions like the broom, only on an institutional level.

I suggest that a religious gesture, the Sign of the Cross, became the corollary within Ivan's court of the dog head-and-horse symbol of his raiding outside it. Two factors contributed to the enhancement of the affectivity of this already charged religious symbol. First, the gesture was implicated in events that Ivan faced in the early years of his dynasty: He had to strengthen "the prestige of the dynasty," and he had to secure "succession for his heir."[164] Sergei Bogatryev suggests that with the help of "spin doctor" Metropolitan Bishop Makarii, they resorted "to the cultural resources of the church" and were able to manifest a "delicate compromise between secular and ecclesiastical authorities"[165] to shore up the dynasty's foundation. One manifestation of this was the establishment of church liturgical and ritual protocol via a Church proceeding in 1551,[166] which included strict instructions for how to make the two-fingered Sign of the Cross.[167] The distinction had implications: The two-fingered sign was used throughout the early church and replaced by the three-fingered cross quite late in Byzantine history; the Russians regarded their gesture as more ancient.[168] This was important because proving the antiquity of Ivan's genealogy in dynastic and ecclesiastical contexts was essential for confirming "Ivan's title of tsar."[169]

The second factor that intensified the affectivity of the sign for Ivan came from the actual form of the gesture, which was made with the extended index and middle fingers; this union signaled the simultaneity of the spiritual and the physical; it was a gesture that bore witness to and safeguarded a covenant with an ineffable source. As one follower put it, "'the Sign of the precious Cross, this excellent sacrament of the faith, teaches us how to know a mystery.'"[170] The mystery, signified by this highly symbolic expression, implies the presence of something wholly separate but also tangible and pervasively present. I propose that the concept of connection with an unseen ineffable presence may be seen as a religious analogue of a psyche's unconscious awareness of an unspeakable secret. The "economy of two natures" in one substance[171] matches the grammar of Ivan's raids. Endowed with salvific power, the symbol is an antidote for the union of his parents. Salvation (for Ivan) lies in the symbol's capacity to decontaminate the charged affect of (the concept of) coupling.

This decontaminating function of the sign is what exempts Ivan from psychic reorganization. The two-fingered gesture allows him to reveal the secret of his parents' union while simultaneously disguising it in the garb of religious discourse. On the one hand, it evokes *chistit'*, "cleansing" and "purification," a concept and word that are part of the father's preservative lexicon in *The Return*. On the other, words associated with the gesture obscure meanings that relate to ill-gotten gains. The word "finger," *palets*, in its meaning as one of the digits on a hand, possesses other meanings as well: specifically, "pilfer," "steal," or "thieve," *vorovat.*

Keeping in mind the unifying potential of shared religious culture, we can imagine how heavily this symbol may have weighed within Ivan's monastic order itself, especially in light of the oaths sworn by the brotherhood to protect Ivan and "finger," *ukazyvat'*, those who slander and betray him. In other words, Ivan's devotional practices, complete with their decontaminating charge, were likely transmitted to his brotherhood; I suggest that the tight supervision of this population through an enforced monastic regimen based on vows of loyalty effected the transmission of Ivan's structure of mind to his followers. That is, he transmitted to them, through religious symbolism and its linguistic correlates, an unconscious obligation to protect his secret. This is an example of how individual and collective experience can be critically linked through the machinery of preservative repression.

The Collective Transmission of Ivan's Phantom

Ivan IV ruled Russia for more than fifty years. Just as the extraordinary length of his reign gave it an enduring historical significance, his ruling idiom also made an indelible impact on collective processes of Russian self-fashioning.[172] It is no coincidence that it resonates with the rules that guide expression in Zvyagintsev's film; its grammar yields a new way of looking at heretofore intractable questions about the source of collective cultural identity. It is a tool for parsing the intersection between secrets, collective memory, cultural identity, and history.

One such intersection can be found in a defining, yet profoundly perplexing, event of modern Russian history, the 1653 religious Schism, or *Raskol.* This refers to the eventual institutionalization in the mid-seventeenth century of two distinct orders of Russian Church practice. The rupture occurred when the Patriarch Nikon of Moscow imposed reforms intended to bring Russian Orthodox practice more consistently into alignment with the practices of the other Eastern churches.[173] More specifically, Church officials were looking to correct "certain divisive and erroneous innovations" that had crept into Orthodox liturgical practice.[174]

One example of an "erroneous innovation" was the two-fingered Sign of the Cross, which we saw differed from the three-fingered form used throughout the rest of the Eastern Orthodox world. The seventeenth-century Church saw such Russian accents as intrusions on Orthodox practice,[175] which required *rooting out.* Implicit in this judgment was the belief that the rites established by the Church Council in 1551 were *tainted*, divergent from those of the true pan-Eastern Orthodox lineage, "the true and full [*vsesovershenu*] faith."[176] It is not farfetched to claim that the reforms demanded a *decontamination* of Russian practice.

I have italicized some words in the preceding paragraph to call attention to the Church's rhetoric of justification and to demonstrate how that rhetoric unwittingly and cryptically, but powerfully, impugned as illegitimate Ivan IV in his equation with, and representation of, Russia itself. The words and concepts of the denunciation resonate deeply with Ivan's own unconscious preoccupations, and I will argue that this resonance was a causative factor in the violent resistance to the reforms, as well as the forms, which this violence—often self-directed—took.

In short, the Church condemned rites that it had previously sanctified in a text solicited by Ivan to shore up—to the point of historical revisionism—his own legitimacy. This is a clear, if perhaps unconscious, link between Ivan's problematic origins and the rites of the Russian church. The classification of these Russian sanctified rites as "innovations" brands them as (inadvertent) by-products, outgrowths off of the main trunk of an established tree. In sum, the implication that Ivan's faith was tainted implied that his political legitimacy was tainted too: that his rule, like the two-fingered Sign of the Cross, was a consequence of deviance.

Historians are puzzled by the intensity of the popular reaction to these reforms. Some perceived the rigidity of those who opposed them as evidence of stubbornness or lack of intellectual sophistication and reflective of the conservative spiritualism that characterized the targeted rites.[177] Thus, the term Old Believers to designate those faithful who refused to accept the symbolic substitutions mandated by the reforms.[178] Sergei Zenkovsky connects the Old Believer stance to a collective need for the stability of time-honored religious practice. He links the resistance of the Old Believers to the intense suffering of the years that followed Ivan IV's death.[179] These "massacres," "conflagrations," and other traumas, including the *intrusion* into Russia by the Polish and Lithuanian military, and even the occupation of land acquired during Ivan IV's imperial expansion, created a reliance on Orthodoxy as a steadfast source of order in a chaotic world.

I find this persuasive. Yet, Old Believer resistance may be understood too in terms of preservative repression. From this perspective, the Church's rejection of the two-fingered Sign of the Cross as tainted might be unconsciously experienced as a defamation or betrayal of what Ivan stood for and therefore of Ivan himself. Old Believers in fact did decry the intentions of the Church as betrayal and treachery.[180] The Church's defamatory rhetoric threatened the integrity of a collective unconscious in which the spiritual and affective weight of a religious gesture had become fused with its decontaminating function as enacted by and under Ivan. In other words, castigating this practice as a diversion from sanctioned Church rituals was a threat to the integrity of a hidden covenant between Ivan and his followers.[181]

Many Old Believer families are loosely identified as Cossacks;[182] their ancestors cooperated with Ivan IV to conquer the Khans; they served as standing guards or musketeers for Ivan's Moscow palace, the *strelt'sy*, who were also essential to the operation of Ivan's *oprichnina*.[183] There was a critical link between the men who participated in Ivan's monastic observances and the Old Believers.

I cannot take this exploration any further here. But I suspect that the rhetoric and the specific acts of resistance undertaken by Old Believers may be understood as symbolic language pointing to an elided problematic history that they are unconsciously obligated to preserve. The possessed quality of their behavior is of particular interest in this regard. Ritual prohibitions of foreign products, such as potatoes and tea or of paper currency because it bore the image of the Antichrist, may indeed have "helped to reinforce a sense of cohesiveness within the Old Believer community and against the world at large."[184] But *The Return* has sensitized us to how resistance around eating may also be read metaphorically as a sign pointing to problematic self-fashioning. The "fiery" spirit attributed to Old Believers may also be a function of the collective memory of Ivan.[185] The inclination toward self-immolation as a means of resistance among extreme Old Believers recalls the collective memory of Ivan's self-destructive fiery temper, illustrated in the folk song "The Taking of Kazan."—Not surprisingly, the folk song is closely related to Old Believer Cossack traditions. Future inquiry along these lines might uncover other lexical clues that explain the extremity of the Old Believer resistance, which has been compared by one scholar to the suicidal actions of the Jones cult.[186]

The Return was released twelve years after the fall of the Soviet Union; twelve years is (coincidentally?) the amount of time the father has been away. At twelve years old, Russia was approaching adolescence, a time when social transformations require painful processes of reorganization. The dissolution of the Soviet collective identity, which was retroactively rendered shameful, recapitulated the collective affective experience of the Old Believers in the face of the Russian Church's negation of sixteenth-century liturgical practice. *The Return* is a response to this affective experience. Zvyagintsev portrays a nameless Russian family organized around the need to decontaminate a staining secret. It is a haunting portrait precisely because the affective experience depicted is so central to that of the Russian collective unconscious. The resonance of the film with Ivan IV and his place in Russian collective memory, as well as with the traumatic Schism, endows the film with its powerful mystical aesthetic.

Notes

1 Erica Abeel, "Return of the Prodigal Father; Andrey Zvyagintsev Talks About 'The Return.'" *Indiewire*. (2004).
2 Zvyagintsev himself calls attention to Tarkovsky's influence as evidenced in the epigraph that opens this chapter. The points of similarity, according to the director, lie "In his attitude toward the rhythm and flow of time. A dream-like pace." Ibid. See also Anaïs Cabart "Andrei Zvyagintsev's *The*

Return: A Tarkovskian Initiation," *Close Up* 1.2 (2013): 52, who states that the film is full of "visual quotations or homage" to Tarkovsky.

3 Donato Totaro, "Time and the Film Aesthetics of Andrei Tarkovsky," *Journal of Film Studies* 2.1 (1992): 26.

4 Andrew Sarris, "Oedipal Drama, Russian Style: Zvyagintsev's The Return," *The Observer* (2/2004).

5 See, for example, Barnaby B. Barratt, "Fathering and the Consolidation of Masculinity: Notes on the Paternal Function in Andrey Zvyaginstev's The Return," *Psychoanalytic Review* 102.3 (2015): 347–364. Psychoanalytically oriented, Barratt's focus is on the "(mis)alliance between the actual and the symbolic father (both of whom are always both present and absent in psychic life)." See also Kim Dillon, "The Emerging Identity as Expressed Through Russian Art House Cinema," *Verges: Germanic & Slavic Studies in Review* 2.1 (2013): 1–9; Terrence McSweeny, "The End of Ivan's Childhood in Andrei Zvyaginstev's The Return (2003)," *International Journal of Russian Studies* 2.1 (2013): 95–108; Merle Molofsky, "The Return," *The Psychoanalytical Review* 91.6 (2004): 853–859, who more specifically states that the father's definition of manhood is "the manhood of exigency, a readiness for hardship and disaster," 855; and Yana Hashamova, "Resurrected Fathers and Resuscitated Sons: Homosocial Fantasies in The Return and Koktebel" in Helena Goscilo, Yana Hashamova eds., *Cinepaternity. Fathers and Sons in Soviet and Post-Soviet Film* (Bloomington: Indiana University Press, 2010), 169–190.

6 Many of the works cited earlier voice this sentiment, but it receives extended attention in Andrada Fătu-Tutoveanu, "'The Return of the Sacred': Implicit Religion and Initiation Symbolism in Vozvrashchenie (2003)," *Journal for the Study of Religions and Ideologies* 14.42 (2015):199–230; Brygida Pawlowska-Jadryzyk, "Murky Images, The Poetics of Intertextual Dissonance in the Apocryphal Films of Andrei Zviagyntsev," *Załącznik Kulturoznawczy* 2 (2015): 240–255.

7 See especially the sophisticated analysis offered by Philip Cavendish "The Return of the Photograph: Time, Memory and the Genre of the Photo-Film in Andrei Zviagintsev's *Vozvrashchenie* (The Return)," *The Slavonic and East European Review* 91.3 (2013): 467.

8 Ibid., 466.

9 Ibid., 468.

10 Peter Steiner and Sergej Davydov, "The Biological Metaphor in Russian Formalism: The Concept of Morphology," *SubStance* 6.16 (1977): 154. Cf. the metapsychological notion of a "kernel" *yadro*, as secret, in Abraham and Torok's metapsychology.

11 Klaus-Dieter Seemann and N. W. Ingham, "Genres and the Alterity of Old Russian Literature," *Slavic and East European Journal* (1987): 254–255.

12 The word "Sunday," *voskresen'ye*, is a near rhyme of the word in the film's title, *Return*, *vozvrashcheniye*, providing strong linguistic evidence that the events depicted in the prologue establish the context for understanding the particular intrapsychic conflict that triggers the father's return.

13 Tony Hunt, "The Rhetorical Background to the Arthurian Prologue: Tradition and the Old French Vernacular Prologues," *Forum for Modern Language Studies* 6.1 (1970): 1, states that the prologue was "designed to familiarize the audience . . . with the subject . . . and with the circumstances [leading to] the action, i.e., it was expository."

14 Vladimir Nabokov, *Nikolai Gogol* (New York: New Directions, 1944), 4; cited in Magdalena Vintrova, "Olfactory Images and Creation of Meaning

in Gogol's 'The Nose' and *Rushdie's Midnight Children*," M.A. Thesis (2004) A & M University, 25.

15 Vintrova, "Olfactory Images," 24–26.

16 Ibid.

17 Cf. Barratt, "Fathering," who claims that the tower scene presents "an archetypal test of bravado and masculinity," 207. See also Merle Molofsky, "The Return," *The Psychoanalytic Review* 91.6 (2004): 853–859, who emphasizes Ivan's adolescence.

18 Irina Anisimova, "The Terrors of History: Revolutionary Gothic in "Mother Earth" by Boris Pilniak," *The Slavic and East European Journal* 55.3 (2011): 376–395. Robin Aizlewood links the word to a "poetics of disorientation" and "demonic possession"; "'Besy,' Disorientation and the Person," *The Slavonic and East European Review, Personality and Place in Russian Culture* 88.1/2 (2010): 304, 308. Cf. James Smethurst: "Gothic-influenced texts contain a past event involving an unrightful and violent usurpation which constrains the actions of succeeding generations. This familial original sin is often passed down through the bloodlines of both the sinners and the sinned against" in James Smethurst, "Invented by Horror: The Gothic and African American Literary Ideology in *Native Son*," *African American Review* 35.1 (2001): 29, cited in "The Terrors of History," 381.

19 Within the less-than-30-second dialogue between Ivan and his older brother Andrei on the tower platform, Andrei precludes speech about descending twice. The rationale for this prohibition is the avoidance of being called a "goat": "do you want to be called a goat"? (. . . *chtoby tebja kozlom nazyvali?*)

20 Betrayal is symbolized by a billy-goat's horns, which are "given" to the husband by his wife or her illicit lover, *rogatii kozyol*. The visual image of boys' in their underwear cum swimming briefs atop the tower reinforces the sexual focus of the subtext, a detail that we will see becomes important in our process of reconstructing the secret.

21 Caroline Humphrey, "Dangerous Words: Taboos, Evasions, and Silence in Soviet Russia," *Forum for Anthropology and Culture* 2 (2005): 374. In Soviet prison slang the term was used to emphasize the condition of betrayal (akin to that performed by an adulteress) to refer to prisoners who chose to align with Soviet authorities against the prison population. The emasculating condition of a cuckolded husband seems to underlie the contemporary usage of the term in Russian *mat* lexicon to refer to homosexuals.

22 Victor Erofeyev, "Dirty Words," *The New Yorker* (September 15, 2013).

23 S. A. Smith, "The Social Meanings of Swearing: Workers and Bad Language in Late Imperial and Early Soviet Russia," *Past & Present* 160 (1998): 172. See also Felix Dreizin and Tom Priestly, "A Systematic Approach to Russian Obscene Language," *Russian Linguistics* (1982): 233–249.

24 Dreizin, Priestly, ibid., 234.

25 He tells her that he would have died of fear had she had not come (*Esli by ty ne prishla, ja by umer*), and she is perplexed by his apparent surprise at her presence. "Darling, what are you talking about? I'm here with you" ("*Nu, chto ty, milen'kij Nu Chto ty govorish' ja by umer.*")

26 Nicolas Abraham and Maria Torok, *The Shell and the Kernel: Renewals of Psychoanalysis*, vol. 1, trans., Nicholas Rand (Chicago: University of Chicago Press, 1994), 175–176.

27 Tatiana Tiaynen, *Babushka in Flux: Grandmothers and Family-Making between Russian Karelia and Finland* (Tampere University Press, 2013).

28 Edward L. Keenan, "Ivan the Terrible and His Women," *Russian History* 37.4 (2010): 345.

29 Terence McSweeney, "The End of Ivan's Childhood," 7, notes how the "silence of the grandmother is palpable." The transcendent quality and power of Galina Popova's silent performance as the Babushka has been noted by her colleagues as well as by critics; Natalia Vdovina, the actress who plays the mother, states that her own performance was much influenced by Popova's.

30 There are fascinating connections between the tropes used to convey the drama embedded in *The Return* and folkloric paradigms identified as vernacular expressions of religion in Russia. See Alexander Panchenko's "How to Make a Shrine with Your Own Hands" in Marion Bowman, A. Lo Valik, Ulo Valik eds., *Vernacular Religion in Everyday Life: Expressions of Belief* (London: Routledge, 2014), 50–57, for an incisive analysis of a paradigm whose structure includes components to those used in the film. See, for example, his discussion of the tale of fratricide committed by St Ioann, who kills St Iaokv, which includes details such as wood burning ovens and watery burials. In another variant, the elder brother is inspired to murder as a result of his witnessing a sacrificial act committed by the father, suggesting "the guilt of one or the other parent." Yet another version implicitly castigates the mother—whose absence from home opens the space for the fratricide to transpire—as the implicit source of the crime.

31 Cf. the Russian proverb "through fire and water," *itti v ogon' I v vodu*, which is used in oaths that promise to protect someone or to swear allegiance to the completion or execution of a particular event. According to Louis Menashe, "Review," *Cineaste* 29.2 (2004): 27, Zvyagintsev suggests that the fireplace aligns with "traditional symbols of femininity."

32 McSweeney, "The End of Ivan's Childhood," suggests that the father who returns is not a "New Testament . . . Christ, rather a more severe Old Testament figure demanding respect and obedience"; Vladimir Strukov, "The Return of Gods: Andrei Zviagintsev's "Vozvrashchenie (*The Return*)," *The Slavic and East European Journal, Special Forum Issue: Resent, Reassess, and Reinvent: The Three R's of Post-Soviet Cinema* 51.2 (2007): 340.

33 Karen Armstrong has discussed how scholars responsible for assembling the New Testament offered teleological interpretations of the *Old Testament* story of Abraham and Isaac, which rendered the latter text a forerunner of the sacrifice of Christ. See Armstrong, *The Bible* (New York: Grove Press, 2007), 106, 150. Vladimir Strukov, "The Return of the Gods," 340, also notes the reversal of the religious references to suggest that the film offers an "interpretation of the myth from the point of view of historical time."

34 Cf. Brygida Pawłowska-Jądrzyk, "Murky," 241, who suggests that "religious symbolism should be understood as more universal, archetypal."

35 Sturkov, "The Return of Gods," 337, claims that the absence of the "two mourning figures . . . indicates the father/s/Christ solitude and the shift of the director's attention towards the father relationship with his sons/apostles."

36 According to Priscilla Hunt, the folds are also evocative of Andrei Rublev's painting *Troiska*, in which "the drapery of garments refers to different modalities of the divine motion . . . indicative of embodiment of the spirit." See "Andrei Rublev's Old Testament Trinity Icon in Cultural Context," *The Trinity-Sergius Lavr in Russian History and Culture: Readings in Russian Religious Culture* 3 (2005): 113.

37 Leo Steinberg, *The Sexuality of Christ in Renaissance Art and in Modern Oblivion*, rpt. (Chicago: University of Chicago Press, 2014), 81, 1–5, discusses the representation of Christ's outlined genitalia beneath covers.

38 Ágnes Pethő, "The Tableau Vivant as a 'Figure of Return' in Contemporary East European Cinema," *Acta Univ. Sapientiae, Film and Media Studies* 9 (2014): 51–76, suggests that visual quotes function as "powerful agent[s] in generating metanarratives." Her analysis of Zvyaginstev's reproduction of Mantegna's painting argues that

> it becomes not only a clearly marked vantage point that doubles the reference frame of the otherwise realistic narrative, suggesting the possibility of an allegorical reading, but it also makes the viewer prepared for further, less obvious biblical motifs or cinematic quotations, and initiates an intricate play between images and media.
>
> 59

Brygida, "Murky," 247, discusses the "interdiscursive links and references" to religious art that characterizes Zvyagintsev's oeuvre.

39 Irene Earls, *Renaissance Art: A Topical Dictionary* (New York: Greenwood Press, 1987), 46.

40 The word "return" in Russian, *vozvrashchenie*, also means "resurrection." The film unfolds over six days; the father's submergence occurs on Friday suggesting that his symbolic return occurred on Sunday when Ivan's fantasy was triggered. Like Christ, he returned from a state of repression.

41 This insight was inspired by Esther Rashkin's analysis of in "The Interred Sign, *L'Intersigne* by Auguste de Villiers de L'Isle-Adam," *Family Secrets and the Psychoanalysis of Narrative* (Princeton: Princeton University Press, 1992), 78.

42 Menashe, "Review," 26, praises this sequence as "wonderful psychological realism."

43 Julius Schnorr von Carolsfeld, *Abraham Sacrificio de Isaac*. For more on Carolsfeld, see *German Masters of the Nineteenth Century: Paintings and Drawings from the Federal Republic of Germany*, The Metropolitan Museum of Art, New York (New York: The Metropolitan Museum of Art, 1981). Carolsfeld's illustrations were critiqued as "complex and cluttered, lacking in harmony of line and symmetry."

44 Panchenko, "How to Make a Shrine," 56.

45 Ibid., 58. Panchenko, 21–22, discusses David Damrosch's claim that this parental triangle bears traces of narrative genres whose origins lie much earlier than the historical period during which Genesis came into being. His argument that the Bible appropriated the narrative tropes in order to introduce "Israel's 'one Lord' into the conversation" is evocative as a metaphor for collective self-fashioning processes.

46 Don Seeman, "'Where Is Sarah Your Wife?' Cultural Poetics of Gender and Nationhood in the Hebrew Bible," *The Harvard Theological Review* 91.2 (1988): 103–125. See also Harvey Goldberg, "Cambridge in the Land of Canaan: Descent, Alliance Circumcision, and Instruction in the Bible," *Journal of Near Eastern Studies* 24 (1996): 9–34. Genesis 22:13 identifies a "ram caught in a thicket" as the object of substitutionary sacrifice. Of significant interest is the translation of this phrase in the Russian Synodal Text, *i vot, pozadi oven, zaputavshijsja v chashhe rogami svoimi*, which also seems to resonate with a similar context. The word "thicket," *zaputavshjsja*, is connected to a lexical chain of words meaning "hidden," "covert," and "clandestine," while the word "caught," *chashhe*, is synonymous with "hard put to it," "messed up," and "entangled," and even "embarrassed," *rasterjannyj*.

47 Sara's sexual fidelity to Abraham is challenged twice when he identifies her as his sister which resulted in her being "taken" into the Pharaoh's and

Abimelech's houses, respectively. See Genesis 12:11–15; 21:22. Abraham's acceptance of the substitutionary sacrificial ram, in this vein, might be seen as his submission to the authority of preservative repression; the object of sacrifice at once conceals and reveals the secret.

48 For analyses that read the dinner scene as evocative of the da Vinci's *Last Supper*, see Terrence McSweeney, "The End of Ivan's Childhood," 100; Kim Dillon, "The Emerging Identity," 6; Ágnes, Pethő "The Tableau Vivant," 60; see also Vladimir Strukov, "The Return of the Gods," 338, who claims that "[i]n *The Return*, the mise-en-scène of the Last Supper is peculiar in its careful geometrical orchestration of people and objects: the brothers sit at opposite sides of the table and the father is between them facing his wife and mother."

49 Priscilla Hunt, "Andrei Rublev's Old Testament Trinity Icon in Cultural Context," 102. Cf. Denys Kondyuk, "Sensing and Longing for God in Andrey Zvyagintsev's The Return and Leviathan," *Religions, Film and Lived Theology* 7.7 (2016): 1–16, identifies "the absence of eye contact and death as a visual means of presenting transcendental relation"; and Strukov, "The Return of the Gods,' 336, who sees in the three men a composite figure of one: "In *The Return* the three male figures constitute a hierarchy of age and authority based on their maturity and represent three stages in a man's life: Ivan-childhood, Andrei-adolescence, and the father-adulthood."

50 Zvyaginstev's interest in Rublev was demonstrated in his insistence that his young actors view Tarkovsky's celebrated film on the artist.

51 Strukov, "The Return of the Gods," 336.

52 Anton Chekhov, "The Cherry Orchard" in Peter Carson, trans., *Anton Chekhov Plays* (New York: Penguin), 2002.

53 Cited in James N. Loehlin, *Chekhov: The Cherry Orchard* (Cambridge: Cambridge University Press, 2006), 9. Cf. Loehlin's comment that Chekhov's plays make "moment to moment [interpretive] demands, and refuse, in the same way, to yield definitive answers to the largest problems they pose," Ibid.

54 Cf. the Russian proverb "to sit in a puddle," *sest' v luzhu,* "to be duped," "to put one's foot in it," "to get oneself in a mess," which also resonates with these connotations.

55 Expressions of hunger occur four times, three voiced by Ivan and one by the father; the physical act of ingestion is represented five times, all of them communal except for a quick shot of Andrei eating bread alone when Ivan and the father find him after a three-hour search. Eating is denied or delayed for Ivan four times.

56 The repetition of this kinship reference verbally echoes Genesis 22 in Abraham frequently uses the word "son" to address Isaac.

57 Cf. the use of the word "bread" in Russian *mat* locutions to refer to a "face" and "female genitalia," *hlebalo* and *hlebal'nik* which reinforces these connotations.

58 Nancy Condor, "Knowledge (Imperfective): Andrei Zviagintsev and Contemporary Cinema," Birgit Beumers, ed. *A Companion of Russian Cinema* (John Wiley & Sons, 2016): 571, argues that this "inversion" is a signature cinematographic technique of the director.

59 Anais Cabart notes how birch trees figure in the film's landscape and suggests that they symbolize renewal. See "Andrei Zvyaginstev's The Return," 52.

60 *"Ham chervil nuzhny zdeshnjaja ryba na hleb ne pojdet."*

61 Strukov, "The Return of the Gods," 339, views in this scene a reference to Salvador Dali's (1904–1989) Christ of St. John of the Cross (1951), which views the crucifixion from above. Specifically, he sees the director's allusion

to the triangulation of the cross by Dali, a reference to the Holy Trinity, as an indication that the director presents the conflict between "the figures of the father and his sons" as eschatological. Irina Novikova, "Death and Dying: Making Sense of Life in Post Soviet Cinemas," Kate Woodthorpe, ed., *Layers of Death and Dying* (Oxford: Inter-disciplinary Press, 2007), 19, sees in the scene a "rigid discourse of masculinity or a 'gender corset', meant to discipline a boyish body and consciousness in compliance with certain schemata of a man's behavior."

62 Laura A. Janda and Olga Lyashevskaya, "Grammatical Profiles and the Interaction of the Lexicon with Aspect, Tense, and Mood in Russian," *Cognitive Linguistics* 22.4 (2011): 737.

63 The injunction "wait," *podozhdat'*, appears in the speech of the father consistently throughout the film in contexts of thwarted eating.

64 The sleigh-like manner by which the father was transported calls to mind the Russian proverb "to get into someone's else's sleigh," *saditsia ne v svoi sani,* which means "to occupy a position or post for which one may not yet be suited," an appropriate description of Andrei and Ivan's initiate status.

65 Cf. the Russian proverb *verevki vit' (out of someone)*, which literally means "to weave the ropes," that is, to have someone's will subjugated to full control, so that it is possible to make them do anything.

66 McSweeney, "The End of Ivan's Childhood," 105, argues that the father's death has "proved a catalyst to propel [the boys] into manhood."

67 Helena Goscilo and Yana Hashamova, "Fathers and Sons in Soviet and Post-Soviet films," 170–171; 185; McSweeney, "The End of Ivan's Childhood," Fatu-Tutoveanu, "The Return of the Sacred."

68 Nancy Condor, "Knowledge (Imperfective)," 574, suggests that this effacement is a signature cinematographic technique seen throughout Zvyagintsev's films.

69 Philip Cavendish, "The Return of the Photo," 488. In n. 36, Cavendish explains that the song was recorded during field trips to the Soviet Union in 1989 and 1990; it was released on CD in 1995 by Smithsonian/Folkways as a collection, *Old Believers: Songs of the Nekrassov Cossacks.* The annotations provided by Margarita Mazo and Olga Velichkina help contextualize the performances within broader ritual practices. The term Cossack is generally used to refer peoples who inhabited Russian land south of Moscow and Ukraine.

70 Ibid.

71 Alexander Fuljushkin, *Ivan the Terrible: A Military History* (Frontline Books, 2008), 36.

72 Ibid., 37.

73 Ibid. Cavendish's observation that Tarkovsky also inserted a Cossack folk song in his film *Nostalgia* (1981) suggests a level of intertextuality that aligns with the dominant aesthetic patterns of the film.

74 Maureen Perrie's excellent review of the literature on the "image of Tsar Ivan" provides a concise and accessible introduction into the complex forces and multitude of factors that must be considered in historical reconstruction, although her specific focus is on the image of Ivan in Russian Folklore. See *The Image of Ivan the Terrible in Russian Folklore* (Cambridge: Cambridge University Press, 2002), 1–27, 35 *et passim.* See also idem., ed., *The Cambridge History of Russia: Volume 1, From Early Rus' to 1689* (Cambridge: Cambridge University Press, 2006). For general histories of the reign I have relied on the following sources, which have been richly supplemented by deeper analyses of various themes: Isabel de Madariaga, *Ivan the Terrible: First Tsar of Russia* (New Haven: Yale

University Press, 2005), aims to dispel the aura of elusiveness surrounding "Ivan the man and ruler," xiv; Andrei Pavlovich Pavol and Maureen Perrie, *Ivan The Terrible* (London: Pearson, Longman, 2003), provide a balanced synthesis of much of the recent scholarship on the reign in their narrative; Robert Payne and Nikita Romanoff's *Ivan the Terrible* (New York: Cooper Square Press, 2002) offers details plumbed from sources associated with Ivan's governing idiom, which will figure significantly in the following discussion.

75 Charles J. Halperin, "Ivan IV's Insanity," *Russian History* 34.1 (2007): 207–218, provides a concise summation of the "psychiatric" approaches and concludes that there is need for more rigor in defining what constitutes "insanity." He also emphasizes the need to reconcile any such "diagnosis" with a historical understanding of Ivan's reign, concepts that are too frequently conflated to the detriment of psychoanalytically inclined studies. See also, idem., "Royal Recreation: Ivan the Terrible Goes Hunting," *Journal of Early Modern History* 14 (2019): 293–316; Richard Hellie, "What Happened? How Did He Get Away with It?: Ivan Groznyi's Paranoia and the Problem of Institutional Restraints," *Russian History* 14.1 (1987): 199–224; David B. Miller, "Official History in the Reign of Ivan Groznyi and Its Seventeenth-Century Imitators," *Russian History* 14.1 (1987): 333–360; Edward L. Keenan, "How Ivan Became 'Terrible'," *Harvard Ukrainian Studies Rus' Writ Large: Languages, Histories Cultures: Essays Presented in Honor of Michael S. Flier on his Sixty-Fifth Birthday* 28.1.4 (2006): 521–542; John Fennell, "Ivan IV as Writer," *Russian History* 14.1 (1987): 145–154; Valerie A. Kivelson's reflective metahistorical essay on scholarship on sixteenth-century Russia discusses the challenges of scholars of this era to "set aside normative judgments, aiming to reconstruct a Muscovite logic from within." See "On Words, Sources, and Historical Method: Which Truth about Muscovy?" *Kritika: Explorations in Russian and Eurasian History* 3.3 (2002): 490.

76 Ann Kleimola, "Review. *Ivan the Terrible: First Tsar of Russia*. By Isabel de Madariaga. New Haven, CT: Yale University Press, 2005," *The Journal of Modern History* 79.4 (2007): 951.

77 Edward L. Keenan, "Ivan the Terrible and his Women," *Russian History* 37.4 (2010): 322–359.

78 Ibid., 326.

79 Ibid., 342.

80 A conflict emerged from the fact that "Solomoniia did not easily accept her fate" and resisted tonsure. Isolde Thyret, "'Blessed is the Tsaritsa's Womb': The Myth of Miraculous Birth and Royal Motherhood in Muscovite Russia," *The Russian Review* 53.4 (1994): 487, n. 37.

81 Keenan, "Ivan the Terrible and his Women," 337.

82 Ibid., 345.

83 Isolde Thyret, "Blessed Is the Tsaritsa's Womb," 484.

84 Ibid., 489.

85 Ibid., 486.

86 Charles J. Halperin, "The Concept of the Russian Land from the Ninth to the Fourteenth Centuries," *Russian History* 2.1 (1975): 33–35. Halperin claims that the term Rus' referred to the cult of the clan of the Moscow princes, which later was extended to refer to the subjects of its princely domain.

87 Ibid.

88 Ibid., 33.

89 Ibid., 31.

90 Smith, "The Social Meanings of Swearing," 170.

91 Isolde Thyret, "Blessed Is the Tsaritsa's Womb," 486. Payne and Romanoff talk of "augeries," *Ivan the Terrible*, 10.
92 Thyret, op cit., 479–496.
93 De Mariaga, *Ivan the Terrible*, 39; Payne and Romanoff, *Ivan the Terrible*, 14.
94 For struggles during the early Regency and Ivan's minority after his mother's death, see Payne and Romanoff, op cit., 33–42.
95 Keenan, "Ivan the Terrible and his Women," 338–339. Cf. Pierre Gonneau, "The Many Deaths of Ivan the Terrible and Their Interpretations," *Mundo Eslavo* 13 (2014): 77, suggests that the historical sources that describe the establishment of a council were "rewritten" at the behest of Ivan "in order to substantiate the thesis that his father chose his mother as regent." Mikhail Krom, "The 'Widowed Kingdom' The Political Crisis in Russia in the 1530s and the 1540s," *Russian Studies in History* 53.1 (2014): 21, suggests that the idea of a will is something Elena Glinsky propagated after Vasily's death, questioning if there ever actually was one, 21.
96 Ibid., 18; de Madariaga, *Ivan the Terrible*, 39.
97 Ibid., 4, n. 1; de Madariaga, *Ivan the Terrible*, 40. Payne and Romanoff say that Elena Glinsky appointed him to the high-ranking position of Master of the Horse and the Boyar Council, *Ivan the Terrible*, 33.
98 De Madariaga, *op cit*; Payne and Romanoff, *op cit*, 33, states that foreign diplomat Sigismund von Herberstein "wrote that Elena was impatient to get rid of her uncle because he blamed her for her liaison with her favorite."
99 John Fennell, ed. *Prince AM Kurbsky's History of Ivan IV* (Cambridge University Press, 2008) 9, n. 4; Isabel de Madariaga notes that these arrests were made amidst the wails of Ivan, *Ivan the Terrible*, 41.
100 I refer to the correspondence between Ivan IV and Prince Andrey Kurbsky (1528–1583). The seventeenth-century provenance of the texts in which this is preserved catalyzed a vigorous debate about how to use these sources for historical purposes. Although the problematic absence of sixteenth-century texts that could verify the attribution of the texts to Kurbsky and Ivan has not been resolved, I am persuaded by John Fennell—the translator of the *Correspondence*—who has argued that the language surround found in Ivan's epistles is so consistent in their idiosyncrasies that he believes they are easily recognizable as unique to Ivan IV (Fennel, "Ivan as a Writer," 146). In particular, Fennell's description of the awkward syntax, "conjunctionalist conditions," incongruence among tenses and infinitives, not to mention puns, Russian *mat*, evokes the veiled lexical strategies that drive *The Return's* cinematographic idiom to invite a similar type of investigation. Toward this objective, I translate several examples of his writing style by listening as well as reading the written language. I suggest that the incomprehensibility of some of his locutions and syntax might be more deeply understood as containing words that hide. My understanding of the controversy was immeasurably helped by Charles Halperin's retrospective account of the twenty-five-year debate over the provenance and historical value of the letters, "Edward Keenan and the Kurbskii-Groznyi Correspondence in Hindsight," *Jahrbücher für Geschichte Osteuropas* H. 3 (1998): 376–403; Halperin, 388, notes that the letters may have been orally composed, which reinforces the idea that we may hear something pressed between the words of Ivan's convoluted language. For linguistic analysis of Ivan's language, see John Fennell, "Textology as a Key to the Study of Old Russian Literature and History," *Text* (1987): 157–166. See also, idem., ed. and trans., *The Correspondence Between Prince A. M. Kurbsky and Tsar Ivan IV of Russia, 1564–1579* (Cambridge University Press, 1955).
101 De Madariaga, *Ivan the Terrible*, 166.

102 The letter was sent in 1564; Fennell, *Correspondence*, ix.
103 Fennel, *Correspondence,* 181.
104 Ibid. Kurbsky's criticism that Ivan's speech resembles that of babbling old women summons up the role of elder women, *baba*, as "ones who know" with regard to pagan fertility practices. See William F. Ryan, *The Bathhouse at Midnight: An Historical Survey of Magic and Divination in Russia* (Penn State Press, 1999), 82.
105 Fennell, *Kurbsky's History,* 3. Ivan later acknowledges as much when he refers to a child's apprehension capacities: "For this is clear, you were still young in years but, however, you can know of it."
106 Fennel, Correspondence, 77.
107 "Vessels," *sodno*; "container," "*sudno*," are synonymic with "bedpan," and "bed-warmer," *grelka*. Ryan, *The Bathhouse at Midnight*, 267, n. 286, links gold with pagan fertility practices.
108 De Madariaga, *Ivan the Terrible*, 63, suggests that these fires "may have fostered an incipient paranoia."
109 Ibid.
110 Recall that the word "fire," *ogon'*, is semantically connected to the words "smudge," "blight," and "stain," the latter of which is used frequently in Ivan's first epistle to Kurbsky, when he repeatedly denies having any stain or blight on his hands (or on the threshold of churches).
111 Ibid., 216. Ivan's letter to King Sigismund Augustus was written in the name of Prince I. D. Bel'sky, whom Sigismund entreated to defect.
112 Alexander Leonidovich, *Ivan the Terrible as a Religious Type: A Study of the Background, Genesis and Development of the Theocratic Idea of the First Russian Tsar, and his Attempts to Establish 'Free Autocracy' in Russia* (PhD Dissertation, Fordham University 1988), 141–142.
113 In contemporary Russian *mat*, the word "fur" is used in the sense of "skin," to denote "prostitute," and the [instrument for] masturbation.
114 An analysis premised on the concept of the phantom also allows us to transcend an implicit binary approach in which psychosis is seen as the "other side of the coin" of effective rule, or as a corruption of it, or as a deviation from a spiritual or social norm. Backward reading obviates treating psychosis and governing as opposing semiotic systems. See Halperin, "Ivan IV's Insanity," and "Royal Recreation," 294.
115 John Fennell, "Ivan IV as a Writer," 147.
116 Ibid., 75.
117 Ibid., 72–73.
118 Cf. Russian *mat, palka*, rod, penis—"stick"; *vstavit palku*, "to copulate," literally "to insert the stick." Payne and Romanoff cite this passage to illustrate how unceremoniously Ivan was treated after his mother's death, *Ivan the Terrible*, 39.
119 De Mariaga, *Ivan the Terrible*, 42.
120 Fennell, *Correspondence*, 76–77, n. 3, "Unfortunately this presumably heavenly ironical joke of Ivan is syntactically almost unintelligible. The train of thought appears as follows: The Shuisky's (and the boyars) had made a practice of having vessels made from the gold and silver of the royal treasure and inscribing their parents' names on them as though they were family possessions. Would it not, Ivan asks, have been a shade more honest had Shuisky exchanged a genuine heirloom, such as his ancient fur coat, for a new one from the royal wardrobe, sold the new one with the money bought gold and silver vessels which they might then call family possessions?"
121 Norman W. Ingham, "The *Groza* of Ivan *Groznyi in Russian Folklore*," *Russian History* 14.1 (1987): 230.

122 Ibid., 230–231.

123 Ibid. Maureen Perrie, *The Image of Ivan the Terrible*, 32, discusses the historical implications of his work and that of scholars who "explain the differences in Ivan's image in terms of the different social groups in which the folklore allegedly originated."

124 Ibid., 227.

125 Ibid., 232.

126 Ibid.

127 Ibid.

128 Charles J. Halperin, "Contemporary Russian Perceptions of Ivan IV's Oprichnina," *Kritika: Explorations in Russian and Eurasian History* 18.1 (2017): 95.

129 Ibid., 121–122.

130 Ibid., 95. See also Richard Crummey, "Ivan the Terrible," *Windows on the Russian Past*, eds. Samuel H. Baron and Nancy W. Heer (Columbus: American Association for the Advancement of Slavic Studies, 1977), 57–74.

131 Isabel de Madariage, *Ivan the Terrible*, 146, citing Russian historian N. M. Karamzin.

132 Halperin, "Contemporary Russian Perceptions," 95.

133 De Madariaga, *Ivan the Terrible*, 179–180.

134 Halperin, "Contemporary Russian Perceptions," 95.

135 Yanov, Alexander. *The Origins of Autocracy: Ivan the Terrible in Russian History* (Berkeley: University of California Press, 1981), 67.

136 Halperin, "Royal Recreation," 294; and idem., "Ivan IV's Insanity," 216.

137 Halperin, "Contemporary Russian Perceptions," 95, 100.

138 "Did Ivan IV's *Oprichniki* Carry Dogs' Heads on Their Horses?," *Canadian-American Slavic Studies* 46.1 (2012): 64.

139 Halperin, "Contemporary Russian Perceptions," discusses this from perspective of records on land transactions, 99–105; See also, Robert O. Crummey, "Ivan IV: Reformer or Tyrant?" in *Reinterpreting Russian History, ed. Daniel H. Kaiser and Gary Marker* (New York: Oxford University Press, 1994), 162–163, for the division of large estates into smaller *oprichik* plots and state terror; de Madariaga notes how land seizure diminished the power of heredity nobility, *Ivan the Terrible*, 255–260; see also, Andrei Pavlov and Maureen Perrie, *Ivan the Terrible*, 155–156, 161–162.

140 Priscilla Hunt, "Ivan IV's Personal Mythology of Kingship," *Slavic Review* 52.4 (1993): 769–809.

141 Ibid., 770.

142 Ibid., 772.

143 Ibid., 808–809.

144 Ibid.

145 Charles Halperin, "Royal Recreation," 294.

146 William Derbyshire, "Verbal Homonymy in the Russian language," *Canadian Slavonic Papers* 9.1 (1967): 137.

147 The term "mite," derives from a parable in the New Testament. In the passage, which warns of the pretense of scribes who "make long prayers" in the New Testament, an impoverished widow gives away her last two coins to the Temple (Mark 12: 41–44 and Luke 21: 1–4).

148 Keenan, "Ivan the Terrible and His Women," 340.

149 Ibid.

150 Ibid.

151 Fennell, *Correspondence*, 71.

152 Ivan goes on to describe Elena's vulnerability with the image of her engulfed in flames, which intimates a link between her threadbare state and

the Moscow fire, when her mother and brothers were accused of manipulating the dynasty. Ibid. Cf. Mikhail Krom, "The Widowed Kingdom," who suggests that Ivan was elevated to the throne "by the merest whim of fate," 16.

153 Ann M. Kleimola, "The Duty to Denounce in Muscovite Russia," *Slavic Review* 31.4 (1972): 71.

154 Yanov, *The Origins of Autocracy*, 67.

155 Alexander Leonidovich, "Ivan the Terrible as a Religious Type," 152–153, claims that *oprichniki* could marry, and they did not keep a traditional monastic diet.

156 "Did Ivan IV's *Oprichniki* Carry Dogs' Heads on Their Horses?," 65; Hunt, "Ivan's Personal Mythology," 798; Leonidovich, "Ivan the Terrible as a Religious Type," 154.

157 Victor Erofeyev, "Letter from Moscow: Dirty Words: The Unique Power of Russia's Underground Language," trans. Andrew Bromfield, New Yorker, September 15, 2003.

158 Halperin, "Dogs' Heads," Ibid., 42, 44–49.

159 De Madriaga includes this description in her account of Ivan's notoriously brutal attack on Novgorod in 1570, *Ivan the Terrible*, 247.

160 de Madriaga, *Ivan the Terrible*, 247; Perrie, Pavolov, *Ivan the Terrible*, 150.

161 Fennell, *Kurbsky's History*, 3–4.

162 A. M. Kleimola, "The Duty to Denounce in Muscovite Russia," *Slavic Review* 31.4 (1972): 759–779. Cf. 767n. 31, "In the 16th century the landholding members of the cavalry, were recruited from all social milieus, including Cossacks, peasants, and even slaves." Serge A. Zenkovsky, "The Russian Church Schism: It's Background and Repercussions," *The Russian Review* 16.4 (1957), 38, remarks on the inclusivity of Ivan IV's most repressive instrument, the *oprichniki*, among whom could be found "Germans and Other West Europeans."

163 Carolyn Pouncy, "Missed Opportunities and the Search for Ivan the Terrible," 323; Perrie and Pavlov, *Ivan the Terrible*, 115–116.

164 Sergei Bogatyrev, "Reinventing the Russian Monarchy in the 1550s: Ivan the Terrible, the Dynasty, and the Church," *The Slavonic and East European Review* (2007): 292.

165 Ibid. Cf. Hunt, "Ivan IV's Personal Mythology," 776.

166 Ibid. See also Donald Ostrowski, "The Moscow Councils of 1447 to 1589 and the Conciliar Period in Russian Orthodox Church History" in *Tapestry of Russian Christianity: Studies in History and Culture*, Nickolas Lupinin, Donald Ostrowski and Jennifer B. Spock, eds., (Columbus, OH: Department of Slavic and East European Languages and Cultures and the Resource Center for Medieval Slavic Studies, The Ohio State University, 2016), 121–155. See also, Jack E. Kollmann, "The Stoglav Council and Parish Priests," *Russian History* 7.1/2 (1980): 65–91.

167 Robert Button, The Theology of Ritual and the Russian Old Rite: "The Art of Christian Living" (PhD Dissertation, University of Exeter, 2015), 92 cites "'On the Sign of the Cross'" (abridged from the psalter printed under the Patriarchate of Patriarch Joseph of Moscow) in the Old Orthodox Prayer Book, 335. This prayer book explicitly states that "in the context of the Crucifixion of Christ, the Sign of the Cross is sacramental, incorporating us into the mystery of the economy of salvation through its specific symbolicity: 'the Sign of the precious Cross, this excellent sacrament of the faith teaches us how to know a mystery.'"

168 Timothy Ware, *The Orthodox Church: An Introduction to Eastern Christianity* (London: Penguin, 1993), 122.

169 Bogatryev, "Reinventing the Russian Monarchy," 292.

170 Robert Button, "Theology of Ritual," 92.
171 Ibid., 293.
172 Hugh Graham, "How Do We Know What We Know about Ivan The Terrible (A Paradigm)," *Russian History* 14.1 (1987): 194, discusses how historical song cycles about Ivan the Terrible illustrate how deeply the ruler's sack of Novgorod had "sunk into popular consciousness."
173 Ibid., 161, 171–174.
174 Paul Meyendorff, *Russia, Ritual and Reform: The Liturgical Reforms of Nikon in the 17th Century* (Crestwood, NY: St Vladimir's Seminary Press, 1991), 45.
175 Robert Button, "The Theology of Ritual and the Russian Old Rite," 7.
176 Crummey, *Old Believers in a Changing World* (DeKalb, IL: Northern Illinois Press, 2011), 78.
177 Michael Cherniavsky, "Old Believer and the New Religion," 3, n. 10.
178 Sergei Bogatyrev, "Reinventing the Russian Monarchy," 271–293.
179 Ibid.
180 Robert Crummey, *Old Believers in a Changing World*, 78.
181 Cf. Serge Zenkovsky, "The Russian Church Schism," 41, who shows that the Muscovite church challenged the discriminatory authority of the Patriarch and tsar on the grounds that Muscovite practices were "an inseparable part of the Russian Orthodoxy, not just a religion but a way of life."
182 Cherniavsky, "Old Believer and the New Religion," 4.
183 Zenkovsky, "The Russian Church Schism," 44–46; 49; Cherniavsky, "Old Believers and the New Religion," 4–5, n. 16.
184 Nadieszda Kizenko, "The Church Schism and Old Belief" in Abbott Gleason, ed., *A Companion to Russian History*, Vol. 10 (John Wiley & Sons, 2009), 151.
185 Georg Michels, "The Violent Old Belief: An Examination of Religious Dissent on the Karelian Frontier," *Russian History* 19.1 (1992): 207, 219–222.
186 Zenkovsky, "The Russian Church Schism," 51 and Thomas Robbins, "Religious Mass Suicide before Jonestown: The Russian Old Believers," *Sociology of Religion* 47.1 (1986): 1–20.

Bibliography

Abeel, Erica. "Return of the Prodigal Father; Andrey Zvyagintsev Talks about 'The Return.'" *Indiewire*. (2004).

Aizlewood, Robin. "'Besy', Disorientation and the Person." *Slavonic and East European Review* 88 (2010): 291–308.

Anisimova, Irina. "The Terrors of History: Revolutionary Gothic in "Mother Earth" by Boris Pilniak." *The Slavic and East European Journal* 55.3 (2011): 376–395.

Apresjan, Valentina. "The Myth of the 'Russian Soul' Through the Mirror of Language." *Folklorica* 14 (2009): 91–121.

Armstrong, Karen. *The Bible*. Grove Press. 2007.

Bartlett, R. "Michels at War with the Church. Religious Dissent in Seventeenth-Century Russia." *Journal of Ecclesiastical History* 52.3 (2001): 566–567.

Barratt, Barnaby B. "Fathering and the Consolidation of Masculinity: Notes on the Paternal Function in Andrey Zvyagintsev's *The Return*." *The Psychoanalytic Review* 102.3 (2015): 347–364.

Beumers, Birgit. Ed. *A Companion of Russian Cinema*. John Wiley & Sons. 2016.
Bogatyrev, Sergei. "Reinventing the Russian Monarchy in the 1550s: Ivan the Terrible, the Dynasty, and the Church." *The Slavonic and East European Review* (2007): 271–293.
Boststein, Leon. "From Russia with Mozart." *American Symphony Orchestra Program Notes (2006).*
Button, Robert. *The Theology of Ritual and the Russian Old Rite: "The Art of Christian Living."* PhD Dissertation. University of Exeter, 2015.
Cabart, Anais. "Andrei Zvyagintsev's The Return: A Tarkovskian Initiation." *Film and Media Studies* 1.2 (2013): 51–62.
Cavendish, Philip. "The Return of the Photograph: Time, Memory and the Genre of the Photo-Film in Andrei Zviagintsev's *Vozvrashchenie* (*The Return*, 2003)." *Slavonic & East European Review* 91.3 (2013): 465–510.
Chekhov, Anton. "The Cherry Orchard." Peter Carson, trans. *Anton Chekhov Plays*. Penguin. 2002.
Cherniavsky, Michael. "The Old Believers and the New Religion." *Slavic Review* 25.1 (1966): 1–39.
Condor, Nancy. "Knowledge (Imperfective): Andrei Zviagintsev and Contemporary Cinema." *A Companion of Russian Cinema*. Ed. Birgit Beumers. John Wiley & Sons, 2016. 565–584.
Crummey, Robert O. *The Formation of Muscovy 1300–1613*. Routledge, 2014.
———. "Ivan the Terrible." *Windows on the Russian Past*. Eds. Samuel H. Baron and Nancy W. Heer. American Association for the Advancement of Slavic Studies, 1977. 57–74.
De Madariaga, Isabel. *Ivan the Terrible*. Yale University Press, 2005
de Montebello, Philippe. "Introduction to German Masters of the Nineteenth Century: Paintings and Drawings from the Federal Republic of Germany." *Metropolitan Museum of Art, New York*. Ed. Harry N. Abrams, 1981.
Derbyshire, William W. "Verbal Homonymy in the Russian Language." *Canadian Slavonic Papers* 9.1 (1967): 131–139.
De Sherbinin, Julie W. *Chekhov and Russian Religious Culture: The Poetics of the Marian Paradigm*. Northwestern University Press, 1997.
Dillon, Kimberley Alexandra. "The Emerging Russian Identity as Expressed through Russian Art House Cinema." *Verges: Germanic & Slavic Studies in Review* 2.1 (2013): 1–9.
Dreizin, Felix and Tom Priestly. "A Systematic Approach to Russian Obscene Language." *Russian Linguistics* 6 (1982): 233–249
Earls, Irene. *Renaissance Art: A Topical Dictionary*. ABC-CLIO, 1987.
Erofeyev, Victor. "Dirty Words." *The New Yorker* (September 15, 2013).
Fatu-Tutoveanu, Andrada. "'The Return of the Sacred': Implicit Religion and Initiation Symbolism in Zvyagintsev's *Vozvrashchenie* (2003)." *Journal for the Study of Religions and Ideologies* 14.42 (2015): 198–230.
Fennell, John. *Prince AM Kurbsky's History of Ivan IV*. Cambridge University Press, 2008.
———. "Ivan IV as Writer." *Russian History* 34.1/4 (1987): 207–218.
———. *The Correspondence between Prince AM Kurbsky and Tsar Ivan IV of Russia: 1564–1579*. Ed. John Fennell. University Press, 1955.

———. "Textology as a Key to the Study of Old Russian Literature and History." *Text* (1987): 157–166.
Filjushkin, Alexander. *Ivan the Terrible: A Military History*. Frontline, 2008.
Graham, Hugh. "How do We Know What We Know about Ivan The Terrible (A Paradigm)." *Russian History* 14.1 (1987): 179–198.
Gonneau, Pierre. "The Many Deaths of Ivan the Terrible and Their Interpretations." *Mundo Eslavo* 13 (2014): 75–87.
Graffy, Julian. "The 'Return.'" *Sight & Sound* 14.7 (2004): 64–64.
Gritten, David. "The Director Who Came in from the Cold." *The Daily Telegraph* (2004): 22.
Halperin, Charles J. "Did Ivan IV's Oprichniki Carry Dogs' Heads on their Horses?" *Canadian-American Slavic Studies* 46.1 (2012): 40–67.
———. "Ivan IV's Insanity." *Russian History* 34.1 (2007): 207–218.
———. "Royal Recreation: Ivan the Terrible Goes Hunting." *Journal of Early Modern History* 14.4 (2010): 293–316.
———. "Edward Keenan and the Kurbskii-Groznyi Correspondence in Hindsight." *Jahrbücher für Geschichte Osteuropas* H. 3 (1998): 376–403.
———. "The Concept of the Russian Land from the Ninth to the Fourteenth Centuries." *Russian History* 2.1 (1975): 29–38.
———. "Administrative Discretion in Ivan IV's Muscovy." Russian *History* 33.2 (2006): 429–446.
———. "Contemporary Russian Perceptions of Ivan IV's Oprichnina." *Kritika: Explorations in Russian and Eurasian History* 18.1 (2017): 95–124.
Hashamova, Yana. "Resurrected Fathers and Resuscitated Sons. Homosocial Fantasies in The Return and Koktebel." *Cinepaternity. Fathers and Sons in Soviet and Post-Soviet Film*. Indiana University Press, 2010. 169–190.
Hellie, Richard. "What Happened? How Did He Get Away with It?: Ivan Groznyi's Paranoia and the Problem of Institutional Restraints." *Russian History* 14.1 (1987): 199–224.
Humphrey, Caroline. "Dangerous Words: Taboos, Evasions, and Silence in Soviet Russia." *Forum for Anthropology and Culture* 2 (2006): 374–396.
Hunt, Priscilla. "Andrei Rublev's Old Testament Trinity Icon in Cultural Context." *The Trinity-Sergius Lavr in Russian History and Culture: Readings in Russian Religious Culture* 3 (2005): 99–122.
———. "Ivan IV's Personal Mythology of Kingship." *Slavic Review* 52.4 (1993): 769–809.
Hunt, Tony. "The Rhetorical Background to the Arthurian Prologue: Tradition and the Old French Vernacular Prologues." *Forum for Modern Language Studies* 6.1 (1970): 1–23.
Ingham, Norman W. "The *Groza* of Ivan *Groznyi in Russian Folklore*." *Russian History* 14.1 (1987): 225–245.
Keenan, Edward L. "How Ivan Became 'Terrible.'" *Harvard Ukrainian Studies* 28.1/4 (2006): 521–542.
———. "Ivan the Terrible and His Women." *Russian History* 37.4 (2010): 322–359.
Kehr, Dave. "Review." *New York Times* (2/6/2004).
Kistova, Anastasia V. and Alexandra V. Kushnareva. "Forming All-Russian National Identity in the Process of Artistic Image Development. Analysis of the Artistic Painting by Vasily Ivanovich Surikov Boyarynya Morozova."

Journal of Siberian Federal University, Humanities & Social Sciences 12.4 (2011): 1669–1683.

Kizenko, Nadieszda. "The Church Schism and Old Belief." *A Companion to Russian History*. Ed. Abbott Gleason. Vol. 10. John Wiley & Sons, 2009. 145–161.

Kivelson, Valerie A. "On Words, Sources, and Historical Method: Which Truth about Muscovy?" *Kritika: Explorations in Russian and Eurasian History* 3.3 (2002): 487–499.

Kleimola, Ann. "Review. *Ivan the Terrible: First Tsar of Russia.* By Isabel de Madariaga. New Haven, CT: Yale University Press, 2005." *The Journal of Modern History* 79.4 (2007): 951.

Kollmann, Jack E. "The Stoglav Council and Parish Priests." *Russian History* 7.1 (1980): 65–91.

Krom, Mikhail. "The 'Widowed Kingdom' The Political Crisis in Russia in the 1530s and the 1540s." *Russian Studies in History* 53.1 (2014): 13–27.

Kondyuk, Denys. "Sensing and Longing for God in Andrey Zvyagintsev's The Return and Leviathan." Religions, Film and Lived Theology 7.7 (2016): 1–16.

Leonidovich, Leonidovich. *Ivan the Terrible as a Religious Type: A Study of the Background, Genesis and Development of the Theocratic Idea of the First Russian Tsar, and His Attempts to Establish 'Free Autocracy' in Russia.* PhD Dissertation. Fordham University, 1988.

Loehlin, James N. *Chekhov: The Cherry Orchard.* Cambridge University Press, 2006.

Janda, Laura A. and Olga Lyashevskaya. "Grammatical Profiles and the Interaction of the Lexicon with Aspect, Tense, and Mood in Russian." *Cognitive Linguistics* 22.4 (2011): 719–763.

de Madariaga, Isabelle. *Ivan the Terrible: First Tsar of Russia.* Yale University Press. 2005.

Maslova, Elena, and Giuliano Bernini. "Sentence Topics in the Languages of Europe and Beyond." *Empirical Approaches to Language.* Eds. Georg Bossong and Bernard Comrie. Mouton de Gruyter, 2006. 67–120.

McSweeney, Terence. "The End of Ivan's Childhood in Andrei Zvyagintsev's *The Return* (2003)." *International Journal of Russian Studies* 2.1 (2013): 95–108.

Menash, Louis. "Review." *Cineaste* 29.2 (2004): 25–27.

Meyendorff, Paul. *Russia, Ritual and Reform: The Liturgical Reforms of Nikon in the 17th Century.* St Vladimir's Seminary Press, 1991.

Michels, Georg. "The Violent Old Belief: An Examination of Religious Dissent on the Karelian Frontier." *Russian History* 19.1 (1992): 203–229.

Michelson, Patrick Lally. "*The First and Most Sacred Right*": *Religious Freedom and the Liberation of the Russian Nation, 1825–1905.* PhD Dissertation. University of Wisconsin, 2007.

Miller, David B. "Official History in the Reign of Ivan Groznyi and Its Seventeenth-Century Imitators." *Russian History* 14.1 (1987): 333–360.

Molofsky, Merle. "The Return." *The Psychoanalytic Review* 91.6 (2004): 853–859.

Nabokov, Vladimir. *Nikolai Gogol.* New York: New Directions, 1944.

Novikova, Irina. "Death and Dying: Making Sense of Life in Post Soviet Cinemas." *Layers of Dying and Death.* Ed. Kate Woodthorpe. Interdisciplinary Press, 2007. 13–22.

Ostrowski, Donald. "The Moscow Councils of 1447 to 1589 and the Conciliar Period in Russian Orthodox Church History." *Tapestry of Russian*

Christianity: Studies in History and Culture. Eds. Nickolas Lupinin, Donald Ostrowski and Jennifer B. Spock. Department of Slavic and East European Languages and Cultures and the Resource Center for Medieval Slavic Studies, The Ohio State University, 2016. 121–156.

Panchenko, Alexander. "How to Make a Shrine with Your Own Hands: Local Holy Places and Vernacular Religion in Russia." Eds. Marion Bowman, Ulo Valk. *Vernacular Religion in Everyday Life: Expressions of Belief*. Routledge, 2014. 42–62.

Părău, Călina. "Through the 'Eye of the Machine': Poetics of the Inhuman in Andrey Zvyagintsev's films." *Ekphrasis. Images, Cinema, Theory, Media* 1.15 (2016): 129–138.

Pavlovich Pavol, Andrei and Maureen Perrie. *Ivan The Terrible*. Pearson: Longman, 2003.

Pawlowska-Jadryzyk, Brygida "Murky Images, The Poetics of Intertextual Dissonance in the Apocryphal Films of Andrei Zviagyntsev." *Załącznik Kulturoznawczy* 2 (2015): 240–255.

Payne, Robert and Nikita Romanoff. *Ivan the Terrible*. Rowman & Littlefield, 2002.

Perrie, Maureen. *The Image of Ivan the Terrible in Russian Folklore*. Cambridge University Press, 2002.

———. *The Cambridge History of Russia: Volume 1, From Early Rus' to 1689*. Vol. 1. Cambridge University Press, 2006.

Pethő, Ágnes. "The Tableau Vivant as a "Figure of Return" in Contemporary East European Cinema." *Acta Universitatis Sapientiae, Film and Media Studies* 9.1 (2014): 51–76.

Pouncy, Carolyn. "Missed Opportunities and the Search for Ivan the Terrible." *Kritika: Explorations in Russian and Eurasian History* 7.2 (2006): 309–328.

Rashkin, Esther. *Family Secrets and the Psychoanalysis of Narrative*. Princeton University Press, 1992.

Reed, Walter L. *Dialogues of the Word: The Bible as Literature According to Bakhtin*. Oxford University Press,1993.

Robbins, Thomas. "Religious Mass Suicide Before Jonestown: The Russian Old Believers." *Sociology of Religion* 47.1 (1986): 1–20.

Ryan, William F. *The Bathhouse at Midnight: An Historical Survey of Magic and Divination in Russia*. Penn State Press, 1999.

Rzhevsky, Nicholas. *The Cambridge Companion to Modern Russian Culture*. Cambridge University Press, 2012.

Sarris, Andrew. "Oedipal Drama, Russian Style: Zvyagintsev's The Return." Observer (2/2004).

Seeman, Don. "'Where is Sarah Your Wife?' Cultural Poetics of Gender and Nationhood in the Hebrew Bible." *Harvard Theological Review* 91.02 (1998): 103–125.

Seemann, Klaus-Dieter and N. W. Ingham. "Genres and the Alterity of Old Russian Literature." *Slavic and East European Journal* (1987): 254–255.

Shevchenko, Olga. *Crisis and the Everyday in Postsocialist Moscow*. Indiana University Press, 2008.

Smith, Kathleen E. *Mythmaking in the New Russia: Politics and Memory during the Yeltsin Era*. Cornell University Press, 2002.

Smith, S. A. "The Social Meanings of Swearing: Workers and Bad Language in Late Imperial and Early Soviet Russia." *Past & Present* 160 (1998): 167–202.

Steinberg, Leo. *The Sexuality of Christ in Renaissance Art and in Modern Oblivion.* University of Chicago Press, 2014.

Steiner, Peter and Sergej Davydov, "The Biological Metaphor in Russian Formalism: The Concept of Morphology." *SubStance* 6.16 (1977): 149–158.

Strukov, Vladimir. "The Return of Gods: Andrei Zviagintsev's" "*Vozvrashchenie (The Return)*." *The Slavic and East European Journal* (2007): 331–356.

Tiaynen, Tatiana. *Babushka in Flux: Grandmothers and Family-Making between Russian Karelia and Finland.* Tampere University Press, 2013.

Terras, Victor. *Handbook of Russian Literature.* Yale University Press, 1985.

Thyret, Isolde. "Blessed Is the Tsaritsa's Womb": "The Myth of Miraculous Birth and Royal Motherhood in Muscovite Russia." *The Russian Review* 53.4 (1994): 479–496.

Totaro, Donato. "Time and the Film Aesthetics of Andrei Tarkovsky." *Revue Canadienne D'études Cinématographiques/Canadian Journal of Film Studies* (1992): 21–30.

Vintrova, Magdalena. *Olfactory Images and Creation of Meaning in Gogol's "The Nose" and Rushdie's Midnight's Children.* Masters Thesis. Texas A&M University, 2004.

Von Carolsfeld, Julius Schnorr, *Abraham Sacrificio de Isaac. German Masters of the Nineteenth Century: Paintings and Drawings from the Federal Republic of Germany.* The Metropolitan Museum of Art, 1981.

Ware, Timothy. *The Orthodox Church: An Introduction to Eastern Christianity.* Penguin, 1993.

Zenkovsky, Serge A. "The Russian Church Schism: Its Background and Repercussions." *The Russian Review* 16.4 (1957): 37–58.

4 Imperial Legacy, Aborted Mourning, and the Meaning of Horror in Kim Jee-woon's *A Tale of Two Sisters*

Kim Jee-woon's 2003 psychological thriller *A Tale of Two Sisters* (*Janghwa Hongyreon,* literally *Rose and Lotus*)[1] broke domestic box office records in Korea, and, simultaneously, its phenomenally successful debut on American screens—a first for the Korean film industry—marked Korea's entrance into the global theater of international cinema. The film received both popular and critical praise for its unique cinematic voice, which is quintessentially uncanny, a taut amalgamation of the familiar and the strange.[2] The uncanny is evoked by Kim's exquisite attention to cinematic detail, reflected in both his sets and in patterns of repeated imagery,[3] as well as his orchestration of light and shadow, not to mention the interplay of color schemes that shape and nuance the narrative. The complex interweaving of these strategies garnered Kim status as a provocative, original, and important index of South Korean cultural production.

As has been the case with the preceding analyses, my interpretation of *A Tale of Two Sisters* rests on the premise that these details are linked by embedded networks of lexical coherence that symbolize a silenced shameful saga; it also assumes that once the secret is uncovered, it will yield a new vantage point for construing the film's implicit cultural critique. Kim's film was a vanguard of a new cultural aesthetic that emerged as a result of Korea's growing international engagement. A majority of critics view this aesthetic, known as the "Korean Wave," *Hallyu*, as exemplary of the transnational cinema aesthetic that we discussed in Chapter 1.

A defining characteristic of *Hallyu* cultural aesthetic is its "hybrid" quality,[4] which refers to the intermingling in a product of "domestic" and "foreign" elements. Kim's dexterous comingling of global visual language (which evinces an extraordinary degree of cineliteracy) with components of Korean horror cinema marks the film as inherently transnational. Kim's deployment of this hybrid idiom to represent the dissolution of a young Korean woman's mind, moreover, can easily be seen to allegorize the unraveling of a national consciousness as a result of globalization.[5]

Research on *Hallyu* is animated. Some view the cultural phenomenon as a response to tensions arising from a clash between traditional aesthetic values and rapid economic, political, and social transformation; they suggest that the aesthetic negates the impact of Japanese colonial cultural repression.[6] *Hallyu* objects, in this view "appropriate and articulate global popular cultural forms to express . . . [repressed] local sentiment."[7] The power of the critique does not derive simply from the amalgamation of these disparate forms of representation but rather from its implicit construction of a "third" culture in and of itself.[8] This perspective is premised on cultural theorist Homi Bhabha's understanding of hybridity as "an interpretive and reflective mode [of representation] in which assumptions of identity are interrogated."[9] In this vein, *Hallyu* "third space" has been interpreted as an aesthetic that subversively challenges the domination of global cultural trends as opposed to merely intermingling with them.[10]

Hallyu and *A Tale of Two Sisters,* as its hallmark cinematic expression, are thus constituted in part by the way they interrogate the assumptions driving Korean collective identity. The notion of repeated trauma as a result of continual subjugation by outside forces, such as China, then Japan, and then the United States post-World War II, has lead critics to link Korean identity formation to collective reckonings of historically experienced transformations that have yet to be assimilated. Interpretations of Kim's idiom suggest that he allegorizes the collective displacement and alienation that occurred from the beginning of the twentieth century, when Japan imposed colonial rule (1910–1945); to the subsequent geopolitical split of the Korean peninsula; through the harsh and repressive autocratic rule; and, finally, to the rapid democratization spurred by a state invested in establishing a narrative of (Western defined) progress and development.[11] The following analysis does not reject the valuable insights offered by these discussions, but the specificity of the linguistic networks that undergird my interpretation of the film allows for a radically different explanation for how the film engages with particular collective historical experiences.

My use of the word "radical" is not meant sensationally; rather, it reflects my break with the regnant perspective that the film's denouement provides us with an *aha* revelatory flashback, which explains the source of the protagonist Bae Su-mi's psychic disintegration. Most analyses of the film approach the coda as an uncomplicated representation of the affective circumstances that triggered her hallucinations when she returns home after a stay in a psychiatric ward. The crux of the scenes' content is segment informs us that Su-mi's mother hung herself inside a clothes bureau and was unwittingly discovered by Su-mi's younger sister, Su-yeon, who subsequently died as a result of her effort to release the stranglehold, which caused the bureau to fall and crush her. Taken as a flashback, the scenes imply that Su-mi's delusions derive from personal guilt catalyzed by her apprehension that she may have prevented Su-yeon's death.

I do not deny that the devastating deaths of a beloved mother and sister, combined with a postmortem sensation, however irrational, of a missed potential for preventing them, could lead to severe psychological distress as the psyche attempts to assimilate the grief. However, the presence of Eun-joo, a longtime medical colleague of Su-mi's father, Bae Moo-hyeon, and Su-mi's mother's nurse raises questions about the representation's truth value: because we have just learned that Eun-joo was cast as the stepmother in Su-mi's delusions, it seems counterintuitive to accept this version of Eun-joo as distinct from Su-mi's previous projections. Indeed, the fact that the segment includes an observation of Eun-joo that Su-mi did not witness, coupled with the fact that Eun-joo's acts essentially stage the crime that Su-mi accuses herself of having perpetrated—not doing anything to prevent Su-yeon's death,[12] implores an alternative explanation.

I argue that Su-mi's guilt is not a function of her own life experience; rather, the affect that saturates her loss derives from an ancestor's unutterable culpability in the death of a child, which was transmitted unwittingly, as an encrypted secret, to Su-mi's unconscious. I will demonstrate how her "return home" may be construed as a fantasy that is triggered by the words of a psychiatric doctor who seeks explanation for her catatonic state.[13] This cause-and-effect structure sheds light on the film's implicit tripartite segmentation, with its prologue, central fantasy mimesis, and concluding segment that comments on the fantasy that precedes it, exactly like Andrey Zvyagintsev's *The Return*.[14] In a *Tale of Two Sisters*, the beginning of the third narrative segment—in which the so called flashback appears—is marked by a blackout right after Kim reveals to the audience that what has just transpired in the house are projections of Su-mi's deranged psyche.[15] This economical demarcation encourages us to view the third segment as a revenant, a metanarrative comment on Su-mi's saga in the house, in the same way that Zvyagintsev's photojournalistic denouement in *The Return* provided another optic for understanding the mimesis of the journey that precedes it.

The notion that the scene depicting Su-yeon's death is part of a flashback assumes chronological movement: Su-mi is first in the hospital; then released and returned home; finally, she is re-institutionalization after a relapse, when she discovers that Eun-joo has not been physically present with her in the house.[16] The idea of a fantasy, however, suggests instead that Su-mi never physically leaves the hospital. The third segment represents Eun-joo's car ride to the haunted house, ostensibly from the hospital replicates Kim's representation of Su-mi's supposed trip from hospital to home, which initiated the fantasy segment of the film. The rapid alternation of scenes that depict Eun-joo being haunted at the house with shots of Su-mi in her hospital calling for Su-yeon suggests that Eun-joo's presence in the house is yet another delusion; the film urges us to view the third segment not as a flashback but as a representation of Su-mi's unreliable point of view. It suggests, in other words, that the drama portrayed in the third segment is also a hallucination. Questioning the truth value of the denouement allows us to see more clearly how Eun-joo's characterization allegorizes a shameful individual, family and national collective experience that was shut up and not talked about.

The Phantom and the Korean Culture-Bound Psychological Concept of *Han*

Our inquiry into psychic haunting in the Korean context implores consideration of the Korean culture-bound psychological syndrome *han*[17] and its most prominent symptom *hwabyŏng*.[18] Scholars define *han* as a cultural construct that involves feelings of regret due to injustices caused by family members[19] or, on the collective level, by repeated traumatic experiences of colonization.[20] Symptomatically, *hwabyŏng* is manifested somatically "as a feeling of something pushing-up in the chest, palpitation/heart-pounding, respiratory stuffiness/oppression, a mass in the epigastrium or chest, dry mouth, insomnia, and anorexia."[21] Soyoung Suh cites a reference to this illness in court records as early as 1603 to claim that its status as "Korea's 'national illness'" is historically justified.[22]

There is consensus that Korean *han* is catalyzed by cultural and social norms attendant upon a "face-saving culture" that demands that individuals prioritize the preservation of harmonious social relationships above the expression of personal grievances. This institutionalized form of silencing is a central axis of Confucian shame-based social practices that are rooted in affective values governed by family relations. Primary among the affective rules is the "unquestioning loyalty" and filial submission expected of each family member; this logic also underlies the relationship between the state and society.[23] Transgression of those "psychological bonds" leads to an "existential anxiety."[24] The psychic discomfort caused by *han* is existentially a "struggle to obey."[25]

As a social construct of unexpressed suffering, the transgenerational transmission of *han* nonetheless functions as a social mechanism that intrinsically offers the possibility for eventual restitution of the injustice experienced when interpersonal bonds were transgressed.[26] This differs from the phantom, which conceals both the shameful affect and the traumatic event itself. A descendant who inherits a secret *does not know and cannot share or express* it through grievances, such as petitions for justice or even literary and filmic endeavors.[27] One of the intellectual objectives of this chapter is to suggest that our understanding of *han* may be refined if considered alongside Kim's film. His overt engagement with blocked expression and generational breakdowns in signification makes it clear that he envisions transgenerational trauma as a fundamental component of the Korean collective psyche;[28] however, his film refracts the experience of *han* as a symptom of preservative repression, specifically. Reading from the film *back to culture* will uncover a heretofore unrecognized line of traumatic historicity that deepens our understanding of *han* as a cultural mind-set underlying Korean cultural identity and production.

The film signals its narrow perspective of *han* with the changes made to a conventional spectral trope for *han* haunting. The trope, a spectral female figure, is identified almost universally by critics as a representation of a *wŏnhon,* that is, a postmortem female who returns to the living driven by "vengeance" against those responsible for her unjust death. The classical story of *Rose and Lotus*, upon which the film is loosely based, tells how the characters are forced to commit suicide and haunt local magistrates until the stepmother's coercion of their deaths is uncovered and justly punished; these acts make them paradigmatic *wŏnhon* figures. But when a female apparition appears at the end of Su-mi's nightmare on the first night of her "return" to the house,[29] the apparition's countenance is different from conventional cinematic representations of *wŏnhon.* While Kim's spectral figure shares the features of long black hair and a downward tilted head (staples in representations of vengeful female ghosts in gothic-inspired Asian horror films), it is distinguished by his substitution of a black robe for the conventional white one, which is ubiquitous in such films. On the semiological level, this sartorial transmutation denies the *wŏnhon* a primary signifier of purity and chastity, which denoted her status as mistreated and hence mitigated the violence she perpetuates (postmortem) in order to sustain audience empathy (Figure 4.1).[30]

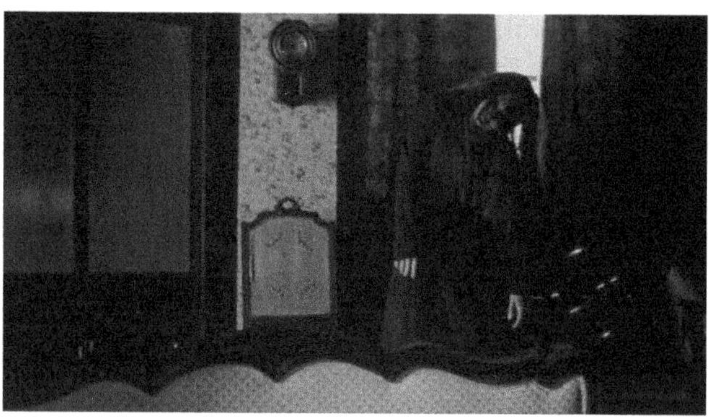

Figure 4.1 Black-robed female apparition.

Kim's wardrobe change tacitly announces a refashioning of the *wŏnhon* figure's connotative meaning and foreshadows the film's emphasis on disrobing and dressing. The sartorial shift suggests that this *wŏnhon* is of a different order than those who return to execute revenge. Visual clues, such as the angle of Su-mi's head and hair in the hospital when we first meet her, link her to her mother's death; the same dangling head is a feature of the *wŏnhon* apparition. Is the apparition a version of Su-mi's mother? If so, why does she return? The scenes preceding the spectral arrival of the *wŏnhon* show us a nightmare: A sequence of images depicts a story of an adolescent girl whose hand is bloodied when she reaches out to touch Su-mi's mother's forearm; these images are interspliced with images of Su-mi's restive sleep. The segue from an image of the girl's bloody hand back to the bloody source, the mother's arm, reveals a bloody string that dangles from the mother's red stained, white dress sleeve.

These fragmented images evoke a scenario that implicates mother and adolescent girl in an act of violence.[31] The apparition, who appears after Su-mi apprehends this unconscious knowledge, can now be concretely identified as a representation of Su-mi's mother's secret. The motif of a bloody string of the dream is repeated, this time in the form of blood streaming down the apparition's leg. This image is followed immediately by the abrupt descent of a disembodied hand alongside the blood. The imagery resonates with that of the dream to provide a gruesome gloss on the blood motif: It evokes dismemberment and wounds inflicted on a baby in utero.

The possibility that the *wŏnhon* figure is a phantom who returns to ensure that Su-mi preserves a secret about her mother and a dismembered child is strengthened by other elements. Eun-joo identifies herself as Su-mi's mother "in this world" and implies that this role involves "oversight" and the containment of "sordid" figures, which requires her to "live on with you girls."[32] This emphasis of her role as overseer suggests that she is the human extension of the apparition, the phantom who returns to ensure that unconscious knowledge remains concealed. Eun-joo attempts to establish a grammar for existing in the house. Her concern with Su-mi's "manners," "habits," or "tricks"; her efforts to contain what Su-mi "tells" Moo-hyeon; and her insistence that it is her job, and not Su-mi's, to put the father's washed and folded undergarments in their rightful spot all point to her role as psychic censor.

The object of censorship is made clear in a conversation between Su-mi and Eun-joo about the latter's treatment of Su-yeon. Su-mi confronts Eun-joo who is in the kitchen drinking tea and reading, and is incredulous that this behavior would go on in her father's presence. Eun-joo retorts that Moo-hyeon lacks agency to *solve* or *resolve problematic issues*.[33] The dialogue about solutions and resolutions is linked lexically to Eun-joo's act of reading as well: The word *p'ulda* is a homograph whose semantic range links the verb "to read" with chains of verbs that denote acts of dissolution, untangling, untying, and unraveling. These linguistic relationships evoke the deliberate termination of a fetus.

Acknowledging that the apparition is a phantom requires us to reassess Eun-joo's status as a stepmother. Every commentary I have read assumes Eun-joo is Moo-hyeon's wife. But I find no evidence in the film's intricate and detailed networks of coherence to confirm this. Without completely dismissing a romantic tension between the two, the film takes great pains to reflect other reasons for a close relationship between them. She is present in old photographs, seemingly shot by Su-mi's own mother since they were found among her belongings, which reveal a long-term academic and professional association. Relinquishing the idea of Eun-joo's status as Su-mi's "real" stepmother opens up a perspective that sees in her characterization a symbol, a piece of Su-mi's mother's saga, which Su-mi is unconsciously obligated to preserve. This then yields a clearer perspective of the relationship between the two "monster-mother" tropes[34] deployed in the film: Whereas the *wŏnhon's* "return" figures the psychic summoning of Su-mi's mother's secret, the "stepmother" is a convenient construct for disguising the mother culpable in the death of a child.

Prelude to the Prologue

We have already identified problematic mourning of maternal and sororal losses as the specific psychic reorganization that the fantasy is called upon to resist. Su-mi's fantasies allow her to give voice to the haunting drama that obstructs her self-fashioning through lexical distortion. The opening frames of this phantom film offer clues for deciphering the way the cinematographic idiom calls attention to the secret inscribed within it.

The first visual is a black screen upon which production credits are projected. A lilting, waltz-like score accompanies the opening credits. The triple meter and its evocation of rotating movements[35] foreground a context of inexorable interchange suggestive of transgenerational haunting, while the three-quarter rhythm foreshadows a relational dynamic propelled by implicit links between three out of four people.[36] The acoustic motif composed by Lee Byong-woo extends throughout the filmic text.

After four frames, a new image replaces the black screen to serve as a backdrop for the projection of cast and, finally, the film's Korean title, *Rose and Lotus*. The new backdrop is a detail of the renowned textile designer William Morris's "Blackthorn." "Blackthorn" was made into wallpaper by J. H. Dearle in 1892 and appears on the walls of Su-mi's kitchen, where much of the action of the film takes place.[37] The design is a central visual figure of the film, not to mention the source of its dramatic play with greens and reds, but it also sketches, via embedded lexical and semiological networks, the context of the secret that haunts Su-mi (Figure 4.2).

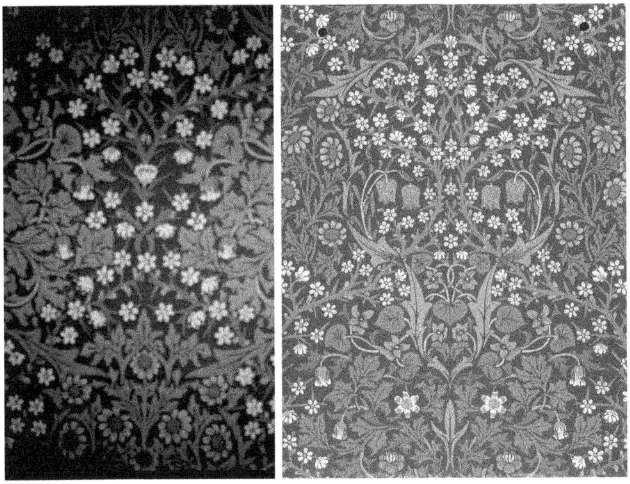

Figure 4.2 William Morris design "Blackthorn" with humanoid figure and skull; the latter is courtesy of "Victoria and Albert Museum, London."

Consider first the object of depiction, the blackthorn tree (*Prunis spinose*), known especially for its propensity "to inosculate," that is, "conjoin," with other trees. The print depicts thick intermeshing branches, leaves, and flowers; it is infused with an unmistakable fecund sensibility that is highlighted in Morris's celebration of the blackthorn flower's reproductive organs: the stamen; the pollen producing part of a flower; and the carpel, or female reproductive organ, consisting of an ovary, a stigma, and a style, which are woven into an extended fallopian motif reminiscent of Guillermo del Toro's fig tree in *Pan's Labyrinth.* A lexical link that connects the word "flowers," *kkottŭl* (which refers to the seed-bearing part of the flower, including reproductive organs, petals, and sepals), to a semantic chain of words related to "menses," *wŏlgyŏng*, heightens the sexual overtones. From one perspective, the design's fecundity, conveyed in the lush contrast produced by the intermixing of bright red petals and vibrant green stems and leaves, colors associated with marriage and the generative energy of spring (lunar New Year), augers successful conception and reproduction. From another perspective, the spatial arrangement of the white flowers may be seen to delineate the product of such a union, a baby, which is suggested by its semblance of a humanoid shape, with head and outstretched arms and legs as if it is emerging from the green foliage.

Alongside these auspicious connotations of birth, the dense and luxurious lines and textures of the design also call to mind erotic "paintings of spring flowers," *chunhwado,* which depict disrobed women or couples engaged in intercourse, and thus intimates a sense of impropriety. The sense of indecorum is heightened by another pattern formed also by white flowers that entangle with the blood-red flowers to form a simulacrum of a "skull," *dugaegol:* The lines of the stamens, curved downward by the weight of heavy, hanging petals, along with the border of the swerving leaves and branches from which the stamens emerge, delimit, like a "cage," *gol*, eye sockets, while the entanglement of leaves and flowers that underlie the white flower pattern demarcates the skull's cheek and jaw line. These postmortem intimations assume greater significance when considered alongside the unformed feet and hands characteristic of the gingerbread man shape: Together, they conjure more pointedly a fetal death. We shall see that these overtones find reverberation in the film's visual attention to images of bloody sacs; sanguine threads; and disembodied hands, feet, and legs. The verb form of the word "skull," "to skull," or "to beat the head," *mŏrirŭl ttaerida,* by the same token, tacitly anticipates the multiple acts of hitting and beating (doll heads) that occur in the film.

The relationship between the white flower patterns that evoke the antithetical concepts of life and death, and the spatial design of conjoined leaves, branches, and flowers in which they are embedded presages the lexical means by which the abortion will be concealed. A semantic network organized around synonyms of the verb "conjoin," and "scarf" (to join the ends of two pieces together by notching them so that they fit over or into each other,) *gyŏrhaphada*, such as the verb "to scarf," *dŏpta,* which denotes acts of "covering over," "overspreading," and "slime," and the verb "to scarf," *ipta*, meaning "pull on," "incur," and "to be in mourning," linguistically insinuates how the design conceals within itself a saga of an abortion.

Kim deploys the classic technique of dissolve to depict the disassembly of the white flower from the thick green and red mesh; cinematographically, this "saturates" the "Blackthorn" design to intimate that the fetus may have been disengaged from the womb via means of solvents. This dissolve also functions as a segue; the technique indicates the passage of time and in so doing identifies the flow or transmission of the saga concealed within the design as a causative agent of Su-mi's subjective experience. The homophonic link between the words "saturate" and "impregnate," *p'ohwashik'ida,* reinforces this perspective. Morris's rich "Blackthorn" design provides a gloss for the film's vision of Su-mi's dissociative status. The design also serves as a semiotic model for the lexical symbols and strategies that transformed the unutterable event into an encrypted secret; like a "matrix" or "shape," *mohyŏng,* the design is a metaphor for the source of the entire shameful saga that flows from it: the "uterus" or "womb," *chagung*, a synonym of the words "shape," "model," and "matrix."

The Prologue

The internal lexical structures unveiled in the imagistic prelude of *A Tale of Two Sisters* yield a potent interpretive tool for interpreting the film's inaugural representation of Su-mi. The orchestration of images and disembodied sounds in the scene, set in a psychiatric institution, gains greater clarity in light of the semantic networks tacitly articulated in the "Blackthorn" design. For example, the creaky "rasp," *ch'ojo*, of a heavy metal door that initiates the prologue sustains the reproductive connotations of "Blackthorn" via homonymy: The sound *ch'ojo* also refers to a young woman's first menses. In similar fashion, the static shot of a ceramic basin filled with water that ripples in response to the impact of the noisy door closure visually echoes the wavy movements of Morris's dissolved design to emphasize the reverberating affect of adolescent transformations. Sounds of disembodied "footsteps," *balchaguk*, bracketed by the opening and closing of raspy doors, reinforce the sense of an unseen but felt presence of a silenced shameful drama whose "traces" and "vestiges," *balchaguk*, have been transmitted as a psychic "legacy," *yusan*.

The psychic legacy alluded to receives fuller adumbration by the image of a pair of disembodied "hands," *son*, immersed in the basin's water. The ritualistic nature of the handwashing, three splashes on each hand, evokes a context of ablution; because, later in the film, Su-yeon directly quotes from the New Testament, it is possible that the ritual washing tacitly alludes to Mathew 27:24, in which Pilate cleanses his hands in front of Jesus and a crowd in order to consecrate his defensive denial of responsibility for turning over the fate of a life to someone else. The word *son* is homophonic; other meanings of the word include "loss," "blow," "descendants," and "wandering evil spirit," all of which suggest that the handwashing represents the transmission of a psychic legacy about an "abortion" or "miscarriage," *yusan*, which must be denied and washed away.

When we see how the film re-members the basin, the hands, and the acoustic element that resonates with women's reproductive cycles into the persona of a male doctor, *ŭisa*, whose primary interest is in excavating from Su-mi language that will allow him to ascertain the extent of her grasp on her identity, we begin to comprehend how his extractive "intention," *ŭisa*, implicitly implicates a doctor in the abortion. The synonymic connection between the word "basin," *bunji*, the word "poison," *dok*, and the latter word's other meaning, "dock," whose significance as an important spatial marker related to the shameful saga becomes increasingly clear, further intimates a doctor's complicit involvement. This connection would explain Su-mi's reaction to the psychiatrist, whose efforts to extract the kernel of her identify would be experienced as a fatal threat to preservation of a status quo.

To be sure, Su-mi's entry into this scene, announced acoustically with another raspy squeak and clang of a door's opening and closing, followed by the sound of footsteps while the doctor washes his hands, reveals her already to be zombie-like. But the concurrent representation of the doctor drying his hands with a towel, an act of "desiccation," *marŭda*, that evokes connotations of "divestment," or "cutting out," *marŭda*, offers compelling linguistic evidence that this sight was a catalyzing factor for the production of a fantasy. Lexical reinforcement is found in the doctor's rejoinder to Su-mi's silent response to his greeting, which asks how she is (or from whence she came). Although on the surface, the doctor appears to offer encouragement for her to speak—*ja gŭrŏm, uri yaegi; jom haebolkka*, "let's try to talk a bit"—his placement of a tape recorder, *girokkye*, on the table, after switching it on as he speaks, more pointedly identifies that what's on the table for attempted discussion involves a "storage" of "memory," *giŏkryŏk*. For Su-mi, the doctor cryptically communicates the target of his memory retrieval via the lexical strategies of avoidance that we have uncovered thus far. For example, his verb "try," *haeboda,* is synonymous with a word that means "settle," "fix up," "clear," "figure out," and "untangle," all verbs that are connected by an implicit objective to resolve (or dissolve) a complicated affair, *haegyŏrhada*. Moreover, said affair is implied in the phonetic structure of the locution "[let] us talk," *uri aegi*, which could also be *heard* as referring to a "baby," *agi*. Pressed within the doctor's words, we hear a distorted reference to a stored memory of an affair concerning a baby, which had to be "untangled," "figured out," and "cleared up" (with the aid of a doctor).

These lexically disguised references to a stored memory appear throughout the doctor's unintended monologue; every time he urges Su-mi to speak, we hear the word "baby," and his repeated requests that she "look," *boda,* at the family photo, tacitly threatens to "expose," "reveal," "set forth," and "uncase," *boda,* her secret—the source of her identity that the doctor seeks to extract. Relentless in his digging for information, he presses Su-mi to speak specifically about "that day."[38] His repetition of the verb "to talk about" sustains the implicit "baby" discourse throughout the scene; locutions such as "give your speech to me," *jul su issŭlkka,* tacitly point again to the doctor's complicity with regard to what happened to the baby. The word *jul*, used here in its verb form meaning "give," is also homophonic; the range of its signification, including the words "string," "line," "streak," "ancestor," and "rasp," uncannily resonates with the bloody string motif that appears throughout the film. Here, the word *jul* connects the doctor's disembodied hands with other disembodied limbs, as well as embryonic tropes, which incriminate the "umbilical cord," *t'aetchul* ("placenta" + "string") as a figure for natal murder. (Figure 4.3).

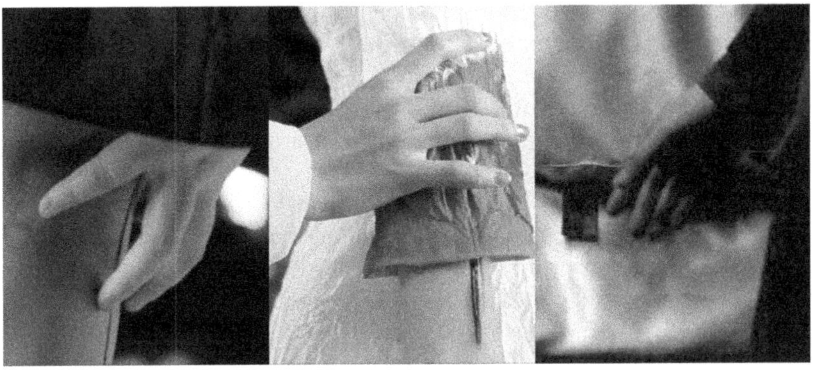

Figure 4.3 Bloody string motif imagery.

This subtext explains why Su-mi is unable "to give" the doctor the words that he requests. Giving him the words (from "talk") means giving him the baby; this speech transaction is impossible because it conflicts with Su-mi's unconscious obligation to preserve a secret about her mother's culpability in an abortion. Indeed, in light of the strong possibility that a doctor is implicated in the secret (for which more evidence will be adduced later), giving the baby to the doctor would have been tantamount to revealing the secret she is charged to deny.

Su-mi cannot respond to the doctor's invitation to identify herself because her identity derives from an unconscious knowledge that she is obligated to conceal from her own awareness. Caught between unconscious yearning for psychic expansion to begin the slow, painful process of mourning but prevented by an equally powerful unconscious force whose role is to guard against these very inclinations, Su-mi's psyche has only one alternative: to create a fantasy that allows her to continue to remain silent while at the same time acting out or staging the content of the secret and the conditions that led to its silencing

The Homecoming Fantasy

Kim relies on the trope of the haunted house to figure Su-mi's fantasy. It is a common metaphor for a deranged psyche; the fragile structure of a house that is "prone to agitation" is an apposite metaphor for representing threats to psychic integrity.[39] The object that transports her "back to her house," the "vehicle," *yongaek*, also carries overtones that resonate more specifically with "solvents" or "solutions" that "resolve" problems (like the one the fantasy is called upon to resist). These insinuations are heightened through Kim's establishment shot once the vehicle has arrived at the house. The camera lingers on the car's "tire," while Su-mi's disembodied foot extends from the vehicle's door. While one critic has critiqued the shot as "fetishistic,"[40] an alternative explanation is suggested by the image of a "tire," which preoccupies the camera right before the disembodied foot emerges. The word *t'aiŏ* is a near rhyme of the word "fetus," *t'aea*.

The implications of this inexact rhyme are reinforced when we step back to see how Kim's angle represents Su-mi's foot as the marker of her descent and departure from the vehicle; the gesture, in other words, tells us something about her arrival at "home." For example, the word *bal*, "foot," is a homophone whose other meanings, "informing on others" and "bad habit," evoke a negative context of public exposure and shame. The image of the disembodied "foot" associates the home with an aborted fetus, while the word "foot" links it to scandal. Su-mi's foot's descent from the vehicle stages the withdrawal or "departure," *ital*, secession from a maternal body.

Su-yeon's immediate desire to eat after she too emerges from the car suggests that Su-mi's gestures require (psychic) digestion. Significantly, she sets her sights on the "ground-cherry," (*physalis alkekengi*) *kkwari*, which makes itself available for eating as parts of the plant naturally detach or secede. It took Su-yeon a couple of attempts before she found the fruit, which was used medicinally in Korea as a diuretic, to reduce inflammation and also to promote labor.[41] A sexual subtext emerges when Su-yeon forcibly breaks open the inflated calyx of the ground-cherry to find its fruit; the Korean term for the hymen membrane, "cherry," *ch'ŏnyŏmak*, is a conventional signifier for virginal chasteness (Figure 4.4).

I understand the calyx to be a symbol of the womb, the receptacle where a baby was conceived and then aborted. The fruit's purgative effect points to the impossibility of swallowing or assimilating this saga.

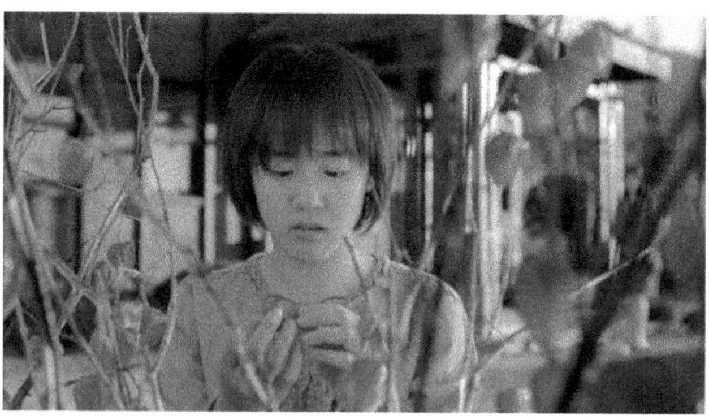

Figure 4.4 Su-yeon eating the ground-cherry seed.

The constellation of meanings attached to the ground-cherry establish a context that encompasses virginity, sexual intercourse, and conception and induced labor, all of which are communicated through a symbolic system that associates horticultural and human reproductive systems. Su-yeon cannot ingest the ground-cherry "seed" because the word "seed," the origins of "child," *jason,* is contaminated by the secret of the mother's abuse of a fetus. The overlap between seeds, origins and babies, and Su-yeon's inability to swallow suggests that Su-yeon herself is a symbol in Su-mi's fantasy that points to a piece of their mother's concealed drama. In light of Su-yeon's birth order, she is the youngest or "baby" of the family, which is emphasized in Su-mi's infantilizing treatment of her, the possibility arises that Su-yeon is symbolically linked to the aborted fetus.

If Su-yeon symbolizes the aborted fetus, it yields a more precise optic for understanding Eun-joo's symbolic role. The simultaneity of Su-yeon's first menses and Eun-joo's period connects them via reproductive processes; this reinforces our earlier conjecture that Eun-joo's characterization is a disguised version of the mother who was culpable of abusing the fetus. Her consistent mistreatment of Su-yeon in Su-mi's fantasy dramatizes Su-mi's mother's abuse of her fetus. The fantasy, which ostensibly tells the story of how and why Su-yeon died, may now be seen as a disguised account of the abortive act committed by their mother against her first baby, an event whose very occurrence was silenced.[42] This logic also elucidates Su-mi's denial of Su-yeon's death: It is symptomatic of her unconscious filial obligation to *preserve a baby's death as unknown*. Acknowledging Su-yeon's death threatens the integrity of a psyche organized around the disavowal of the loss of a baby.

Symbolic Significance of Eun-joo, Sun-kyu, and Moo-hyeon

Eating scenes comprise a significant cinematographic mechanism for conveying information about the secret inscribed within *A Tale of Two Sisters*. In the three eating scenes during which conversations occur, none of the women ever complete a meal, highlighting the impossibility of psychic assimilation. Lexical overtones that link the three eating scenes to the secret are amplified by Kim's compositional strategy, which stealthily sharpens their symbolic orientation through the intervening scenes that connect them. For example, Eun-joo alludes to the need for extensive "preparations" for the meal she plans to cook to celebrate the girls' return, when she welcomes the girls to the house. On one level, she obliquely communicates that (psychic) preparation is a necessary component of eating, similar to preparing for a test or trial; is Su-mi capable of adhering to a grammar that makes any word contaminated by the secret unavailable for psychic digestion?

The possibility of a trial becomes stronger when we hear Eun-joo admonish the girls' choice to go to the (lake) "dock," *dok*, directly upon their arrival, before entering the house to change into more suitable clothing. As a structure that facilitates transportation from land to water, docks resonate with the film's interest in transformations of states of being, from solid to dissolution; we've seen how the word *dok* is also a homophone with a range of meanings that together point to substances to cause and contain an abortion. Eun-joo's critique, and the umbrage she takes, is thus more pointed than conventional disappointment on the part of a parent toward inadvertent disrespect shown by a child.

Eun-joo incriminates the clothing that the girls wore to the dock as inappropriate. We have seen how the wardrobe change of Kim's *wŏnhon* apparition signaled its different referential status from conventions. Eun-joo links the dock to problematic garments (and processes of disrobing and dressing); her following comments on meal preparation suggest that clothing issues are a topic whose ingestion is also problematic.[43] Eun-joo's forced cheeriness conveys the duplicity of her character; her "welcome," *hwanyŏng*, has all the warmth of her apparitional avatar, the *wŏnhon*: *hwanyŏng*, a homophone, also means "phantom," "ghost," "shadow."

Eun-joo's duplicity extends to Su-mi's experience once she is shooed upstairs by Eun-joo. Su-mi discovers a clock, whose frozen hands represent the "layered, noncoinciding temporalities in operation within the film."[44] She apperceives duplication in the form of diaries and multiple dresses of the exact same fabric and shape, which hang in the wooden wardrobe. This piece of furniture elicits revulsion because it is the site of her mother's and sister's deaths; other reasons are suggested by lexical links: The word "wardrobe," *otchang*, a synonym of *ŭisangsil*, "wardrobe room" or "clothing shop," also carries a proprietary connotation, in the sense of "legacy," *yusan*, the same word used to refer to a miscarriage, or abortion.

Disoriented by the duplicity, Su-mi later accuses Eun-joo for her hand in touching "someone else's things," while they are eating the dinner promised by Eun-joo. The ostensible topic of conversation between them is whose job it is to arrange (the father's) clothes and undergarments. Su-mi's indictment indicates that wardrobes are linked to inappropriate "touching" and "placement" of "clothes." Eun-joo's vague reply that, as for the wardrobe, "it is as I had done it before," moreover, suggests that temporal duplicity is a function of her coexistence with Su-mi's mother's adolescent self.

The comment elicits from Su-mi a declaration: Su-mi states that she will not eat dinner with "that man," referring to her maternal "uncle," *samch'on*, Sun-kyu. Su-mi refers to a previous topic of conversation between Eun-joo and Moo-hyeon before the latter left the table. Eun-joo expresses her interest in having dinner with Sun-kyu and his wife, a visit that we learned about earlier when Moo-hyeon related having extended the invitation during a phone conversation. Eun-joo goes on, adding that it would be a pity not to see them since they have arrived and don't live far, and they haven't been in contact for a long time. As we shall see shortly, these spatiotemporal references foreshadow the setting of a memory involving Su-mi's mother and her younger brother that Eun-joo will recount in a dramatic dinner scene sequence. Moo-hyeon's response that he will "sort out," *chŏngnihada*, (the visit) would not warrant reflection if were not that during the phone conversation he also reassures his listener that Sun-kyu's visit will be fine, he will handle it. What is it about Sun-kyu's visit that needs handling by Su-mi's father? And how does it help us discern their symbolic significance in Su-mi's fantasy?

Su-mi uses the definite article "that," *kŭ*, to refer to Eun-joo and Sun-kyu. One explanation for this convergence can be derived from the fact that, as we shall see, both of them were implicated in acts that brought family shame. However, when Eun-joo prunes the denotative meaning of the locution "that man" to refer narrowly to biological relations, it smells like a ploy to exclude other possible connotations. Pointing out how Su-mi's term of reference is inappropriate because Sun-kyu is in fact her maternal uncle, Eun-joo substitutes a biological connotation of "uncle" that precludes the possibility of using the term to designate men of a parent's generation who are intimate with but not necessarily biologically connected to the family.

While there is no doubt that Sun-kyu is indeed Su-mi's maternal uncle, and that he was part of the saga, in light of Moo-hyeon's involvement with Sun-kyu's visit, the possibility arises that in Su-mi's fantasy, the word "uncle" refers not to a sibling of a parent, but an intimate friend of Su-mi's mother's father (Su-mi's maternal grandfather.) Eun-joo parries Su-mi's efforts to give expression to some unconscious knowledge about an "uncle," and therefore alerts us to her need to keep his identity concealed. This preservative zeal is also seen later on when Eun-joo denies Moo-hyeon's capacity to resolve issues related to the abuse of babies, and she exhibits similar preservative instincts when she diverts Su-mi from "waking up" her dad to tell him about Su-yeon's abuse.

Eun-joo's concern with maintaining Moo-hyeon's unconscious status intimates agitation around the issue of a father's knowledge about a daughter's grief. Keeping a father unaware, in other words, emerges as a distinct component of the concealed drama. This interpretation would help account for the blurring of lines that might yield a consistent pattern of Moo-hyeon's characterization. Figuring out how Moo-hyeon fits with the other symbols is challenging precisely because there is inconstancy in his representation. Sometimes Moo-hyeon appears unconscious and unresponsive to his surroundings. His dumbfounded response to a character's epileptic seizure raises doubt about his credentials as a doctor. Su-mi questions why he can't understand the source of her agony even though, she insists, it is right in front of him. Moo-hyeon's blindness suggests that he figures someone whose relation to the drama must remain inaccessible.

It may be that Moo-hyeon's enigmatic characterization represents the way he symbolized different men for Su-mi's mother. In addition to his role as someone who is unaware, Moo-hyeon is also cast in two other distinct but by no means mutually exclusive roles: that of the psychiatrist and that of the abortionist. These identities hinge on our recognition that he was trained in medicine, which is established by the photos encrypted among Su-mi's mother's memorabilia.

When Moo-hyeon confronts Su-mi about her delusions, he plays the role of the psychiatrist who pressed Su-mi to distinguish herself from other members of the family. Other examples that demonstrate an association between him and the psychiatrist include Su-mi's criticism that Moo-hyeon is constantly wanting to unravel the source of her grief; repetitive shots of Moo-hyeon dispensing antipsychotic medication also reinforce the link.

At the same time, there are instances when Moo-hyeon seems to assume the identity of the abortionist. In one kitchen scene, Su-mi, having discovered bruises on Su-yeon's arms, accuses Eun-joo of abuse. Eun-joo, placidly drinking tea and reading a book, replies that Su-yeon deserved it. Recall that Eun-joo is the incarnation of that dimension of Su-mi's mother who participated in the shutout and excluded act. When Su-mi, incredulous, asks how Eun-joo could engage in such behavior with her father present, Eun-joo retorts that he is incapable of "resolving the issue." This conversation is crosscut with images of Moo-hyeon shaving; represented as a shaver, that is, as someone who cuts or severs something off of the body, *kkakta*, Moo-hyeon belies Eun-joo's words.

Details in this mise-en-scène, such as Eun-joo's uneaten cookie and the assortment of tea vessels on the table, deepen this subtext. The word *saram*, a homophone that means both "cookie" and "baby," intimates the presence of the secret. Lexical links that connect the word tea "vessels" with "embryo" and "womb," *pae*, also point to the "issue," or "offspring," *chasik*, that needed resolution. Su-mi angrily rids the table of the cookies and tea vessels, refusing to submit to Eun-joo's insistence that she remain blind to unconscious knowledge about abuse; the wide arc of her arm movement that "sweeps," *somyŏl*, them cryptically stages the "extinction," "dissolution," and "demise," *somyŏl*, of a fetus.

Su-mi's hysterical command, at another point, that Moo-hyeon refrain from "touching" her with his "sordid hands," also implies an association between the father and someone who had a hand in the abortion. At times his diction, too, subtly resonates with this context. For example, when he stands up from the dinner table to excuse himself, he tells Su-mi that she is exhausted so she should delay "bringing order," *chŏngnihaeya*, to the tableware until the following day. A sexual subtext is suggested by a synonymic link between the words "dishes" and "receptacles," *kŭrŭt*, the objects Moo-hyeon has identified as needing to be cleaned up and ordered, and the word for calyx, *kkotpatch'im*, which is related to contexts of broken hymens and conception, as per Su-yeon and the ground-cherry seed. Moo-hyeon's comment uncannily evokes a statement heard by Su-mi's mother, which set the time an abortion would take place.

The foregoing discussion has established that we must understand the Bae family members not in terms of their familial relation to Su-mi, but in terms of how they symbolize with the figures implicated in her mother's shameful trauma. With these identities in mind, we are prepared to decipher the cataclysmic dinner scene whose extended duration reflects its centrality for understanding the film.

The Dinner Scene

All of the foregoing associations receive their fullest development in the family dinner attended by Moo-hyeon, Eun-joo, Sun-kyu and his wife Mi-hee. During this scene, Eun-joo presents herself as someone who has access to a family recollection involving the youthful behavior of Sun-kyu. Eun-joo articulates a distorted account of the conditions of public scandal that led to the encryption of a shameful experience. The information conveyed points to the ventriloquized status of Eun-joo's speech; her character enunciates memories of Su-mu's adolescent mother about an unutterable event that transpired. Surprisingly, this linguistic slippage has not received the close interrogation it deserves. Rather, Eun-joo is understood to be addressing her own younger brother.[45]

The scene's opening is exquisitely orchestrated; it establishes a cadence that strongly resonates with the internal structures of lexical coherence uncovered thus far. Attendant upon the visual image of Eun-joo's hands that insert a CD into a player, we hear a rapid sequence of sounds, first a doorbell, then a chorus of stringed instruments, playing the opening *tutti* of Wolfgang Amadeus Mozart's Violin Concerto #5. The convergence of the elements augurs an approach to human behavior that pays close attention to nuances in pitch, not to mention the rhythms of speech and behavior. The acoustic aggregation from a single bell chime to the fullness of multiple violin voices evokes the collective relational dynamic of a lineage secret, while it also foreshadows the public as an agent of its silencing. Indeed, the insinuation of the *tutti* music, which diffuses the resound of the chime, imputes an agency that echoes public turmoil;[46] the synonymy between the word "music" and "the hue and cry" of collective sentiment, *taesodong*, reinforces this.

The "stringed instruments" recall the bloody "strings," *jul*, motif; the near homophony of the words "instruments," *akki*, and "baby," *agi*, moreover, especially when heard within the context of sounds drowning out other sounds, also reverberates with a drama of conception and dissolution. As the genre of music whose notes shape the ambience of Eun-joo's following performance portends, the "violin concerto," literally "song of the violin and concerted beats," implicitly classifies her upcoming monologue in terms of an orchestrated articulation of a saga wrought by collaborative forces that still resounds and plays in the psyche of later generations.

Eun-joo's status as a cipher for Su-mi's abortionist mother is sartorially reinforced by her bright red top, ruffled with layers that encircle her neck like the petals of the red flowers in the Morris design. This design, of course, appears again as the backdrop of the dinner drama. Kim depicts Su-mi watering an array of green plants, which reanimates the visual play of reds and greens reminiscent of horticultural and biological reproduction. The plants' absorption of the water, moreover, implicitly points to an experience of serious humiliation: The "linguistics of eating and drinking" in Korean refers to suffering wrought by shame in terms of swallowing water.[47] Eun-joo's botanic wardrobe, which renders her a figurative recipient of her watering, cryptically stages an experience of intense humiliation suffered as a result of public bobbery evoked so viscerally by Mozart's *tutti*.

A close-up shot of a morsel of meat that has been dissembled from a cooked fowl, *sae*, serves as a visual segue from the scene in the front hall to the kitchen. Kim's fixation on the cooked bird narrows our focus to the "excavated," "investigated," "scraped," and "carved," condition of the meal's culinary masterpiece. The perspective, which is refracted through a wine glass into which a thin red stream of wine is being poured, visually alludes to the bloody string motif. Lexical reverberations of a similar order connect the word "fowl" or "bird," *sae*, and its synonym, "baby," *salam* (via the word *saekki*, "kid," "bastard," and "cord"), to offer a more precise, albeit lurid, indication of the intrapsychic drama whose assimilation is attempted in the dinner scene. The word "fowl" functions as a cryptonym that hides the word "baby"; it also, via homonymic relationship between the word "bird" and "new," *sae*, links the "stepmother" ("new mother") with "new born." Although conventional belief in the medicinal properties of the flesh of fowl imbues it with curative potential, it is rendered impotent within the linguistic surround of the lineage secret (Figure 4.5).

Once Su-mi finishes carving the fowl and serving it, she addresses Sun-kyu and regales him with an account of events that took place in the neighborhood where Su-mi's mother and he grew up; the film suggests this location was the same house where they are now gathered. References that situate the house "down from" Seoul, and Eun-joo's own references to ploughs and "new roads" as features of the terrain where the events of her memory transpired, point to a time before the southern part of the peninsula was completely modernized, a trend that was

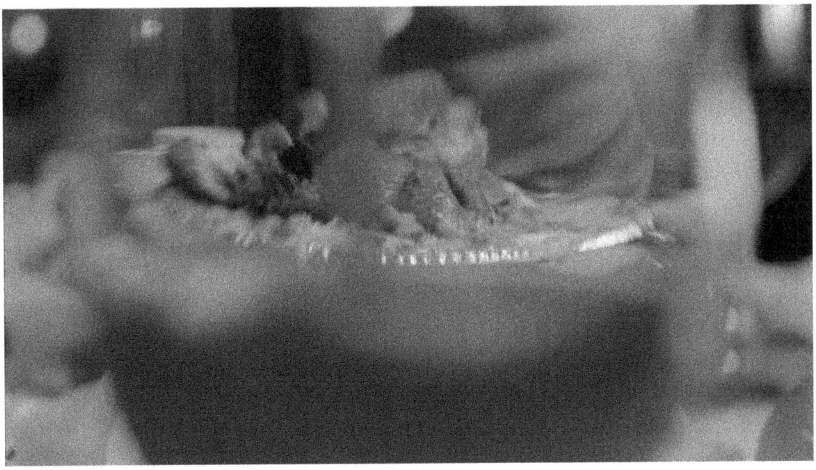

Figure 4.5 Red wine stream and carved "fowl"/"baby."

catalyzed in the early 1960s. The film also intimates that Sun-kyu and his wife Mi-hee still live in the vicinity of this property, or family legacy. The broader implications of aligning a family history with the trajectory of national modernizing patterns will be discussed later. What first demands elucidation here is how the recollections spoken by Eun-joo link collective and personal memories on the familial scale.

Eun-joo accomplishes this by juxtaposing two distinct stories that are interrelated discursively through their shared focus on Sun-kyu's behavior. In the first account, Sun-kyu's actions are depicted by a sequence of verbs that recapitulate the consequences of a desire to go fishing: seizing, jumping, drowning, hanging, as well as the topsy-turvy effect these acts had on the entire community. There are implicit regenerative and sexual connotations associated with fish, which derive from Chinese literary conventions: The expression "fish and water together," which appears in Chinese and Korean sources,[48] for example, refers to a harmonious romantic relationship. With this in mind, Eun-joo's tale of Sun-kyu's efforts to "jump," *ttwiŏ*, into a small creek, in order to "catch" or "seize," the "fish," cryptically points to an act of sexual intercourse. At the same time, this lexical constellation intersects with another that hinges on the homophony between the verb "jump," *ttwiŏ*, and the verbs "pulsate," "kick," "splash," "bound" (as in tied up), all of which refer to acts that culminated in Sun-kyu's near drowning. From intercourse, the narrative turn toward Sun-kyu's retrieval of something that thrashed about, literally, "hanging," "dangling," *hŏujŏkkŏrigo*.

The evocation of thrashing and dangling calls to mind the image of Su-yeon's jerky hand extending from inside the wardrobe where she was trapped, which Eun-joo witnessed and silenced. This link between

Su-yeon's twitching hand and the jiggling meat retrieved by Sun-kyu suggests that what Eun-joo cryptically, albeit viscerally, narrates is the spasmodic movements of a late-term fetus. She goes on to state that Sun-kyu's retrieval of this "meat" triggered in the neighborhood community tumultuous paroxysms, the collective tempest anticipated by Mozart's *tutti*.

The events of the second memory recounted by Eun-joo, which specifically refers to Sun-kyu as a preadolescent boy, *ŏril*, seem to have transpired at an earlier time. From the "funny story" of Sun-kyu's fishing exploits, the monologue turns to a collective memory of a "crazy fellow" *michin saram*, who strips off his clothes in response to rain; this propensity made him the laughing stock of the neighborhood. The combination of precipitation and the removal of clothing alludes to the classical expression "clouds and rain," *kurŭmgwa pi*, a conventional metaphor for sexual intercourse in traditional Chinese and Korean literature. This sexual subtext suggests that this second narrative in fact glosses the first.

The episodic quality of the second account is expressed through a rapid sequence of verbs. Yet, whereas the first story makes repeated reference to the second person pronoun you, *niga*, to clearly delineate Sun-kyu as the subject of the actions, the second, longer narrative is less rigorous to the point that the subject is dropped out of two sentences. While such "drops" are contextually sanctioned when they can be easily worked out, successful interpretation of context is dependent on the frame provided in the discourse itself. Frequently a dropped subject will be understood as referring to the subject who has established the domain of discourse, which in this context, would refer to Eun-joo (as Su-mi's adolescent mother).

For example, following a detailed description about "that man" who, suddenly, in the face of precipitation, threw off his clothes and "violently jumped," *magu ttwiŏ* (the same verb used to describe Sun-kyu's water plunging act), "around the newly paved road," the subject of the following verb, "participated, attended," *tanida kŭraetch i,* is dropped. The gap suggests it occludes the identity of the participant, Su-mi's mother. The subject-less sentence extends to the following predication, which refers to "exhaustion," *p'igon*, and a retreat to home, *chibŭro*. Eun-joo and Moo-hyeon both referr to Su-mi's "exhaustion" as a consequence of her "homecoming." Eun-joo's ventriloquized account implicates both in a shameful experience; it identifies Su-mi's mother as having engaged in someone's naked antics.

Eun-joo sums up this narrative, like she did with the first, with a reference to public reaction. Her description that the villagers grabbed their "stomachs" (and "womb" and "fetus"), *pae,* with laughter at these events, linguistically places Su-mi's mother and her fetus at the core of the collective hilarity. Laughing manically, Eun-joo concludes her narrative by returning to the subject of Sun-kyu, where she refers to him in the third person. Eun-joo remarks that Sun-kyu ended up emulating the man and ran alongside him "in concerted rhythm, beat," which caused revulsion in their mother. Eun-joo looks to Sun-kyu for communion in this mirth, but he flatly denies any memory of the events she recounted. Sun-kyu, whose actions may have catalyzed the scandal, is the paradigmatic filial son, who fulfills without question (memory) his obligation to preserve the family's shame. This quality is hinted at in his name, which includes the Sino-Korean word *sun,* "to obey, to submit to, to go along with."

Eun-joo asks Sun-kyu if his impoverished memory is due to madness. Her insinuation is self-referential. It implies that madness and repression are linked for Su-mi's mother; it suggests that the only way for her to sustain her psychic integrity in the wake of these events was through preservative repression of her own memory of them. The prevalence of enclosed cases, such as wardrobes and the boxes containing Su-mi's mother's memorabilia, reinforces the notion that Su-mi's mother's memories were put in a special storage compartment, a crypt. When Su-yeon invokes a chant, "*t'arit'ak'um,*" immediately upon discovering a small picture of her mother, we get a more precise glimpse of the mother's psychic status: The odd locution is the transliteration of words articulated by Jesus when he "raised the dead [female] child to life by a word of power."[49] Su-yeon's attestation that her mother transmitted this locution to her, just as they are pouring over the boxed objects treasured by their mother as she grew up, implies the locution is encrypted memorabilia.

In other words, Su-mi's mother denied the death of her firstborn child as well as the events that led up to its conception at that time. Instead of accommodating the loss by rearranging the psyche, she fantasized that the lost object itself was

> 'magically' taken into the psyche and preserved in an 'instrapyschic crypt.' The structure of the crypt prevents the psyche from integrating the loss (and thereby disintegrating the subject), protects the secret from exposure, and maintains the (fictitious) integrity of the debased object [the baby], thereby allowing the subject to deny the loss ever occurred.[50]

Inasmuch as Su-mi's mother was able to deny the death of her eldest daughter, it was because her psyche was tricked into believing that the latter continued to live—*dead but alive*—within a psychic crypt.

Understanding that the saga was psychically encrypted before its transmission as a secret illuminates a logic that links the specters who reveal themselves to Su-mi. Aside from the first apparition, all others wear green clothes: The adolescent girl, who bloodied her hand in Su-mi's nightmare, wears pale green clothing; another specter, also an adolescent female, who appears twice in the kitchen after the dinner, wears a green dress with blue trim; the specter in a fetal position under the sink also is an adolescent girl who wears the same dress, green with blue trim, but it is covered with a dark red slime, reminiscent of a placenta. (Figure 4.6)

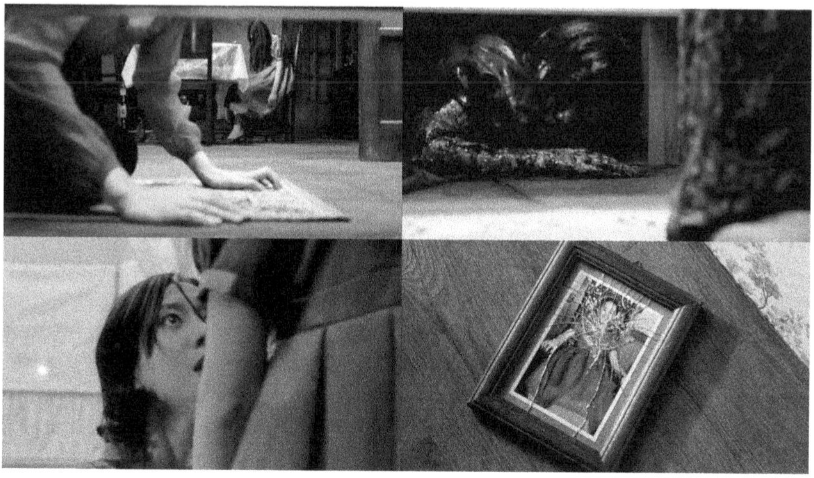

Figure 4.6 Apparitions of the incorporated aborted baby and the cracked photo of Su-yeon.

The key to uncovering the significance of this semiotic pattern lies in yet another image of a green dress: the framed photo of Su-yeon when she was a young toddler. Eun-joo knocks the picture when she backs out of the room after having witnessed Su-yeon's jerking hand, and it falls to the floor, fragmenting the glass. Because we know that Su-yeon is a symbol of the fetus, the sartorial overlap compels us to see the specters also as representations, but of a different order.[51] The specters are different embodiments of the fetus who had lived, dead but alive, encrypted in Su-mi's mother's psyche. This explains the symbolism of the dream, where the adolescent-aged fetus incarnates the mother's culpability; it also makes sense of the specter under the sink, who now appears as the fetus itself. As for the last spectral form, it appears twice, right before and right after the climactic scene of the dinner sequence. The repetition calls attention to their bracketing function, framing our focus on what transpires between the time of their manifestations.

The climactic scene depicts Eun-joo reaching for a hair clip that is lying on the floor close to the location of the fetus specter. The scene is fraught with tension; first, it follows Eun-joo's invocation of madness and repressed memory, which triggered an epileptic seizure in Sun-kyu's wife, Mi-hee. While Mi-hee is on the floor flailing and gasping, unable to give voice to her experience, we are shown her low line of vision. It is through Mi-hee that we first see the specter's existence. The audience's awareness, and their recognition that Eun-joo remains incognizant of it, is a driving factor of the scene's horror. As with all mises-en-scène, Kim's overdetermined attention to detail in this scene suggests that there is a deeper context that would explain more fully the form and content of his specific representation of the dinner scene sequence.

Earlier, Su-mi had given Su-yeon the clip, which had been among the memorabilia encased in the locked boxes that Su-mi retrieved from the family estate's stores, their legacy, *yusan*. Through the use of phantasmagoric imagery, the climax reconfigures the implications of Su-mi's gesture for a psyche structured by the abortionist context. Her act haunts because through it she unwittingly transmitted a piece of her mother's "encrypted" memory to Su-yeon. Moreover, the word denoting the object of transmission, "clip," *k'ŭllip*, is cognate with the verb "clip," *k'ŭlliphada;* within the context of the drama, the word "clip" as hairclip becomes a word that obscures semantic associations of the verb "clip," such as "resect," "exscind," and "disbranch," all of which evoke abortive acts. Su-mi's unwitting transmission of their mother's encrypted memory mirrors the way the daughters were "handed" the secret.

This subtext is refracted in the central image of the spectral scene: the intersection of Su-mi's hand with the specter's disembodied one. These details speak. Kim stages the interaction in terms of a conflict over possession of the clip. Eun-joo's fixation on the object is represented as curiosity, her facial expression reflects an attempt to make sense of its existence after the confusion produced by Mi-hee's seizure, not to mention Sun-kyu's rejection of her account of other "encrypted" memories. This chaos, which was catalyzed by Eun-joo's memories, simulates the tumult that ensued when a shameful family affair became public. In this way, we can read Eun-joo's inclination to retrieve the clip as a recapitulation of Su-mi's mother's own psychic efforts to reconstruct unconscious knowledge about the abortion and her culpability so that the fetus can be named, buried and mourned. That she was not able to accommodate the "incidence" (*nakha*, also "downfall") of public and family shame, catalyzed her descent into madness; this chain of affective experiences is intimated by the specter's location under the sink's basin, the latter object of which recalls the psychiatrist's handwashing and its attendant associations with poison and solvents.

The specter's motive for retrieving the clip is to preserve and conceal the secret, the source of its "life." If the union of hands cryptically instantiates the abortive act, it also situates it within a context of psychic fragmentation. Translated into language, Eun-joo's reaching act tacitly comments on these psychic consequences: The verb "reach," *mich'ida*, is a homograph that also means "to go crazy" and "lose one's reason."

To conclude the film analysis, it seems fitting to look more closely at Eun-joo's soliloquy right before the mimesis of the fantasy concludes. The monologue culminates a long sequence of bloody scenes where abortive acts such as beating and cutting are directed toward a huge sac that Su-mi believes contains Su-yeon. By now, we know that the struggle over the bloody sac is a struggle between Eun-joo, as protector of Su-mi's mother's secret, and Su-mi, as the desperate psyche that seeks expansion in order to accommodate it and thereby assimilate her own grief. Every critic that I have read has interpreted this scene as a psychotic rendition of the conversation that transpired "in real life" between Eun-joo and Su-mi in the film's denouement, the third segment, which is presumed to represent a "flashback" scene.

The questionable truth value of the scene, however, yields an alternative perspective. Eun-joo refers to a memory whose traces persist, notwithstanding a lifetime effort to "sweep" it away; to what exactly does she refer? In the "flashback," Eun-joo warns Su-mi that she will regret her impertinence; in the fantasy, Eun-joo's speech is self-referential, however. When she asks Su-mi how she arrived "here," she refers to the house as a crypt, the place where not only the dead but alive fetus lives but also Su-mi's mother, her sister, and figments of the other people who were involved in the drama. Su-mi's arrival at the house as the result of a fantasy, a desperate trick the psyche plays on itself so as to preserve the status quo. Eun-joo's gesture to "end it right here" is thus suicidal; it reflects the direness of Su-mi's psychic disintegration and tacitly points to the psychic conditions that led her mother to hang herself.

Eun-joo speaks as Su-mi's mother and in content and cadence, it sounds like a family injunction, common in premodern Korea, which offers short instructions for proper lineage rules. The "I told you so" inflection recalls Eun-joo's judgmental quip about the sister's neglect to change clothes before going to the dock; both conjure a mother's disapproval. The timbre suggests that the inflection also bears traces of Su-mi's grandmother's, whose response to the public shaming suffered by the family was surely integral to her daughter's incapacity to acknowledge the loss of her baby. Eun-joo's narrative reflects a collective psychology that hinges on maternal repressive forces. The camera's angle, looking up from the perspective of Su-mi lying on the floor, focuses on Eun-joo's womb to concretely locate the source of collective repression; this frame of reference reminds us that the violent interaction between Eun-joo and Su-mi occurs in the recesses of a psychic womb-like tomb (Figure 4.7).

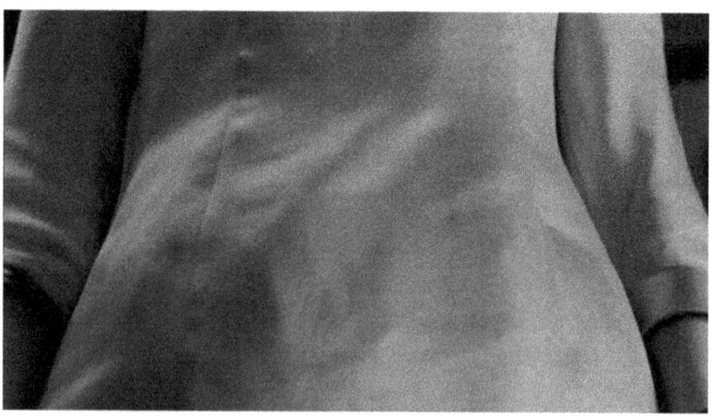

Figure 4.7 Shot of Eun-joo's womb from Su-mi's perspective.

The collectiveness of voices resounding in Eun-joo's injunction raises the possibility that Eun-joo's symbolic function extends beyond the parameters of the film to allegorize collective experiences. The room in which the Red Cross medicine cabinet is stored offers a clue about how Eun-joo's characterization points to an embedded sociohistorical context. As a space where medical procedures involving sharp objects and incisions take place, not to mention a place that stores the antipsychotic medication consumed by the household's women, the clinic may be construed as an interface between fantasy and the "reality" that prompted it. The prominence of the Red Cross image in the background of the violent struggle over the control of the bloody sac and its cord, during which Su-mi's hand is stabbed, suggests we read it as the backstory of the drama.

Although Moo-hyeon's medical profession might account for the presence of the official imprint of the Red Cross in the house, the film suggests it belonged to the previous inhabitant of the house, Su-mi's maternal grandparents. Eun-joo's account referred to the neighborhood as not yet modernized when she grew up; the Red Cross sign indicates the house functioned as a clinic. The sounds of running feet that reverberate among the bedrooms occupied by Su-mi and Su-yeon recall those heard in the prologue and suggest that many people, who were on the move, inhabited the house. The synonymic link between the word "house," *chip*, and the homograph, *yŏgwan*, whose semantic range of meaning includes locales where females live to serve and entertain, such as "rooms for temporary accommodations" or "place for strangers," "hotel," "house of entertainment," and even the figure of a "court lady," provides more context. Japanese architectural features of the house point to its time of construction: during Japan's occupation of Korea from 1910 until 1945.[52]

When we combine these components with the secret that haunts Su-mi, a sociohistorical scenario comes into view: The house evokes an abode that housed women who were abducted and recruited to serve the Japanese military as "comfort women," a euphemism for forced sex slavery.[53] Many "comfort stations," which housed the recruited or coerced women, worked closely with doctors who treated them for venereal disease; these doctors also performed abortions for women who were impregnated in their service.[54] Ninety-five percent of the 200,000 Korean "comfort women" who were recruited and sent abroad to serve Japanese troops came from the southern, rural part of the Korean peninsula,[55] likely because the southern port city of Busan was a transportation crossroads for the forced migrations.[56]

The haunting affect of the house can now be seen as a function of house's elided prehistory, that it was a lodge for those women waiting to be shipped out to their unknown destinations. Brothel operators such as a figure called Kitamura, who brought twenty-two Korean girls to Busan to join more than six hundred others, all of whom were transported to the Burmese front, for example,[57] placed the recruits in houses where they were introduced to the routines of their new positions. In light of the film's preoccupation with domestic "jobs," wardrobe changes, veiled references to sexual jaunts, a "new road," and the idea that Sun-kyu mimicked the actions of the "crazy man," the house emerges as a site of licentiousness, medical practice, and training in domestic service. The Red Cross sign identifies the house as a site of Japan's Korea-based transnational network of sexual slavery.

Many of the trafficked women believed that their work would be to "visit the wounded in hospitals, roll bandages and perform other similar tasks."[58] This potential for working as a nurse was, however, subterfuge. The Japanese deployed the Red Cross' humanitarian image to camouflage the identity of "comfort women," whose gross numbers among Japanese retreating forces in 1945 testified to the extensive reach of the Japanese military brothel system.[59] The last-minute disbursement of Red Cross bands to "comfort women" by the Japanese military as a way to conceal their true "job," moreover, implicated the profession of nursing as complicit in shrouding Japanese sexual slavery. This also impacted the formation of a collective memory of experience under the Japanese regime.

These circumstances suggest an affective and psychic contiguity that links (Su-mi's mother's) individual traumatic memory formation to the traumatic collective memory of "comfort women." Su-mi's last delusions represent Eun-joo as susceptible to haunting by her house's (family) secret. I claim that this susceptibility derives from her identity as a nurse. Eun-joo's character deploys deceptive tactics to ensure blindness rules in the management of the crypt, similar to the strategies used by the Japanese military to conceal the management of their transnational military brothel system. Yet, at the same time, the white uniform of a nurse yielded a necessary camouflage for concealing the sexual nature of the women's service, which facilitated assimilation back into a society that valorizes female purity. Eun-joo's "return" to Su-mi's house allegorizes the return of comfort women to Korea. In Su-mi's hallucination, Eun-joo's horror of the dolls compels her to pull a blood-hued cord that hangs out of the wardrobe doors to symptomatically reenact an abortion.

Eun-joo's self-censorial behavior at the moment she apprehends the near-death of Su-yeon also stages the experience of women who were forced to silence their role as witnesses to coerced abortions. Significantly, second thoughts compel her to return to the scene, but she is thwarted by Su-mi's appearance. Although Eun-joo makes an attempt to draw Su-mi's attention to the sound of the bureau's fall, Su-mi does not follow. Eun-joo's belated inclination to "save" Su-yeon—the baby, as well as her decision to estrange herself from the event, encapsulates a complex affective context that includes desire to relieve and comfort, while it also implies a dissociation from the event, in the face of preservative repression. These associations emerge in lexical patterns as well: the word *tŏrŏjuda,* which means "relieve," "comfort," "give solace," and "save," and its synonym, the homograph, *tteŏnot*, which, in addition to meaning "save," also denotes acts such as "separate," "dissociate," "estrange," and "sever."

The recent trend in Korea to dedicate memorial tablets to the spirit of aborted infants "water children" or "water babies," *suja*, may perhaps be understood as a ritual response to the repressions of comfort women/nurses in an earlier generation.[60] Similarly, the recent proliferation of rituals such as the "auspicious rebirth offering ceremony for an aborted fetus" suggests an attempt to initiate collective practices of mourning in order to make a discursive space where an aborted fetus may be publically grieved.[61]

The specificity of the film's focus on blocked mourning, family shame, and severance tacitly enunciates the concealed psychic experiences of Korean "comfort women." At the same time, the film suggests that the "comfort women's" experience itself is an allegory for Korea's self-fashioning in the aftermath of Japanese colonization: Both "comfort women" and Korea had to reconfigure a sense of self and the place of this self in a changed world. The symbolism of the nurse, moreover, intimates that self-fashioning will require a status quo that balances a disposition toward acts that save, comfort, and relieve, and acts oriented toward an opposite end, to sever, exclude, and shut out family members (including fetuses) who have brought shame to the family, or collective.

For example, Korean nationalists advanced their political positions in terms that countered Japan's assertion that Korea was merely its "wayward sibling." Japan ridicules the Korean collective for its assumed attachment to parent China, which prevented it from evolving as independently and successfully as Japan had; this was the reason for Korea's subjugation, it had to be guided and mentored by Japan.[62] Japan's contempt led to a telling discursive reaction from Korean writers: It is distinguished from other cultural retrievals that attempt to

> regain a purely authentic national culture. . . in turn-of-the century Korea, the culture targeted for expurgation was not that of the immediate colonizing power, as is so often the case with colonies of the West, but that of its neighbor, China. For Korean nationalists, the task of recovery was one of disentangling this hybrid into what they viewed as its component national parts, disavowing one and cherishing the other.[63]

Twentieth-century debates over how to disentangle China from the foundation of Korean collective identity regenerated a centuries-long debate among the intelligentsia over what constitutes the legitimate

"Korean' lineage," which was carried out during the Chosŏn dynasty (1392–1897).[64] In response to the Japanese derision, nationalists *denied Korea had any genealogical relationship with China.*[65] The discursive attempt to expunge from Korean collective memory a familial affiliation whose existence brought shame to the collective resonates with the process of crypt formation represented in *A Tale of Two Sisters;* it also reflects a historical propinquity that may be explained in terms of collective preservative repression.

Historical Extension

Kim relies on two surprise twists to establish new epistemological frameworks for making sense of Su-mi's world: The revelation that Su-yeon is dead and the disclosure that Eun-joo-as-stepmother is also a figment of Su-mi's psyche. The epistemological shifts both concern the necessity for psychic reorganization with regard to the identity of family members, which became blurred and unstable as a result of Su-mi's devastating loss. Kim represents as symptomatic the link between Su-mi's fantasy, which denies Su-yeon's death and the fantasy of Su-mi's mother, which denied the abortion; this angle reveals a genealogical trajectory that has wide-reaching implications for our understanding of national collective memory formation. In particular, the repetition of a symptomatic response to problematic mourning catalyzed by preservative repression yields a potent historical tool. The following discussion will illustrate how a similar responsive pattern may be extrapolated from Korean history as well.

The convocation of epistemological shifts, unstable identity, shame, and problematic mourning exhibited in Kim's masterpiece uncannily resonates with the circumstances of a crisis that befell the Chosŏn dynasty in 1644. The crisis was catalyzed when China, which had been ruled by the Ming Dynasty (1368–1644), succumbed to Manchu forces. The impact of the Ming fall on Korean national self-fashioning processes was shocking and transformative. The Manchu victory was a catalyst for Korean royal instability, which triggered a "search for a new episteme" of kingship to reify Chosŏn political legitimacy.[66] How should Korea, which defined itself in terms of its civilized status within the Sino-centric sphere of influence, proceed when barbaric Manchus undermined the supremacy of Chinese culture? Finding this new center also meant dealing with the shameful dimension of the Ming subjugation and the impact of this loss on Korean national identity.

Korean historian JaHyun Kim Haboush and others have animated the intensity of this search with their in-depth analyses of its manifestation in contemporary discourses. The studies shed a light on Chosŏn processes of collective and political identity formation: All concur the Ming's fall was perceived by Korean elites as a destruction of the boundaries of civilization.

> Concerns [about the rise of the Manchus] extended far beyond the discourse of power, however, and permeated every aspect of the restructuring of [collective] identity. The new order challenged their epistemological foundations, and hence Koreans had to construct a new episteme of the world and the self, one that allowed them to sustain their political beliefs and to maintain their cultural identity.[67]

The historical explanation can be translated into terms of national self-fashioning: The Ming fall required epistemic reorganization in order to establish equilibrium. The materialization of discourses that advance different strategies for reorganization are rich evidentiary sources for understanding what and why particular criteria were deemed essential for demarcating a new center. Of particular significance is the emergence of a competitive discourse that claimed Korea had become the more authentic and superior guardian of Chinese culture in the wake of the Ming's fall. Haboush argues that Korea saw itself as not just a superior guardian, but the *only guardian* of authentic cultural values. As Haboush puts it, "Korea no longer conceived of itself as a part of a larger civilized order, but as a lone entity whose survival as a culture required a separation from the larger, 'corrupt' order that prevailed externally."[68]

The assumption that reorganization of national identity requires enacting the role of vigilant guard to preserve the memory of China's cultural supremacy invites phantomatic interpretation; this position becomes more persuasive in light of the familial structure upon which Chinese-Korean relations were premised and understood: China was "elder brother" to Korea's "little brother."[69] Confucian strategies for sustaining social order based on hierarchical structures of authority imbued these roles with specific attitudinal and affective characteristics, which informed identity formation processes. In this vein, Korea's reaction to the Ming fall may be construed as a reaction to the loss of a family member who has incurred shame. While the affective resonance of familial terms has been noted, and certainly examined from the perspective of how such language was deployed to bolster political claims of legitimacy, I will extend the scope to investigate the specific role played by shame as a catalyzing agent for the particular strategies adopted by the court in response to the traumatic loss of Ming China.

My hypothesis is that the centrality of family terms in the discourses that reflect on Korea's process of epistemic reorganization intimates the existence of a collective secret about a family, the royal Yi family, whose ancestor, Yi Sŏnggye (r. 1392–1408), established the Chosŏn Dynasty. The paradigm of fraternal affinity between Korea and China, which undergirds seventeenth-century Korea's self-proclaimed role as a vigilant guardian of China's cultural memory, is itself a rhetorical product of early Chosŏn dynastic historians, who used it to justify the founding father's usurpation of power from the reigning Koryŏ Dynasty (918–1392).[70]

The problem was that the dynastic claim made by Yi Sŏnggye, a celebrated general who fought for the preceding dynastic ruler, was recognized as based on a blatant violation of "the core political virtue of loyalty to one's sovereign."[71] This transgression "had somehow to be explained away, both to gain legitimacy in the eyes of the Korean political elite and to gain recognition from [newly established] Ming China as a legitimate government."[72] Yi Sŏnggye, and his descendants, deployed history-writing as a potent tool to shape a claim for legitimacy. Historical records constructed a memory of the dynasty's origins oriented toward convincing both audiences "that Yi's overthrow of the previous dynasty was not a usurpation of power, but instead a justifiable transfer of the right to rule, which Koreans, like the Chinese, called the Mandate of Heaven."[73]

Early Chosŏn historians, "insecure" about their legitimacy, searched for a "great founding ancestor," whom they identified as having Shang Dynasty (ca. 1500 B.C.–1046 B.C.) origins. Korean political legitimacy was thus bolstered by a claim to Sino-Korean consanguinity. The ancestor, Kija, was configured as a sage, the innovator of a golden age of civilization;[74] thus Korea was as old and civilized as China, even if its territorial location and size made it peripheral within the Sino-sphere of cultural influence.[75] This rhetorical strategy assuaged Ming China with assurance that Korea would "serve the Great [Older Brother China]," *sadae*, which bolstered political claims on the Korean peninsula.

Ultimately, the dynasty's legitimacy was forged by a political strategy termed "deterritorialized sovereignty" because of the asymmetry in Sino-Korean power relations. While China's regional power and cultural influence is the indisputable source of Korea's conception of sovereignty, and while the structure indubitably facilitated Korea's survival as a distinct political domain, it still begs the question of why the Chosŏn deployed the family analogy, instead of, say, the ruler/minister analogy, which would have been relevant given the established power structures.

The context is that Ming dynasty records confused Yi Sŏnggye's paternity and erroneously blamed him for killing the last four Koryŏ kings. There were serious ramifications as a result of this error, the most urgent being that the Ming founder refused to acknowledge the Yi dynasty as legitimate; there was "overriding anxiety over the Chosŏn court's political legitimacy and a concern with Chosŏn's reputation at the Ming court."[76] Even though "Yi Sŏnggye was not involved with King Kongmin's death, but he and his supporters certainly deposed the latter three monarchs and ordered their deaths." The story of Yi Sŏnggye's treatment of the last ruler of the Koryŏ, King Gongyang, is especially well known. Notwithstanding claims that he "lived out his natural years," King Gongyang was murdered along with his two sons in 1394:

> They were strangled to death under Yi Sŏnggye's royal orders. In the meantime, the Chosŏn court drowned the entire Koryŏ royal family, throwing them into the sea while they were en route to their place of exile. Distant members of the Wang royal clan still at large were hunted down and killed . . . Through these acts, a combination of killings and discursive effacement, the Chosŏn eliminated its Koryŏ predecessors, potential rival claimants to the Korean throne, and vestiges of symbolic loyalty to the Koryŏ past. In other words, efforts by the Chosŏn court was as much an attempt to correct Ming documentation of royal ancestry as it was an attempt to whitewash the bloodshed that surrounded Chosŏn's rise.[77]

The fraternal rhetoric discursively veils Yi Sŏnggye's transgression of the bonds of political loyalty that are required for social harmony; at the same time, the rhetoric conceals the shame experienced by the Ming founder's initial disdain of Yi Sŏnggye's ancestry. Although "these patterns emerged from pragmatic exigencies, they acquired a normative power but only because they were repeatedly used and called upon" for dynastic legitimizing purposes. The "strategy was to create and control a mythology about Korea and its relationship with [China] that could withstand the vicissitudes of imperial politics."[78]

Cultural Haunting

The shameful nature of the Ming's subjugation required that Korea's genealogical relationship with China be reconfigured. One approach was to demote Kija from his central position in Chosŏn legitimizing discourse;[79] this had the effect of loosening the fraternal ties that complicated Korea's repositioning. Controversies over mourning rituals that beset the court reflect serious inquiries into the premise of royal legitimacy, as well as "the standards by which questions concerning the throne could be evaluated."[80] There was unprecedented examination of royal legitimacy within the context of how to publicly express grief over the loss of a stepson, or a stepmother, to cite two specific examples. The crux of the issue is how to mourn royal relations whose ties to the ruler fall outside of ritual protocol, the problem is one of naming. Haboush concludes that mourning ritual controversies reflected state anxiety over its ability to reify its relationship to civilization and its role in a changed world order.

Obsession with filial rank and mourning may also be seen as symptomatic of the problem of *how to ritually mourn China*, whose hierarchical status was compromised by shame. Anxieties over the logic of Korea's inheritance of the Ming's civilizing mantle weighed heavily; they locked the state and local communities in conflict over how best to *guard, preserve, and save* Chinese civilization, but underlying this was also the need to *sever* China from its legitimizing position of eldest brother. Korea's status as second primary son of a family was implicitly transformed to that of the primary son, whose primary objective is to perpetuate the civilizing lineage.[81] Efforts to camouflage the "stench"[82] of these circumstances took different forms. For example, evidence of the court's denial of the Ming fall was manifested in 1730, almost a hundred years after the Manchus defeated the Ming, when Chinese officials discovered contemporary Korean identification plaques, which bore the reign title of the last Ming king.[83]

Of significant interest to this study is how the Korean ancestral pantheon was reorganized to accommodate the founding and last Ming Emperors; this transformed the Ming family status from that of elder brother to that of ancestor. Through the incorporation of the Ming rulers into Korean ancestral cult, the shameful demise of the dynasty was ritualistically commutated into a postmortem existence perpetuated by state-sanctioned royal sacrifices. The incorporation of the Ming rulers into the Korean pantheon as a means to perpetuate the existence of the dynasty strikingly resonates with Su-mi's mother's creation of a crypt to hide the baby whose death had to be denied.

The shame of Chinese relations became a central issue driving Korean nationalists in the twentieth century, who refuted Japanese historians revisionist and scornful account of Korea's cultural evolution.[84] Studies have shown how these discursive echoes deepen our understanding of Korean national identity formation by focusing on the structural similarities in the form and content of the reactions to challenges to Korean sovereignty. Many scholars invoke the concept of *han* to explain the patterned repetition as a product of social and cultural conditions throughout Korean history; Japanese colonial rule reawakened and reactivated "deep seated original wounds."[85]

The construct of *han* may be construed as a narrative schemata for organizing history: It

> underscore[s] the degree to which one's ancestors' tragedies can continue to have an impact on how the living experience themselves in relation to history, and, especially, how the living conceptualize the causes and consequences of misfortune in terms of the past.[86]

If *han* is stimulated, it must be because it relates to a similar past violation of familial bonds. The link between the crises triggered by the Ming collapse and Japanese rule is that they both triggered existential anxiety over collective identity.

While the similarities between seventeenth- and twentieth-century discursive reactions to epistemological crises have garnered much attention, I will conclude this exploration by focusing on another crisis, one that occurred in the eighteenth century, which is also implicated in the chain of *han* transmissions, but which, like *A Tale of Two Sisters*, provides a more precise account of its shape and form.

The earliest textual reference to *han* symptoms, *hwabyong*, appears in the veritable historical records of King Chŏngjo (r. 1776–1800); his symptoms derive from a life trajectory that was shaped by the need to transcend the ignominy and shame generated by the acts and speech of his father, the Heir Apparent, Prince Sado (1735–1762), who was ordered by his father, King Yŏngjo (r. 1724–1776), to commit suicide by entering a wooden chest that was sealed. Prince Sado died of asphyxiation and starvation seven days later. The rationale for the filicide was Sado's madness. The royal policy prohibiting any record or discussion of this encasement, which was enforced to ensure the *preservation* of the Grand Heir, Chŏngjo, and thereby *save* the integrity of the dynasty, required that Chŏngjo be posthumously adopted by the *deceased older brother* of his father, Prince Hyojang (1719–1728), to avoid any criminal implication that could threaten Chosŏn legitimacy.[87] The introduction of this *new father* into Chŏngjo's life, moreover, which precluded the latter from publically and ritually fulfilling his *filial obligation* to his biological father, proved to be the source of his *han* psychosomatic symptoms.

King Chŏngjo was reportedly obsessed[88] with *incorporating ritual offerings* to his biological father as a means to "restore" or "rectify," *chŏng*, his biological "patrilineal ancestor's," *jo*, rank. We've seen how the public display of mourning the Ming founder and last emperors attempted to annul the shame of the Ming's demise; Sado's son envisions a similar strategy. The focus of his compulsion, namely re-interment, also suggests that he identified with his father by means of *encryption*. Recognizing how "the fact that he could not render full honor to his father was a constant signifier of his own compromised ancestry," we can hear a symptomatic logic in Chŏngjo's oft-repeated desire to "abdicate in the name of filial devotion" in order to "obliterate Prince Sado's imperfection and thus retroactively legitimate his ancestry."[89] Chŏngjo's plan to re-stage his father's burial speaks to the memory of his father's physical demise, but it also suggests unconscious knowledge about the concealed source of Sado's psychic affliction.

Whereas dynastic historians who compiled the record of Chŏngjo's reign made public the psychosomatic effects of repression with their account of the king's *hwabyong* symptoms,[90] the private dimension of Chŏngjo's suffering is provided by his mother, a woman who documented her position as an eye witness to and inadvertent participant in the traumatic affairs that threatened the perpetuation of the dynasty. Her accounts, compiled as four memoires, are entitled "Remembrances amidst *han*," *Hanjunok*. Prompted by painful external events that ensued as a result of her decision to not commit suicide in the wake of the "Sado incident," Lady Hyegyong's (1735–1815) record was motivated by her observation that the court's imposed silence was ineffective for putting "those painful memories to rest." She viewed her narrative as a means to fill in the vacuum of words so that linguistic circulation can diffuse the spectral shadow of her husband's death.[91] Her detailed account of the complex conditions that led up to the terrifying event contains vivid descriptions of Sado's symptoms; when read with the concept of the phantom in mind, the symptoms point to haunting by a shameful, unspeakable family saga.

Sado's Phantom

JaHyun Kim Haboush's lively and eloquent translation of Lady Hyegyong's memoires bodies forth in expressive verbal images a litany of psychosomatic and hallucinatory symptoms, not to mention obsessive compulsive behavior and aphasia. Astoundingly, Lady Hyegyong approaches Sado's illness psychoanalytically, suggesting that his symptoms are the result of a deficient bonding between parents and child during Sado's youth.[92] To justify her conclusions, she provides details about Yŏngjo's behavior toward his son as well. Of particular historical interest to us is the fact that Yŏngjo had to deal with serious contentions made by aristocratic families that he poisoned his *elder* reigning *brother*, King Kyŏngjong (r. 1720–1724).[93] These continually resurfacing charges of fratricide and regicide informed, Haboush has noted, Yŏngjo's rigorous efforts to demonstrate his sincerity toward ruling as a filial sage-king. He appropriated the rhetoric of filial piety to shore up his image and self-proclaimed his position as *father* to Korean subjects.[94] This assumption of a paternal rank in order to detract from a shameful fraternal conflict recalls the reorganization of ritual commemoration practices that transformed Ming's fraternal status into a parental one.

Although the picture of early father-son relations portrayed by Lady Hyegyong is not based on her own observation, given that she did not enter the royal family until she was nine years old, in 1774, her ability to correlate early behavior with later symptoms of madness suggests the likely veracity of the information insomuch as it establishes a psychoanalytical logic. Some of the components of her account help us reconstruct Sado's behavior as a distorted representation of the secret he must at all costs preserve; they also include references to Yŏngjo's obsessive compulsive behavior around Sado, as well as the details of Sado's domestic environment, both of which reveal a linguistic surround governed by patterns of avoidance and decontamination. For example, Lady Hyegyong is incredulous that Sado was installed at the age of five in the residence of King Kyŏngjong's second wife, Queen Sonui, and was cared for by the latter's servants, who had been loyal to Yŏngjo's elder brother before he died; the implication is that rumors that the king died by murderous circumstances, which impugn Yŏngjo as the perpetrator, would have been pressed between the lines of his early caretakers.[95]

King Yŏngjo compulsively washed out his ears and mouth after exchanging words with Sado from the gate,[96] suggesting a grammar organized around a regimen of purification rituals. His "fastidious" avoidance of words that "connoted death, such as *sa* (to die) or *kwi* (to return)," his compulsion to change out of clothes worn to his regular audience before entering his chamber, not to mention his distinction between gates that led to pleasant or unpleasant activities, sheds more light on the specific rules governing the system.[97]

King Yŏngjo's aversion to criminal cases, especially trials for murder, is a sensitivity that might be explained by the murmurs linking him to the death of his predecessor.[98] The fact that Yŏngjo did not change his clothes on his way to his son's residence after attending to official business to inquire whether his son had "eaten dinner," combined with the father's habit of washing his ears and throwing the water he used to do this into another courtyard, made it clear, as Sado was heard to say, that for Yŏngjo, Sado was a person "upon whom he washes off his inauspiciousness."[99] Yŏngjo's increasing fury toward Sado after the latter was appointed regent was spurred by the former's displeasure that "Sado's regency did not ease, as he had hoped, the virulent factional tension that he believed was at the root" of persistent rumors about the means by which he ascended the throne.[100] Lady Hyegyong's account does not provide enough information to sketch more clearly the event whose repression appears to have driven Yŏngjo's speech and behavior, but her detailed account of Sado's symptoms offers clues for reconstructing a disguised articulation of its central components.

A link between Yŏngjo's behavior and Sado's madness receives support from the homophonic resonance between the word "ear," *kwi*, and the verb "return," especially in light of the spectral context of the locution "returning spirit or ghost," *kwishin*, which Sado invoked as a source of terror and the cause of his symptoms. According to Lady Hyegyong, this phobia was caused by Sado's first serious episode of psychosis, which transformed Sado in to someone "so different in fact that one could hardly believe that he was the same person." The incident occurred when Sado tried to "command ghosts and spirits," with charms and spells collected in a canonical Taoist scripture entitled the *Jade Spine Scripture* (*Okch'ugyŏng*).[101]

Sado's attraction to this "Taoist recantation text that was favored by blind fortune-tellers" makes sense in light of his psyche's enforced blindness to the presence of a secret. A core scripture for the worship of the Taoist God of Thunder, the text was used by adepts to invoke "celestial *guardians* to *safeguard* the scripture and its *legitimate* holder."[102] (emphasis mine) Help from the Thunder God could only be received through the "recitation of the scripture, visualization of the precious image of [the Thunder God] and chanting of the incantation of the Heavenly King."[103] Lady Hyegyong describes Sado's hallucination of "the thunder god" and says the delusion triggered the metamorphoses of his personality from being "touched" by an illness, to being possessed by it.[104] Sado, like his father, developed a specific aversion to words which offer clues about just what cannot be assimilated and why it elicits such fear. The word *ok*, "jade" for example, is synonymous with *mal*, a homograph whose range of meanings include "horse," "words," "speech," "mouth," "tongue," "steed," and "vocable," together which conjure a scene of utterances and equine (military) matters. This lexicon resonates with the martial representation of the Taoist god of thunder who is called into being via incantations; it also recalls Lady Hyegyong's earlier reference to Sado's obsession with military games, which were encouraged by his caretaker, but which made him fearful about being caught.

The word "spine," on the other hand, conjures "vertebrae," or skeleton bones, markers of death. More context is suggested by Prince Sado's inability to bear the sight of the Chinese graphs for "thunder," and "thunderclap," *p'uk*. Epigraphic analysis of the graph that designates the word "thunder" reveals that the word is a composite of two independent Chinese graphs, arranged vertically, with the word "rain," *pi*, on top and the graph for "field," *punya,* below. The word "rain" is a homograph that also means "mistake" or "fault," while the word "field" is synonymous with *pŏl*, a homograph whose range of connotations include "punishment," "clique," "pain," and "sconce." Together, these words evoke a scene of collective violent transgression that occurred at night.

When these lexical signifiers are read in tandem with the other fearsome graph, "thunderclap," *p'ayŏrŭm,* which too is comprised of two graphs, again the one meaning "rain," above; below, the word *kunju,* "monarch," "brother," "ally," we see that the words Sado avoids adumbrate a scenario of malfeasance involving a brother or monarch. Lady Hyegyong curses the *imsin* year, 1752, for the emergence of Sado's terrible state; earlier she mentions the *sinim* year, 1722, during which a clique known as the Noron, who defended Yŏngjo's royal claim, was put into crisis by a bloody purge. The reverberations between the calendrical dates, whose Korean forms are mirror images of one another, suggest that the harrowing events of the latter may be an unconscious source of Sado's phobias. The purge led Yŏngjo to adopt "taboos and a peculiar gravity that were severe enough to be considered a sickness."[105]

Sado's hallucination and linguistic phobias emerged around the same time that he was made Regent by his father, which required Sado publicly acknowledge Yŏngjo's royal legitimacy. The phobias suggest psychic agitation about this, and, indeed, Sado's inability to carry out his father's orders resembles Hamlet's failure to execute his father's vengeance. Sado's desire to please Yŏngjo and publicly play out filial obeisance to Korea's self-styled father is thwarted by an unconscious knowledge of his father's problematic royal legitimacy.

Lady Hyegyong's several references to foods that Sado cannot ingest alert us to the possibility that what cannot be physically consumed is linked to what cannot be psychically assimilated: The foods cited as inedible are those foods on which certain Chinese words are printed. Lady Hyegyong remarks that although Sado expressed a bright personality in his infant years, upon acquiring language, certain characteristics began to emerge that would lead to symptoms later. Reticence in speech is one example; another is reflected in an anecdote about Sado's avoidance of objects deemed too "luxurious" for possession.[106] While Lady Hyegyong cites this as evidence of Sado's early wisdom and maturity about the perils of greed, one might also conclude that for Sado luxurious items are associated with his royal prerogative, which his unconscious knowledge causes him to doubt.

Yŏngjo's clothing regimen appears in distorted forms in Sado's symptomatic behavior. Yŏngjo's usual habit of entering his living quarters only after changing from the clothes he wore at his regular audience or other public functions reflects an effort to separate public and private attire. This attention to disrobing emerges in Sado's full-blown clothing phobia which, at times, led to fatal consequences.[107] Central themes emerge from Lady Hyegyong's description of the symptoms, such as an agonizing sensitivity to cloth; a preference for the undyed white hemp material used for mourning garb by Korean subjects; and a proclivity to abruptly remove clothing and, subsequently, rape.[108] Sado's penchant for traveling incognito into the villages symptomatically dramatizes his position as an imposter of legitimate rule.

These details reverberate with Eun-joo's account of a madman who, disturbed by *rain*, disrobes abruptly to engage in sexual activity; Sado's shadow may also be seen in the form of a wooden bureau, the source of Su-mi's horror. It evokes the most harrowing detail of Sado's tragic story, the means by which his suicide/murder was executed. The wooden rice chest into which he willingly entered objectifies his condition: It locks him up and thereby conceals the family member whose actions brought shame to the ruling lineage. Meanwhile, the sealed off object himself was the carrier of a secreted crypt that also threatened the perpetuation of the royal line. His suicide enacts the encryption of a family shameful secret while it also cryptically reveals it as the source of his own psychosis.

While a thorough investigation of Lady Hyegyong's memoires, as well as other relevant texts, is necessary to validate this historical interpretation, the route that leads me to it suggests that the concept of the phantom is a powerful heuristic for expanding our understanding of *han* as a cultural construct. The foregoing analysis indicates a historical vector that links early dynastic efforts to conceal the bloody stains of its origins, and the ignominy caused by early Chinese derision of the Yi Sŏnggye's genealogy, to the epistemological crisis that befell Korea when Ming China was conquered by the Manchus; I construe these events as the source of psychic preconditions that explain the dynamic driving Yŏngjo and Sado's destructive relationship. Sado's story demonstrates how preservative repression on the collective level plays itself out on the individual level of a royal prince.

Sado's story line is recursive, not teleological. It is different from *han* oriented narrative schemata that "limit the idea of failure for the Korean... father by providing the potential for closure in the person of the son (or grandson)."[109] Shaped by a haunting deed he did not commit, Sado is unable to redeem the family shame and give it closure. Yet his secret, notwithstanding the efforts of the dynasty to repress it, was transmitted into the collective unconscious. The recurrent metaphorical references to his story in *A Tale of Two Sisters* point to the repercussions of his secret on the collective level to explain why the cognitive and emotional construct of *han* itself emerged as a central, defining dimension of Korean cultural identity. This offers a new vantage point from which to explore the shaping force exerted on Korean self-fashioning and collective memory formation by a shameful dynastic secret.

Notes

1 The film's title derives from the titular names of two sisters whose story is contained in a classic Korean tale dating from the Chosŏn dynasty (1392–1910). The story tells of a greedy and heartless stepmother who implicates her eldest stepdaughter in a framed context of illicit, premarital sex, with the use of a skinned rat made to look like a miscarried embryo in order to force the sisters to drown themselves as a result of the shame and thereby ensure that her son will be the sole inheritor of the sisters' unknowing father's estate. The story continues to relate the postmortem return of the sisters who seek revenge and haunt the local magistrate until an honest official finally listens to what they have to communicate, excavates the alleged fetus and uncovers the treachery of the stepmother. The resolution of this injustice ultimately leads to the punishment of the stepmother and her son and the rebirth of the sisters to their father's new wife. The story's prevalence in Korean culture is paramount; no less than five films have endeavored to portray it. See Peter Lee, ed., *A History of Korean Literature* (Cambridge: Cambridge University Press, 2003), 283. The degree to which Kim's version adheres to or transgresses the original story emerged as an important criterion in Korean critical assessments of the film. I concur with critics who argue that Kim's film should not be construed as a "remake" or even adaptation of the classical tale; viewing the classical precedent as a collective repository of historically transmitted patterns of meaning and symbolic forms representative of cultural knowledge from which Kim draws to tell his tale of two sisters not only respects the structural integrity of the film as wholly distinct and independent of the narrative with whom it shares a tale, but, as will become clear in the ensuing, discussion, recognizing these distinctions yields a novel vantage point for understanding their textual relationship. For an excellent summary of the Korean critical scholarship on the film, see Seo Jeongnam, "Analysis of Changhwa Hongnyon (*A Tale of Two Sisters*)—With a Special Focus on the Narrative and Characters," *Acta Koreana* 14.1 (2011): 73–116.

2 Virtually every analysis of the film mentions its breakthrough aesthetic status; see, for example, Colette Balmain, "Pan-Asian gothic" in Glennis Byron, ed., *Globalgothic* (Oxford: Oxford University Press, 2015), 119–132;

Eunha Oh, "Mother's Grudge and Woman's Wail: The Monster-Mother and Korean Horror Film" in Alison Peirse and Daniel Martin, eds., *Korean Horror Cinema* (Edinburgh: Edinburgh University Press, 2013), 60–72; Leung Wing-Fai, "From *A Tale of Two Sisters* to *The Uninvited*: A Tale of Two Texts" in *Korean Horror Cinema*, 173–187; Jinhee Choi, "A Cinema of Girlhood: *Sonyeo* and the Decorative Impulse in the Korean Horror Cinema" in Jinhee Choi and Mitsuyo Wada-Marciano, eds., *Horror to the Extreme: Changing Boundaries in Asian Cinema*, Vol. 1 (Hong Kong: Hong Kong University Press, 2009), 39–56; Robert L. Cagle, "Diary of a Lost Girl: Victoriana, Intertextuality and A Tale of Two Sisters" in *Korean Horror Cinema*, 158–172; K. K. Seet, "Mothers and Daughters: Abjection and the Monstrous-Feminine in Japan's Dark Water and South Korea's *A Tale of Two Sisters*," *Camera Obscura* 24.2 (2009): 139–159; Katarzyna Ancuta, "Spirits in Suburbia: Ghosts, Global Desires and the Rise of Thai Middle-Class Horror," *Horror Studies* 5.2 (2014): 233–247.

3 Jinhee Choi, "A Cinema of Girlhood," 55; Robert Cagle, "Diary of a Lost Girl," 158; Seo Jeongnam, "Analysis of Changhwa Hongnyon," 100.

4 Youna Kim, ed., *The Korean Wave: Korean Media Go Global* (New York: Routledge, 2013); Beng Huat Chua, "Conceptualizing an East Asian Popular Culture," *Inter-Asia Cultural Studies* 5.2 (2004): 200–221; Youna Kim, "The Rising East Asia 'Wave' Korean Media Go Global" in Daya Kishan Thussu, ed., *Media on the Move: Global Flow and Contra-Flow* (London: Routledge, 2007), 121–135. "Hybridity" is cited as a characteristic feature of *Hallyu* culture on the South Korean Government's website, Korea.net Gateway to Korea; see also Doobo Shim, "Hybridity and the Rise of Korean Popular Culture in Asia," *Media, Culture & Society* 28.1 (2006): 25–44; Woongjae Ryoo, "Globalization, or the Logic of Cultural Hybridization: The Case of the Korean Wave," *Asian Journal of Communication* 19.2 (2009): 137–151.

5 See for example Valentina Marinescu, "Many Faces of Hallyu in the Global World" in idem., ed., *The Global Impact of South Korean Popular Culture: Hallyu Unbound* (Lanham, Maryland: Lexington, 2014), 1–4; Lee, Keehyeung Lee, "Assessing and Situating 'the Korean Wave'(Hallyu) Through a Cultural Studies Lens," *Asian Communication Research* 9 (2005): 5–22; So Young Park, "Transnational Adoption, Hallyu, and the Politics of Korean Popular Culture," *Biography* 33.1 (2010): 151–166.

6 Dooboo Shim, "Waxing the Korean Wave," *Asia Research Institute* 58 (Singapore: National University of Singapore, 2011): 3–21.

7 Woongjae Ryoo, "Globalization, or the Logic of Cultural Hybridization," 142.

8 Jonghoe Yang, "The Korean Wave (*Hallyu*) in East Asia: A Comparison of Chinese, Japanese, and Taiwanese Audiences Who Watch Korean TV Dramas," *Development and Society* 41.1 (2012): 103–147; Doobo Shim, "Hybridity," 39 *et passim*. For the third culture argument, see Jin, "Hybridization of Korean Popular Culture," 148–64, and Woongjae Ryoo, "Globalization, of the Logic of Cultural Hybridization," 143.

9 Homi K. Bhabha, *The Location of Culture* (London: Routledge, 1994), cited in Dal Yong Jin, "Hybridization of Korean Popular Culture Films and Online Gaming" in Youna Kim, ed., *The Korean Wave*, 150.

10 Eun-Young Jung, "Transnational Korea: A Critical Assessment of the Korean Wave in Asia and the United States," *Southeast Review of Asian Studies* 31 (2009): 69–80; Kelly Fu Su Yin and Kai Khiun Liew, "*Hallyu* in Singapore: Korean Cosmopolitanism or the Consumption of Chineseness?," *Korea Journal* (2005): 210.

11 Jinhee Choi, “A Cinema of Girlhood,” 56; Robert Cagle, “The Good, the Bad, and the South Korean: Violence, Morality and the South Korean Extreme Film” in *Horror to the Extreme*, 123–144.

12 Bliss Cua Lim, *Translating Time: Cinema, the Fantastic, and Temporal Critique* (Durham: Duke University Press, 2009), 235, which argues that the film’s spectral aesthetic derives from “immiscible times” through which multiple modes of being are represented to expose an untranslatable trauma, offers a different theoretical route to explain the same similar cinematic phenomenon. My analysis does not assume the traumatic source of the repression to have resulted from dynamic operations but rather to lie in an intrapsychic secret deriving from a previous generation. Cf. David Martin Jones, “Time-Images, Tourism and South Korean History” in David Martin-Jones, William Brown, eds., *Deleuze and Film* (Edinburgh: Edinburgh University Press, 2012), 57, where he claims the film reflects “the confusion over layers of the past” that Anna Powell describes in *Delueze and Horror Film* (Edinburgh: Edinburgh University Press, 2006), 11, as characteristic of the genre: “The past impregnates the present in a haunting which seeks to block the flow of present into the future.” Kim has remarked that “In the structure of the story of the film, there are layers of secrets within the family.” “Deleted Scenes: Secrets,” *A Tale of Two Sisters* DVD.

13 For other interpretations of Su-mi’s “return,” see Seo Jeongnam, “Analysis of Changhwa Hongnyon,” 88; Robert Cagle, “Diary of a Lost Girl,” 165; Leung Wing-fai, “A Tale of Two Texts,” 176; Jinhee Choi, *The South Korean Film Renaissance: Local Hitmakers, Global Provacatuers* (Middleton, CT: Wesleyan University Press, 2010).

14 Alan Hyun-Oak, *The Grammar of Focus in Korean Syntax and Its Typological Implications*, PhD Dissertation, University of Southern California (1985), where he discusses the communicative dynamism in Korean grammatical structures that highlight one part of a sentence as conveying the most important—new—information, which is intensified by lexical focusing devices.

15 Robert Cagle, “Diary of a Lost Girl,” 166; Bliss Cua Lim, *Translating Time*, 236; others have seen it as a flashback, but do not distinguish between the central mimesis and the later, more obvious flashback which represents the source of the trauma, namely the deaths of Su-mi’s mother and sister.

16 Leung Wing-fai, “A Tale of Two Texts,” 176.

17 Bou-yong Rhi, “Hwabyung - An Overview,” *Psychiatry Investigation*, 1.1 (2004): 21. The word *hwabyŏng* is comprised of the word “fire,” *hwa*, to signify pent up anger and the word “illness” or “disease,” *byŏng*. See also, Sung Kil Min, “Hwabyung in Korea: Culture and Dynamic Analysis,” *World Cultural Psychiatry Research Review* 4.1 (2009): 12–21; Myunghan Choi and Hye-A Yeom, “Identifying and Treating the Culture-Bound Syndrome of Hwa-Byung Among Older Korean Immigrant Women: Recommendations for Practitioners,” *Journal of the American Academy of Nurse Practitioners* 23.5 (2011): 228–229.

18 Bou-yong Rhi, “Hwabyung - An Overview,” 21–24. Lee Younghee describes construes *han* as “an invention of Korean culture which Korean people have found valuable in coping with life’s struggles,” *Ideology, Culture, and Han: Traditional and Early Modern Korean Women’s Literature* (Seoul: Jimoondang Publishing Company, 2002), 21. Scholars differ with regard to the latinized form of the Korean term; most use *han*, which I follow, but the Romanization *haan* is also frequently seen.

19 Sang-Chin Choi and Gyuseog Han, "Shimcheong Psychology: A Case of an Emotional State for Cultural Psychology," *International Journal for Dialogic Science* 3.1 (2008): 205–224.

20 Sung Kil Min, "Hwabyung in Korea: Culture and Dynamic Analysis," *World Cultural Psychiatry Research Review* 4.1 (2009): 12–21; Richard Roy Grinker, "Mourning the Nation: Ruins of the North in Seoul," *Positions* 3.1 (1995): 192–223, connects the syndrome to Freud's work on mourning; see also idem, *Korea and Its Futures: Unification and the Unfinished War* (New York: St. Martins Press, 1998), 74, where he states that *han* "expresses both personal and collective losses, violations, and consequent resentment—the tragedies of individuals and collectivities of different sizes and inclusiveness can all be represented with the term *han*." Michael Breen, *The Koreans: Who They Are, What They Want, Where Their Future Lies* (New York: St. Martin's Press, 1998), claims Koreans view the experience as unfathomable to outsiders.

21 Bou-yong Rhi, "Hwabyung - An Overview," 14.

22 Soyoung Suh, "Stories to Be Told: Korean Doctors Between Hwa-Byung (Fire-Illness) and Depression, 1970–2011," *Culture, Medicine and Psychiatry* 37.1 (2013): 83. Although the concept of hwabyung is historically verifiable, it was not until 1994 that it became recognized as a "culture bound syndrome" in the American Psychiatric Association's Diagnostic and Statistical Manual of Mental Disorders (DSM-IV).

23 Sung Kil Min, "Hwabyung in Korea; Christopher K Chung and Samson J Cho, "Conceptualization of Jeong and Dynamics of Hwabyung," *Psychiatry Invest* 3.1 (2006): 46–54, 48.

24 Sang Yil Kim, Young Chan Ro, *Hanism as Korean Mind: Interpretation of Han Philosophy* (Los Angeles: The Eastern Academy of Human Sciences, 1984), 104.

25 Michael Breen, *The Koreans*, 38.

26 Jae Hoon Lee, *The Exploration of the Inner Wounds – Han, American Academy of Religion Series* 86 (Atlanta: Scholars Press, 1994), 20:

> On the other hand, if one has a weak or an immature ego due to serious original wounds formed during the early days of life, the experience of loss is liable to cause one to reexperience the original loss in addition to the current loss. In an attempt to avoid the danger of exposing the original wounds, one represses one's own feelings and ideas, and thus the libido itself.

See also Grinker, *Korea and its Futures*, 78: "*Han* refers to a consciousness of ongoing trauma and a lack of resolution and reconciliation."

27 Jisoo Kim, *The Emotions of Justice: Gender, Status, and Legal Performance in Choson Korea* (Seattle: University of Washington, 2015), examines women's deployment of the concept of "grievance" as a social tool to relieve *wŏnhan* repression; Theodore Jun Yoo, *It's Madness: The Politics of Mental Health in Colonial Korea* (Berkeley: University of California Press, 2016), examines mental illness through the literary and legal representations of emotions, which he understands as cultural interpretations of distress in light of Japanese colonial practices of psychiatry.

28 For a different approach, see Keumsil Kim Yoon and Bruce Williams, *Two Lenses on the Korean Ethos: Key Cultural Concepts and Their Appearance in Cinema* (Jefferson, North Carolina: McFarland, 2015), 4–5, who identify *han* and *jeong* as "cultural words" which, along with others, bring into focus a network of cultural contexts—a "cultural ethos—whose structure

underlies Korean film narrative; Yoon and Williams, ibid., 24, advance the idea that *han* is an "an archetypal reality of the Korean people"; Grinker, *Korea and Its Futures,* 83, construes *han* as "a genealogy of hardship and struggle."

29 Sheng-mei Ma, "Asian Cell and Horror" in Andrew Hock Soon Ng, ed., *Asian Gothic: Essays on Literature, Film and Anime* (Jefferson, North Carolina: McFarland, 2008), 187–209; Eunha Oh, "Mother's Grudge and Woman's Wail: The Monster-Mother and Korean Horror Film," in *Korean Horror Cinema*, 60–72; Ian Conrich, "Gothic Bodies and the Return of the Repressed: The Korean Horror Films of Ahn Beyong-ki," *Gothic Studies* 12.1 (2010): 106–115.

30 Sheng-mei Ma, "Asian Cell and Horror," 198: "The lopsidedness within one's heart is cancelled out when transferred onto the society, particularly the torn bodies of the adversaries."

31 Synonymic chains that link the word "descend" and words related to "ruin," "ruination," *t'arakhada*, may explain the fear generated by the hand's descent.

32 "*Naega chigŭm nŏnedŭrŭl kyŏndyŏnaeya hanŭn kŏt ch'ŏrŏm.*"

33 Cf. Su-mi's resistance against her father's need to "understand," "unravel," *ihae*, that which has not yet been expressed.

34 Eunah Oh, "Mother's Grudge and Woman's Wail."

35 The term "waltz," from German *walzen*, derives from Latin *volvere*, "to turn," "to rotate."

36 Bliss Cua Lim, *Translating Time*, 235, also notes how the leitmotif "unifies conflicting versions of the central traumatic event: different retellings of Su-yeon and the wardrobe and of characters arriving at the house on the fateful day of Su-yeon's death...repetition-in-variance...becomes an auditory analogue for traumatic repetition."

37 Robert Cagle, "Diary of a Lost Girl," 161.

38 "*Gŭ nal ire daehaesŏ jom aegi hae jul su issŭlkka.*"

39 Barry Curtis, *Dark Places: The Haunted House in Film*, (London: Reaktion Books, 2008).

40 Ibid.

41 Christophe Wiart, "Anti-inflammatory Plants" in Wiart, *Ethnopharmacology of Medicinal Plants: Asia and the Pacific* (Totowa, NJ: Humana Press, 2007), 47.

42 Cf. Bliss Cua Lim, *Translating Time*, 239, where she interprets the Eun-joo-as-stepmother figure as the projection of "her self-reproach at her sister's death onto an imaginary stepmother"; and Jin-hee Choi, "Girl Cinema," 55, "Su-mi's aggression toward her stepmother is, in fact, directed toward herself."

43 Cf. Korean expressions for being a target of criticism, which are conceptualized in terms of "eating" (as manifested in the "*mek*- 'eat,'" verbal pattern); see Jae Jung Song, "What (not) to Eat or Drink: Metaphor and Metonymy of Eating and Drinking in Korean" in John Newman, ed., *The Linguistics of Eating and Drinking* (Amsterdam: John Benjamins Publishing, 2009), 210–211.

44 See Bliss Cua Lim, *Translating Time,* 193.

45 See, for example, Seo Jeongnam, "Analysis of Changhwa Hongnyon," 85.

46 Cf. The homograph *ch'aim*, which signifies both "chime" and "rent," and its synonym, the word "rent," *punyŏl*, another homograph with a semantic range devolving on the concept of splitting, such as "rent," "split," "cleavage," and "fragmentation," all of which reinforce a subtext informed by the need to conceal an abortion.

47 Jae Jung Song, "What (not) to Eat or Drink," 211.
48 "*Mulgogiwa muri hamkke.*" Wolfram Eberhard, *Dictionary of Chinese Symbols: Hidden Symbols in Chinese Life and Thought* (London: Routledge, 2006), 124; Ulrike Middendorf, *Resexualizing the Desexualized: The Language of Desire and Erotic Love in the Classic of Odes* (Rome: Istituti editoriali e poligrafici internazionali, 2007), 66, n. 57;158;159. Elsewhere he references how "container images" represent the idea that "sex is motion" in water, ibid., 82. For the association between the female sex organ and fish in Chinese culture, see Zhao Guohua, "China's Culture of Reproduction Worship," *Journal of Popular Culture* 27 (1993): 101–111. Cf. ibid., 105, where he explains that early cultures in China "cherished the concept that children came from food they ate," which encouraged ingestion of foods that evoke female genital qualia.
49 *New Testament*, Mark 5:41.
50 Esther Rashkin, *Unspeakable Secrets and the Psychoanalysis of Culture* (Albany: SUNY, 2008), 43.
51 Cf. Bliss Cua Lim, *Translating Time*, 238, interprets the spectral green-robed figure as a symbol of Su-mi's "unshakeable sense of culpability."
52 Chu-Joe Hsia, "Theorizing Colonial Architecture and Urbanism: Building Colonial Modernity in Taiwan," *Inter-Asia Cultural Studies* 3.1 (2002): 7–23, remarks on the contrast posed by vertical colonial architecture that emphasizes the authority of the colonizers as opposed to the horizontal and dispersed buildings that served as centers of authority in Korea. Jordan Sand, *House and Home in Modern Japan: Architecture, Domestic Space, and Bourgeois Culture* (Harvard University Asia Center, 2005) n. 34, 413, cites "colonial architecture historian Nishizawa Yasuhiko," who points out that housing built in the colonies was "generally more Westernized and of a far higher standard than housing for families of comparable status would have been at home. Nishizawa adduces three reasons for this: the need to create incentives to attract professionals to colonial jobs, the need to display imperial power to subject populations and parity to Westerners through architecture, and the fact that most colonial company housing was built in new districts, where the architecture was conspicuous and called on to set a standard for future construction."
53 Sarah Soh, *The Comfort Women: Sexual Violence and Postcolonial Memory in Korea and Japan* (Chicago: University of Chicago Press, 2008). Christine de Matos and Mark E. Caprio, eds., *Japan as the Occupier and the Occupied* (London: Palgrave Macmillan, 2015), 7, claim that 200,000 comfort women were recruited in Korea.
54 Tessa Morris-Suzuki, "The Forgotten Japanese in North Korea: Beyond the Politics of Abduction," *The Asia-Pacific Journal\Japan Focus* 7.43 (2009): 1–2, 5; and idem., *The Exodus to North Korea: Shadows from Japan's Cold War* (New York: Rowman & Littlefield, 2007).
55 Tessa Morris-Suzuki, "The Forgotten Japanese in North Korea," 5.
56 Ibid., 3.
57 Ibid., 8.
58 Ibid.
59 Tessa Morris-Suzuki, *The Exodus to North Korea.*
60 Frank M. Tedesco, "Rites for the Unborn Dead: Abortion and Buddhism in Contemporary Korea," *Korea Journal* 36.2 (1996): 66.
61 Ibid.
62 Michael E. Robinson, *Korea's Twentieth-Century* Odyssey (Honolulu: University of Hawaii Press, 2007), 36. See also Gi-Wook Shin, *Ethnic*

Nationalism in Korea: Genealogy, Politics, and Legacy (Stanford: Stanford University Press, 2006), 39 *et passim.*

63 Andre Schmid, *Korea Between Empires, 1895–1919* (New York: Columbia University Press, 2002), 11.

64 Hyung Il Pai, *Constructing "Korean" Origins: A Critical Review of Archaeology, Historiography, and Racial Myth in Korean State-Formation Theories* (Cambridge, MA: Harvard University Asia Center, 2000), 113–114. Pai demonstrates that the focus of the debate had been not on the rulers' qualifications or their mandate to rule but on the ethnic origins of the legendary rulers.

65 Sun Weiguo, "Legend, Identity, and History; The Historiographic Creation and Evolution of Tangun Choson and Kija Choson," *Chinese Studies in History* 44.4 (2011): 20–46. Kija, a Shang dynasty (1500–145 B.C.) aristocrat who purportedly fled China and arrived in Korea sometime near the end of the second millennium B.C., was commonly credited, even well before the Chosŏn dynasty, with bringing civilization and Chinese culture to the northern region of Korea. Jae-hoon Shim notes that though records are sparse and inconsistent in places, Kija is generally agreed to have been a sibling of the last Shang king or one of the three wise men of Shang. See Sun, "Legend, Identity and History," 39 *et passim.*

66 JaHyun Kim Haboush and Martina Deuchler, "Introduction" in idem., eds., *Culture and the State in Late Choson Korea* (Cambridge, MA and London: Harvard University Press, 1999), 5.

67 Ibid.

68 Haboush, "Ritual Controversy" in *Culture and State in Late Choson Korea*, 69. See also Kirk W. Larsen, "Comforting Fictions: The Tribute System the Westphalian Order, and Sino-Korean Relations," *Journal of East Asian Studies* 13 (2013): 241.

69 The fraternal structure of "diplomatic ritual" allowed China and Korea to normalize their relationship despite the severe power asymmetry that existed between them. Sino-Korean relations was based on a tributary system in which Chosŏn founders acknowledged Korea's ritual subordination—and accepted Chinese centrality in a universal world order—and thereby garnered protection from external forces and the legitimacy to rule. See Nianshen Song, "'Tributary' from a Multilateral and Multilayered Perspective," *The Chinese Journal of International Politics* 5.2 (2012): 174–176, who argues that the hierarchical Sino-Korean relationship was construed as one of cooperation than one of a continuous struggle over power. Mutual obligations served as parameters within which problems could be solved. Kirk W. Larsen, "Comforting Fictions," questions the extent to which the hierarchy diminished the existence of coercion and raw power amid Sino-Korean relations, but he claims that both sides did adhere to a fiction as a way to preserve the hierarchy without excessive force.

70 Don Baker, "Writing History in Pre-Modern Korea" in *The Oxford History of Historical Writing: 1400–1800*, Grant Hardy Andrew Feldherr, José Rabasa, Daniel R. Woolf, eds. (New York: Oxford University Press, 2012), 104.

71 Ibid.

72 Ibid. The familial terminology used to describe Sino-Korean relations conceals what was a real challenge for Yi Sŏng-gye's claims of authority, his problematic genealogy. Ming historical records reveal that the Ming Emperor did not acknowledge Yi Sŏng-gye as a legitimate sovereign at first.

73 Ibid.

74 Sun Weiguo, "Legend, Identity, and History," 39. Jae-hoon Shim notes that though records are sparse and inconsistent in places, Kija is generally agreed to have been a sibling of the last Shang king or one of the three wise men of Shang.
75 Kyung-Koo, Han. "The Archaeology of the Ethnically Homogeneous Nation-State and Multiculturalism in Korea," *Korea Journal* 47.4 (2007): 14. See also, Gi-wook Shin, *Ethnic Nationalism in Korea: Genealogy, Politics, and Legacy* (Stanford: Stanford University Press, 2006).
76 Wang, Sixiang. *Co-constructing Empire in Early Choson Korea: Knowledge Production and the Culture of Diplomacy, 1392–1592*, (PhD Dissertation, Columbia University, 2015), 158.
77 Ibid., 165–166.
78 Ibid., 172.
79 Sun Weiguo, "Legend, Identity, and History," 20–46.
80 Haboush, "Ritual Controversy," 66.
81 Acknowledging the structural similarity in the form and content of Korean responses to threats of national identity may also elucidate the significance of discursive practices that frame the expulsion of North Korea as the less "legitimate" brother whose shameful acts triggered the Korean war.
82 Ibid., 41.
83 JaHyunKim Haboush, *A Heritage of Kings: One Man's Monarchy in the Confucian World* (New York: Columbia University Press, 1985), 45.
84 Sun Weiguo, "Legend, Identity, and History"; Gi-wook Shin, *Ethnic Nationalism in Korea.*
85 Jae Hoon Lee, *The Exploration of the Inner Wounds*, 20.
86 Roy Grinker, *Korea and Its Futures*, 86.
87 Haboush, trans., *The Memoirs of Lady Hyegyong: The Autobiographical Writings of a Crown Princess of Eighteenth Century Korea* (Berkeley: University of California Press, 1996), 233.
88 Ibid., 25.
89 Ibid., 204–205.
90 Ibid., 24–25. Haboush cites a historical account that states that

> [o]n the first day of his reign, Chŏngjo lamented, "Alas, I am really Prince Sado's son. The Late Majesty made me an adopted son of Prince Hyojang since he thought the main line of the family should be given precedence. Isn't it sad!... though propriety must be strict, human emotion cannot but be expressed."

91 Ibid., 168, details how portions of the *Records of the Royal Secretariat* dealing with Sado were destroyed.
92 Ibid., 246.
93 Ibid., 263.
94 Haboush, *A Heritage of Kings,* 34.
95 Idem., Memoirs, 246–247. This of course is the same set of conditions that I posit led to Ivan IV's haunting in the previous chapter.
96 Ibid., 256.
97 Ibid.
98 Ibid., 257.
99 Ibid.
100 Ibid., 263.
101 Ibid., 265.
102 Maggie CK Wan, "Image and Efficacy: The Frontispieces to the Wanli Emperor's *Yushu jing*," *Artibus Asiae* 75.1 (2015): 47.

103 Ibid., 54.
104 Haboush, *Memoirs*, 265.
105 Ibid., 256.
106 Ibid., 244.
107 Ibid., 281.
108 Ibid., 289, 307–8.
109 Sheila Miyoshi Jager, "A Vision for the Future; or, Making Family History in Contemporary South Korea," *Positions* 4.1 (1996): 50.

Bibliography

Ancuta, Katarzyna. "Spirits in Suburbia: Ghosts, Global Desires and the Rise of Thai Middle-Cass Horror." *Horror Studies* 5.2 (2014): 233–247.

Anderson, Crystal S., et al. *The Global Impact of South Korean Popular Culture: Hallyu Unbound*. Lexington Books, 2014.

Anisimova, Irina. "The Terrors of History: Revolutionary Gothic in 'Mother Earth' by Boris Pilniak." *The Slavic and East European Journal* 55.3 (2011): 376–395.

Baker, Don. "Writing History in Pre-Modern Korea." *The Oxford History of Historical Writing: Volume 3: 1400–1800*, 2012. 103–118.

Balmain, Colette. "Pan-Asian Gothic." Ed. Glennys Byron. *Globalgothic. Oxford University Press,* 2015. 119–132.

Breen, Michael. *The Koreans: Who They Are, What They Want, Where Their Future Lies*. Macmillan, 2014.

Byron, Glennis, ed. *Globalgothic*. Oxford University Press, 2015.

Cagle, Robert L. "Diary of a Lost Girl: Victoriana, Intertextuality and *A Tale of Two Sisters*." Ed. Alison Peirse. *Korean Horror Cinema. Edinburgh University Press,* 2013. 158–172.

———. "The Good, the Bad, and the South Korean: Violence, Morality, and the South Korean Extreme Film." Eds. Jinhee Choi, Mitsuyo Wada-Marciano. *Horror to the Extreme: Changing Boundaries in Asian Cinema*. Hongkong University Press, 2009. 123–144.

Choi, Jinhee. "A Cinema of Girlhood: Sonyeo Sensibility and the Decorative Impulse in the Korean Horror Cinema." Eds. Jinhee Choi, Mitsuyo Wada-Marciano. *Horror to the Extreme: Changing Boundaries in Asian Cinema*. Hongkong University Press, 2009. 39–56.

———. *The South Korean Film Renaissance: Local Hitmakers, Global Provocateurs*. Wesleyan University Press, 2010.

Choi, Jinhee, and Mitsuyo Wada-Marciano, eds. *Horror to the Extreme: Changing Boundaries in Asian Cinema*. Vol. 1. Hong Kong University Press, 2009.

Choi, Myunghan, and Hye-A. Yeom. "Identifying and Treating the Culture-bound Syndrome of Hwa-Byung among Older Korean Immigrant Women: Recommendations for Practitioners." *Journal of the American Association of Nurse Practitioners* 23.5 (2011): 226–232.

Choi, Sang-Chin, and Gyuseog Han. "Shimcheong Psychology. A Case of an Emotional State for Cultural Psychology." *International Journal for Dialogical Science* 3.1 (2008): 205–224.

Conrich, Ian. "Gothic Bodies and the Return of the Repressed: The Korean Horror Films of Ahn Byeong-ki." *Gothic Studies* 12.1 (2010): 106–115.

Creed, Barbara. *The Monstrous-Feminine: Film, Feminism, Psychoanalysis*. Routledge, 1993.

Curtis, Barry. *Dark Places: The Haunted House in Film*. Reaktion Books, 2008.

De Matos, Christine, and Mark Caprio. Eds. *Japan as the Occupier and the Occupied*. Springer, 2015.

Eberhard, Wolfram. *Dictionary of Chinese Symbols: Hidden Symbols in Chinese Life and Thought*. Routledge, 2006.

Grinker, Roy Richard. "Mourning the Nation: Ruins of the North in Seoul." *Positions* 3.1 (1995): 192–223.

———. *Korea and Its Futures: Unification and the Unfinished War*. Palgrave Macmillan, 1998.

Haboush, JaHyun Kim. *A Heritage of Kings: One Man's Monarchy in the Confucian World*. Columbia University Press, 1988.

———. "Constructing the Center: The Ritual Controversy and the Search for a New Identity in Seventeenth-Century Korea." Eds. JaHyun Haboush and Martina Deuchler. *Culture and the State in Late Choson Korea*. Vol. 182. Harvard University Asia Center, 2002. 46–90.

———. *The Memoirs of Lady Hyegyong: The Autobiographical Writings of a Crown Princess of Eighteenth-Century Korea*. University of California Press, 2013.

Haboush, JaHyun Kim, and Martina Deuchler. "Introduction." *Culture and the State in Late Choson Korea*. Vol. 182. Harvard University Asia Center, 2002. 1–13.

Hsia, Chu-Joe. "Theorizing Colonial Architecture and Urbanism: Building Colonial Modernity in Taiwan." *Inter-Asia Cultural Studies* 3.1 (2002): 7–23.

Huat, Chua Beng. "Conceptualizing an East Asian Popular Culture." *Inter-Asia Cultural Studies* 5.2 (2004): 200–221.

Jager, Sheila Miyoshi. "A Vision for the Future; or, Making Family History in Contemporary South Korea." *Positions* 4.1 (1996): 31–58.

Jin, Dal Yong. "Hybridization of Korean Popular Culture: Films and Online Gaming." Ed. Youna Kim. *The Korean Wave: Korean Media Go Global*. Routledge, 2013. 148–164.

Jung, Eun-Young. "Transnational Korea: A Critical Assessment of the Korean Wave in Asia and the United States." *Southeast Review of Asian Studies* 31 (2009): 69–80.

Ju-Yong, H. A., and Joel David. "A Critical Consideration of the Use of Trauma as an Approach to Understanding Korean Cinema." *Journal of Critical Perspectives on Asia* 50.1 (2014): 16–50.

Kim, Alan Hyun-Oak. *The Grammar of Focus in Korean Syntax and Its Typological Implications*. University of Sothern California, 1985.

Kim, Jisoo M. *The Emotions of Justice: Gender, Status, and Legal Performance in Choson Korea*. University of Washington Press, 2016.

Kim, Sang-Yil, and Young Chan Ro. *Hanism as Korean Mind: Interpretation of Han Philosophy*. Eastern Academy of Human Sciences, 1984.

Kim, Youna. Ed. *The Korean Wave: Korean Media Go Global*. Routledge, 2013.

———. "The Rising East Asian 'Wave'." *Media on the Move: Global Flow and Contra Flow*. Ed. Daya Kishan Thussu. Routledge, 2007. 121–135.

Kyung-Koo, Han. "The Archaeology of the Ethnically Homogeneous Nation-State and Multiculturalism in Korea." *Korea Journal* 47.4 (2007): 8–31.

Larsen, Kirk W. "Comforting Fictions: The Tribute System, the Westphalian Order, and Sino-Korean Relations." *Journal of East Asian Studies* 13.02 (2013): 233–257.

Lee, Jae Hoon. *The Exploration of the Inner Wounds—Han*. No. 86. Scholars Press, 1994.

Lee, Keehyeung. "Assessing and Situating 'the Korean Wave'(Hallyu) Through a Cultural Studies Lens." *Asian Communication Research* 2.2 (2005): 5–22.

Lee, Peter. Ed. *A History of Korean Literature*. Cambridge University Press, 2003.

Lee, Younghee. *Ideology, Culture, and Han: Traditional and Early Modern Korean Women's Literature*. No. 18. Jimoondang International, 2002.

Lee, Zuk-Nae. "Korean Culture and Sense of Shame." *Transcultural Psychiatry* 36.2 (1999): 181–194.

Lim, Bliss Cua. *Translating Time: Cinema, the Fantastic, and Temporal Critique*. Duke University Press, 2009.

Ma, Sheng-Mei. "Asian Cell and Horror." Ed. AndrewHock Soon Ng. *Asian Gothic: Essays on Literature, Film and Anime*. McFarland, 2008. 187–209.

Marinescu, Valentina. Ed. *The Global Impact of South Korean Popular Culture: Hallyu Unbound*. Lexington, 2014.

Martin-Jones, David. "Time-Images in Traces of Love: Repackaging South Korea's Traumatic National History for Tourism." *Deleuze and Film*, 2012. 54–70.

Martin-Jones, David, and William Brown. Eds. *Deleuze and Film*. Edinburgh University Press, 2012.

Middendorf, Ulrike. *Resexualizing the Desexualized: The Language of Desire and Erotic Love in the Classic of Odes*. Istituti editoriali e poligrafici internazionali, 2007.

Min, Sung Kil. "Hwabyung in Korea: Culture and Dynamic Analysis." *World Cultural Psychiatry Research Review* 4.1 (2009): 12–21.

Morris-Suzuki, Tessa. "The Forgotten Japanese in North Korea: Beyond the Politics of Abduction." *The Asia-Pacific Journal/Japan Focus Volume* 7.43 (2009): 1–19.

———. *Exodus to North Korea: Shadows from Japan's Cold War*. Rowman & Littlefield Publishers, 2007.

Newman, John, ed. *The Linguistics of Eating and Drinking*. Vol. 84. John Benjamins Publishing, 2009.

Ng, Andrew Hock Soon. Ed. *Asian Gothic: Essays on Literature, Film and Anime*. McFarland, 2008.

Oh, Eunha. "Mother's Grudge and Woman's Wail: The Monster-Mother and Korean Horror Film." Alison Peirse and Daniel Martin. Eds., *Korean Horror Cinema*. Edinburgh, 2013. 60–72.

Pai, Hyung Il. *Constructing "Korean" Origins: A Critical Review of Archaeology, Historiography, and Racial Myth in Korean State-formation Theories*. No. 187. Harvard University Asia Center, 2000.

Park, So Young. "Transnational Adoption, Hallyu, and the Politics of Korean Popular Culture." *Biography* 33.1 (2010): 151–166.

Powell, Anna. *Delueze and Horror Film*. Edinburgh University Press, 2006.

Rashkin, Esther. *Unspeakable Secrets and the Psychoanalysis of Culture*. SUNY, 2008.

Rhi, Bou-Yong. "Hwabyung-An Overview." *Psychiatry Invest* 1 (2004): 21–24.

Robinson, Michael Edson. *Korea's Twentieth-Century Odyssey*. University of Hawaii Press, 2007.

Ryoo, Woongjae. "Globalization, or the Logic of Cultural Hybridization: The Case of the Korean Wave." *Asian Journal of Communication* 19.2 (2009): 137–151.

Sand, Jordan. *House and Home in Modern Japan: Architecture, Domestic Space, and Bourgeois Culture, 1880–1930*. Vol. 223. Harvard University Asia Center, 2005.

Sato, Masayuki, et al. Eds. *The Oxford History of Historical Writing: Volume 3: 1400–1800*. Vol. 31400. Oxford University Press, 2012.

Schmid, Andre. *Korea Between Empires, 1895–1919*. Columbia University Press, 2002.

Seet, K. K. "Mothers and Daughters: Abjection and the Monstrous-Feminine in Japan's Dark Water and South Korea's *A Tale of Two Sisters*." *Camera Obscura* 24.2 71 (2009): 139–159.

Seo, Jeongnam. "Analysis of Changhwa Hongnyon (*A Tale of Two Sisters*)—With a special Focus on the Narrative and Characters." *Acta Koreana* 14.1 (2011): 73–116.

Shim, Dooboo. "Hybridity and the Rise of Korean Popular Culture in Asia." *Media, Culture & Society* 28.1 (2006): 25–44.

———. "Waxing the Korean Wave." *Asia Research Institute* 58 (2011): 3–21.

Shin, Gi-Wook. *Ethnic Nationalism in Korea: Genealogy, Politics, and Legacy*. Stanford University Press, 2006.

Soh, C. Sarah. *The Comfort Women: Sexual Violence and Postcolonial Memory in Korea and Japan*. University of Chicago Press, 2008.

Song, Jae Jung. "What (not) to Eat or Drink: Metaphor and Metonymy of Eating and Drinking in Korean." *The Linguistics of Eating and Drinking*, 2009. 1–26.

Song, Nianshen. "'Tributary' from a Multilateral and Multilayered Perspective." *The Chinese Journal of International Politics* 5.2 (2012): 155–182.

Suh, Soyoung. "Stories to be Told: Korean Doctors Between Hwa-Byung (Fire-Illness) and Depression, 1970–2011." *Culture, Medicine, and Psychiatry* 37.1 (2013): 81–104.

Sun, Weiguo. "Legend, Identity, and History: The Historiographic Creation and Evolution of Tangun Choson and Kija Choson." *Chinese Studies in History* 44.4 (2011): 20–46.

Sung, Kil Min. "Hwabyung in Korea: Culture and Dynamic Analysis." *World Cultural Psychiatry Research Review* 4.1 (2009): 12–21.

Tedesco, Frank M. "Rites for the Unborn Dead: Abortion and Buddhism in Contemporary Korea." *Korea Journal* 36.2 (1996): 61–74.

Wan, Maggie CK. "Image and Efficacy: The Frontispieces to the Wanli Emperor's *Yushu jing*." *Artibus Asiae* 75.1 (2015): 45–79.

Wang, Sixiang. *Co-constructing Empire in Early Choson Korea: Knowledge Production* and *the Culture of Diplomacy, 1392–1592*. Columbia University, 2015.

Wiart, Christophe. *Ethnopharmacology of Medicinal Plants*. Humana Press Incorporated, 2007.

Wing-Fai, Leung. "From *A Tale of Two Sisters* to The Uninvited: A Tale of Two Texts." Alison Peirse and Daniel Martin. Eds., *Korean Horror Cinema*. Edinburgh, 2013. 173–186.

Yang, Jonghoe. "The Korean Wave (*Hallyu*) in East Asia: A Comparison of Chinese, Japanese, and Taiwanese Audiences Who Watch Korean TV Dramas." *Development and Society* 41.1 (2012): 103–147.

Yin, Kelly Fu Su, and Kai Khiun Liew. "Hallyu in Singapore: Korean Cosmopolitanism or the Consumption." *Korea Journal* 45.4 (2005): 206–232.

Yoo, Theodore Jun. *It's Madness: The Politics of Mental Health in Colonial Korea*. University of California Press, 2016.

5 The Religious Specter

Identifying the Intruder in Alejandro Amenábar's *The Others*

When the Chilean-Spanish director Alejandro Amenábar's psychological thriller *The Others* debuted in 2001 to widespread critical and popular acclaim, it not only went on to garner over $209.9 million in gross revenues but also brought the transnational auteur to the forefront of international cinema.[1] Both critics and audiences found his vision, and the surprising "epistemological shift" that concludes the film, extremely compelling. It is the story of a devout Catholic woman, Grace Stewart, who lives with her two children (Anne and Nicholas) in an isolated, dark manor on the previously Nazi-occupied island of Jersey in the immediate aftermath of World War II. Her children are afflicted with xeroderma pigmentosum, a disease characterized by extreme photosensitivity, so the life of the manor is organized by the need to prevent inadvertent exposure to sunlight: Curtains are constantly drawn and rooms are locked with people inside them. When strange phenomena occur—such as the sound of a piano being played from inside a locked room when no one is inside, doors that Grace believes to have been locked being found ajar, and Anne's contention that she has seen four people in the house—the family must deal with the possibility of being haunted by "intruders." The film focuses on Grace's attempt to make sense of the disturbing situations.

Film critics have focused on the "atmospheric, stylish and spooky"[2] aesthetic of the film and also on themes of darkness, which many read as a metaphor for the dark times of Nazi power. Most cite the unforeseen turn of events—namely, Grace's discovery that it is she and her children, and not the "others," who are dead and haunt the house—as an exhilarating dramatic resolution to the intensely constructed suspense of the film; we also learn that their postmortem existence is a result of her having suffocated Anne and Nicholas and then committed suicide.

Academic critics have examined the psychological implications of Amenábar's aesthetic, especially the implicit context of Grace's psychotic break. Many recognize her grief over the loss/death of her husband and concomitant feelings of abandonment, suggesting that these conditions triggered her fatal actions. Discussions of the film frequently reference psychoanalytic theory to explain Grace's unarticulated trauma, especially Freudian notions of the death drive and the uncanny.[3] Anabel Girel's analysis locates the source of psychosis in Grace's relationship to Catholicism; Girel views Grace's acts as resistance against being "haunted by the Catholic."[4]

While these critics share my interest in the connection between Grace's murder-suicide and the film's haunting aesthetic, not one of them connects her psychosis to the "reality" of her blindness to her own existential status as dead, a connection Amenábar has deliberately left obscure. In other words, why do Grace and her children not know that they are dead, especially given that the three other characters in the film—Bertha Mills, the housekeeper; Edmund Tuttle, the gardener; and Lydia, the mute maid—are aware of their postmortem existence? In retrospect of her confused behavior, what are the repercussions of Grace's actions to try to rid "her house" of the "intruders"?[5] Since she is unable to recognize her own existential condition, might there be other aspects of her own identity she is unsure of? Moreover, since her questionable judgment of identity is dynamically interwoven with her zeal to protect "her house" from the light of day and from "intruders," it becomes clear that her ignorance of her own identity is linked to the identity of the "intruders" in the house and to its protection.

The film calls attention to its capacity to conceal and reveal. When considered in tandem with its gothic aesthetic, premised on the idea that the "sins of the fathers [will] be visited on subsequent generations,"[6] the possibility that Grace is haunted by a phantom becomes stronger. As we learned in our analysis of *A Tale of Two Sisters*, the film's revelation of one secret may simultaneously operate as subterfuge, that is, a means to occlude the existence of another secret whose preservation ultimately drives the film's unique patterned form of representation.

From the outset, several elements of the film hint that the secret of Grace's madness may involve a saga other than the one specifically revealed at the end of the film. Anne mentions several times that her mother "went mad," suggesting it is a veiled aspect of the film's secret. This chapter will argue that the film's meticulous presentation of Grace's fantasy stages a secret about an unutterable drama that is quite different from the murder-suicide. The secret of her murder-suicide inscribes within it a story about a concealed intruder whose penetration into a family leads to devastating family shame. This drama is a latent memory of events that Grace did not experience in her own life but which was unwittingly passed into her unconscious through cryptic language and behavior as a gap in the speech of a parent.[7] I understand this silent secret, or "phantom," that Grace receives as the actual source of her psychosis.

The films juxtaposition of two layers, one involving dark and shutout reality and the other being the plane of enlightened awareness, suggests, as we've seen in the three films analyzed earlier, analogues of another juxtaposition: that between the conscious and the unconscious. To identify what lies behind Grace's self-ignorance, we must identify lexical strategies generated by preservative repression. The link between a house choked of light and compartmentalized with locks is meant to represent the topography of Grace's psyche, similar to the way Su-mi's house represented her fractured identity in *A Tale of Two Sisters*. Techniques such as contrasting planes of darkness and light through visual patterns of lighting and shading highlight Grace's struggle between enlightenment and ignorance. These components shape our understanding of how her psyche is compartmentalized and help us discern the trauma that led to its formation.

Grace's penchant for silence ("Silence is something we prize very highly in this house"), which she demands of the three servants who appear at her door at the beginning of the film, indicates a context of preservative repression. Her insistence that her children not speak of a mysterious incident, which we later find refers to the day she went "mad" and killed them and herself, reveals that there is something about Grace that she herself cannot see or know. The consistent repetition of concealment tropes, such as keys and locked compartments, and the urgency to keep the house shut up as tight as a ship against water, moreover, underscores how light, or enlightenment, is perceived as dangerous. When viewed in tandem with the fact that the ostensible reason for these actions involves an *inherited* disease afflicting her children, the possibility emerges that what must be concealed and preserved is connected to issues of genealogy.

This constellation of associations allows us to posit that Grace's inability to distinguish between living and dying is a result of her inheritance of a shameful secret that was transmitted across generations. A close reading of the film will represent Grace's actions, both her psychotic murder-suicide as well as her blindness to her mortality, as a sequel to an ancestral saga. Indeed, a connection between family and the haunting effects of silence is implied in several important scenes of the film. For example, during a homeschool lesson about the persecution of Justus and Pastor at the hands of the Romans, Anne and Nicholas mock the brothers as stupid because they could have lied to the Romans and remained silent about their inner religious beliefs. Infuriated by Anne's insolence, Grace separates them and demands that they memorize a lesson entitled "The House and the Family," in order to understand the repercussions of the denial of faith (in Christ).[8] At this point, Nicholas expresses fear of being left alone lest he see a ghost.

Other scenes that connect haunting and family lineage include two in which conversations about family between Grace and Bertha—which touch on the topics of descendants and ancestors, respectively—are directly followed by auditory manifestations of the intruders' existence. That both conversations end on the topic of the source of Lydia's muteness—a topic of great interest to Grace—moreover, implicates silence as a conduit of the haunting experience. Indeed, Grace's comment regarding Lydia's muteness that "people don't just stop talking; these things are always the result of some sort of trauma" may be construed as a poignant, albeit unconscious, expression of her own position.

The Prologue

As we have seen in each of the films analyzed thus far, the opening segments of phantom films cryptically represent the affective condition that leads to the production of a fantasy. This is the case with *The Others* as well. Although many critics view Grace's bloodcurdling scream, which they assumed to have been triggered by a nightmare, as the initiation of the film's exposition, I argue that what comes before it should not be discounted as inconsequential, even if it seems to be merely an atmospheric place holder for projecting production credits. Amenábar's eerie and ominous first frames, and their acoustic accompaniment by Grace's disembodied voice, are rich resources for reconstructing the secret embedded in the film. Grace narrates a story to her children about beginnings that recalls the faun's disembodied account of Ofelia's origins in *Pan's Labyrinth*. In both films, the opening words establish a background context that glosses the story it precedes.

Grace's first words echo those that opened a popular BBC radio show called "Listen with Mother," which aired during the post-World War II years:[9] "Now, children, are you sitting comfortably? Then I'll begin." The audio quote may be understood ironically, given how the warmth and intimacy it projects contrasts with the horror of the sketches that accompany it. But something else is also communicated by Amenábar's quote, which is that this film implores us to listen as well as watch. The synchronicity of Grace's disembodied narration with these particular images, the film tells us, is important: Images will communicate to us linguistically as well as visually. As this analysis will bear out, listening becomes a crucial means for deciphering the elements of the encrypted drama.

The sketches, apparently from a children's book, appear behind the opening credits as Grace paraphrases, simplistically, the first chapters in Genesis.[10] Macabre in nature, the images—including a marionette holding a violin and hanging limp, head cocked to one side as if its neck has been snapped in a noose; children, wide-eyed with fear; and dark corners and stairways of the manor where the story takes place—extend beyond the narration, lingering beyond speech. Although Grace's narrative seems intent on being comprehensive with regard to God's creation of astral entities, animals, and vegetation, it is noteworthy that her story makes no mention whatsoever of God's creation of humankind, even though the book of Genesis has been understood as a story about origins or "generations," both cosmic, as in heaven and earth, and genealogical.[11]

Because Amenábar's film connects the three issues of silence, family, and haunting, the ellipses surrounding the book of Genesis' focused delineation of genealogical origins seem too pointed to dismiss as a stylistic ambiguity. Indeed, the strategically placed ellipses at the end of this monologue in the screenplay orthographically mark the verbal exclusion. Grace's omission reveals that something about family origins is shut out from her speech. Her narration implores us to extrapolate a drama inscribed in its gaps. With the reference to the book of Genesis, Amenábar has set the film, the family, and the house in a religious context that hints at something darker lurking between the lines.

Grace's scream vocalizes the transition from the prologue to the initiation of a fantasy, a psychic response to the darkness that lurks. Unlike the openings of the other three phantom films, which more precisely delineate the affective condition that summons the fantasy, *The Others* delays clarification until much later in the film. We will see how this is a function of the film's allegorical message; for now, it is enough to see how Grace's scream demarcates a discursive boundary.

Concealed Religious Identity

Two crucial scenes in which direct citation of Genesis figures significantly reinforce the idea that Grace's omission is linked to a denied or excluded reality. As punishment for her perceived deception about witnessing the "intruders," Anne is forced by Grace to read from the Bible. In the first scene, Anne reads aloud the part of Genesis in which Adam and Eve are expelled from the Garden of Eden;[12] in the second scene, Anne reads from the chapter that narrates Abraham's attempted sacrifice of Isaac.[13] The synchronicity between her punishment and trial—she is asked to beg forgiveness of the Virgin Mary for her deceit—and that experienced by Adam and Abraham establish a critical link between family shame and transgression against a parental figure. We have seen how the story of Abraham and Isaac functioned in Andrey Zvyagintsev's *The Return* to allegorize a child whose life is organized by the need to preserve a parent's (or ancestor's). I believe that a similar dynamic is in operation in *The Others*.

Grace punishes Anne because she refused to deny that she had seen the intruders. This disposition resembles the taciturn comportment of the father in *The Return* and suggests that we understand the punishment not only in terms of Anne's (perceived) transgression but as a failure in an unstated trial devoted to strengthening her capacity to deny what she saw. Defending her form of punishment, Grace comments to Bertha that "it's about time [Anne] started to read the Bible." Grace's paraphrase of the text intimates why she believes that Genesis is an appropriate antidote for Anne's stubbornness: For Grace, the text represents the presence of something that is both hidden and exposed. She has faith that by reading the text, Anne will learn how to simultaneously be shown something frightening and made to remain ignorant of it.

What is so frightening in Genesis is intimated by her fanatical protection of her "house," which is more than the upkeep of a physical building or even the restricting of light. Rather, Genesis tells us that her obsession may be read in terms of protecting a lineage that cannot be exposed to view. Even more pointedly, as Genesis suggests, it is not just any lineage that must be hidden from view but a *Jewish lineage*. Thus, the ellipses in Grace's account all but compel us to see that the house that she must protect is her own Jewish lineage. She is haunted by an ancestor's secret about concealed *Jewish* identity.

An interlingual network of female names in the film reinforces this interpretive conclusion. The name of Grace's daughter, Anne, derives from the Biblical Hebrew word for "grace" or "gracious." Additionally, Anne was the Jewish mother of the Virgin Mary and grandmother of Christ. These two facts reveal an intriguing matrilineal chain of Annes, associating a Jewish grandmother with a mother (Grace) and a daughter (Anne). The implication of the commonality of names over three generations reifies the sense that something unknown to a subject in one generation may nonetheless experience something that was secretly known and "within the family house" of a preceding generation.[14] This is especially true in relation to Anne's haunting by an elderly woman, who, we find out later, is a medium conducting a séance and who, at one point, Grace hallucinates is possessing Anne (an important scene about which I will have more to say later).

Grace is also a Stewart, that is, a *steward*. According to the *Oxford English Dictionary*, this is someone who supports, guards, and cares for a *house* in both senses of the word: the physical building her family inhabits as well as its extended meaning in terms of family lineage, the House of Stewart, in which "house" refers "chiefly in biblical use, to a group of people descended from a common ancestor, a race," such as the "house of Israel: the Jewish or Hebrew nation or people." The religious overtones become more pronounced in light of the frequent use of the word "house" to refer to a place of worship, as in a house of prayer. Grace seeks to expel the "intruder" from her *house* and thereby rid her psyche of an unwanted religious affiliation; one connotation of the word "intruder" refers to someone "who enters a religious congregation against the group's wishes." The implication here is that the "intruder" into Grace's house is Jewish. The film climactically reveals the "intruder" into the Stewart house, whose presence Anne apprehends most frequently: the medium who conducts the séance. As the camera pans over her face and upper body while she is in a trance, communicating with the children, without lingering, it nonetheless allows us to see something buried among the busy details of her attire: a brooch of the Star of David. The film thus reveals the haunting experienced by Grace and her children as a function of the physical presence of a Jew into the Stewart household (Figure 5.1).

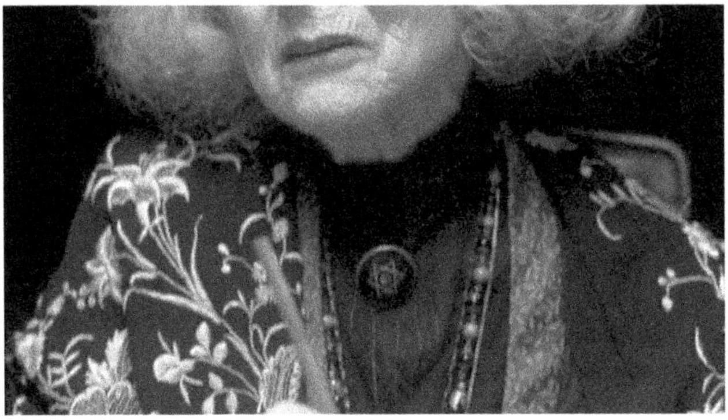

Figure 5.1 Detail of Star of David brooch.

The proper name of the mute housemaid, Lydia, about whom Grace reveals an intense curiosity, suggests the means by which a Jew infiltrated Grace's family line, namely through religious conversion. A "gentile worshipper of the Jewish God," identified as Lydia in the New Testament (Acts 16:14–16), "converted [to Christianity] forthwith, with her *oikos* [family]." She persuaded early proselytizers Paul, Silas, and their other companions to move into her house.[15] This transtextual allusion suggests that Grace identifies with Lydia's trauma-induced muteness because her *name* resonates with other words that are shut out from expression, unutterable words about conversion from Jewish to Christian religious affiliation. Grace's preference for purple hued outfits also intimates identification with the converted Lydia, who was known specifically as a woman who sold purple dye and purple cloth in several texts.[16] Indeed, Grace's sartorial choices may be read as a ciphered staging of an identity marked by conversion.

Proposing that Grace has inherited a Jewish identity that has been silently transmitted to her establishes a vantage point from which to identify, within her acts and speech, linguistic fragments produced in response to a trauma kept secret by the ancestor. For example, her hyper devotion to Catholic dogma assumes extra dimensions in view of the foregoing analysis. Anne's revelation to Grace that the latter's grasp of the concept of "children's limbo" was flawed insinuates the tenuous nature of her Catholic identity. Yet, as we shall see, what defines her identity is not her ignorance of Catholic dogma per se but the disturbing presence within her of an identity transmitted to her as unknowable. Her invocation of the Bible to bolster her adamant rejection of Mrs Mills's suggestion that "sometimes the world of the dead gets mixed up with the world of the living" implicates her Catholic belief system in an unconscious grappling with ghostly figments of her mind that live on—beyond death—in the topography of her psyche.

Listening Clues

Disembodied music is a consistent source of Grace's haunting. Her own assessment that the spectral phenomenon points to "something … not at rest in this house" begs the question of what in the music would elicit a restive presence in her psyche. The music she heard was Frederic Chopin's Waltz in A-flat Major, Op. 69, No. 1—also known as *The Farewell Waltz* because it was composed in response to his fiancé's (Maria Wodzińska's) ultimate decision to reject his offer of marriage. The music links the haunting experience to a context of romantic abandonment, which implies that it speaks to Grace of someone's heartbreak over the end of a relationship. When connected to her references to being abandoned by her servants, not to mention her feelings of abandonment as a result of her family's departure from the island in 1940, as well as Charles, her husband's, departure for war, we begin to see a link between the experience of haunting and desertion. While the film's manifest concern with the secret of Grace's madness seems explained with the denouement's revelation that her psychotic breakdown and subsequent murder-suicide was apparently triggered by the death of her husband, what remains to be elucidated is how her ancestor's Jewishness is specifically linked to a drama of abandonment. A closer examination of Grace's odd and inconsistent reactions to the presence of the "intruders" suggests some answers.

After the musical encounter, she decides to go to the village to ask the local Catholic priest, Father Legrand, to visit the house in order to bless it. This aligns with her unconscious reliance on Catholicism as a means to sustain her unawareness of the existence of a secret (manifested by the music). But given her previous reluctance to leave the house on account of her children, notwithstanding her frustration over the priest's extended absence from the Stewart household, her frenzied insistence on ignoring Mrs Mill's pleas that she not walk out in the fog suggests another hidden motivation for the urgency. Grace's compulsion to brave the fog to seek a "father" in the wake of her exposure (cf. fog, "aftermath," *OED*) to the haunting, melancholic, and nostalgic music associated with romantic dissolution implicates both family and religion as intrinsic to the uncanny affect of her experience. Moreover, these associations between family, religion, and music interconnect with French society.

"Legrand," an ancient patronymic French surname, points to the centuries-old presence of French Catholicism on Jersey Island.[17] Allusions to France and the French language abound in the film. The children state twice that their father is in France fighting the war,[18] which offers an alternative gloss on the link between "father" and "France." Anne also enunciates the French word *monsieur*, complete with a French accent, when she is alone in her room dressed in her First Communion dress. Because this scene segues into the one in which Anne is possessed by the old Jewish woman whom we have seen to be the perceived intruder of the Stewart household, the possibility emerges that Anne's linguistic turn points to the French nationality of the woman whose secret haunts Grace. It suggests, in other words, that when we listen to the film's images, we will also need to hear in French.

The profoundly haunting sounds of a piano emanating from the locked music room late at night suggest that other linguistic and rhetorical elements involving sound, specters, and musical instruments may reveal a logical coherence. This is indeed what I find. For example, the film pays repetitive attention to two silent but visually conspicuous images of a violin and violoncello in scenes in which the effects of haunting are most heightened; the convergence implies that the instruments reverberate with the secret drama of a concealed Jewish identity. Violins are often represented as visual props in representations of Jewish rituals, but this alone does not explain why it would be suffused with a haunting affect. Anne's playful assumption of a French identity yields another possible explanation. Following the clue to listen in French, and bolstered by the frequent site of Anne playing with a marionette (also a word of French origin) to which is attached a violin, we are able to hear in the French word for "violin" the word *viol* (Figure 5.2).

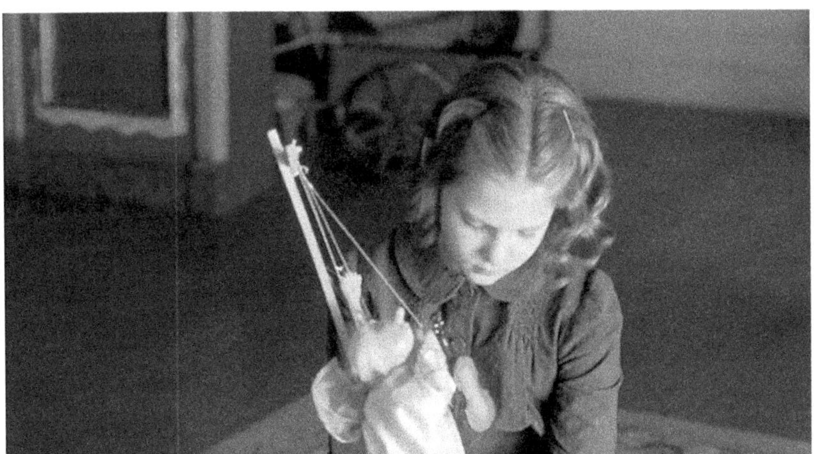

Figure 5.2 Marionette with violin.

Hearing the word *viol* when we see the violin, we are able to uncover the connotation of the word that the image seeks to conceal: *viol*, meaning "violation" or, as a verb, "to violate," as in to violate a law, or to violate (desecrate) a religious order or covenant. Implicit in both meanings is the notion of transgression. This sense is heightened by Anne's transgression of Grace's injunction against sitting on the bedroom floor in her communion dress. Grace's discovery of this transgression and its coincidence with Anne playing with the marionette ultimately trigger Grace's hallucination of the latter's possession.

The word *viol,* understood as "violation," also intimates the religious nature of the ancestor's transgression through an interlinguistic homophone. The French verb for "to violate," *violer*, as well as the past tense of the verb, as in "she violated," *elle a violé*, rhyme with a synonym of the French word for the color purple, *violet*, which we have seen connects Grace to the first Jewish convert, Lydia. The flower, from which the color derives its name, belongs to the genus *Viola* and thus fits into the linguistic chain of signifiers that we have established.

An imagistic cluster of violets and viols appears in a large stained glass window located in the front hall of the Stewart house. Its presence looms in almost every scene that takes place in the hall, and it is the sole object of the lingering camera when Grace, after hearing voices in the "junk room," searches the house for "intruders" by opening up all of the curtains. In a rapid sequence of shots during which rooms are illuminated for a mere second as if a flash went off, the extended duration of the camera's focus on the stained glass window both before and after it is illuminated is noteworthy. Amenábar's camera direction, accentuated by the eerie reverberation of cellos, supports this lexical deciphering of *viol* and violet. If Grace illuminates each room in order to uncover the intrusive presence, it is because haunting her is the tale of her ancestress' internal psychic drama involving a religious conversion (Figure 5.3).

Thus far, we have seen how the mystery of what haunts the Stewart house can be unlocked with the keys provided by the film's ciphered revelations, both imagistic and lexical. Its concern with knowledge that is unspeakable and quests that are unrecognized obliges us to render intelligible what must remain hidden for the characters. The significance of the music imagery lies in part in how it calls upon us to hear that to which the characters are deaf, while it suggests a means to identify the symbol fragments broken off from a haunting secret that is generative of Grace's experience. We can conclude from the foregoing discussion that what is haunting about *viols* for Grace is that they mutely voice her identity as a violator, not only, as the film's surface seems to suggest, as a result of her murderous actions; rather, her transgression is that she is the descendant of a Jewish woman who converted to Christianity and violated religious decorum (*OED*). What has yet to be explained is the

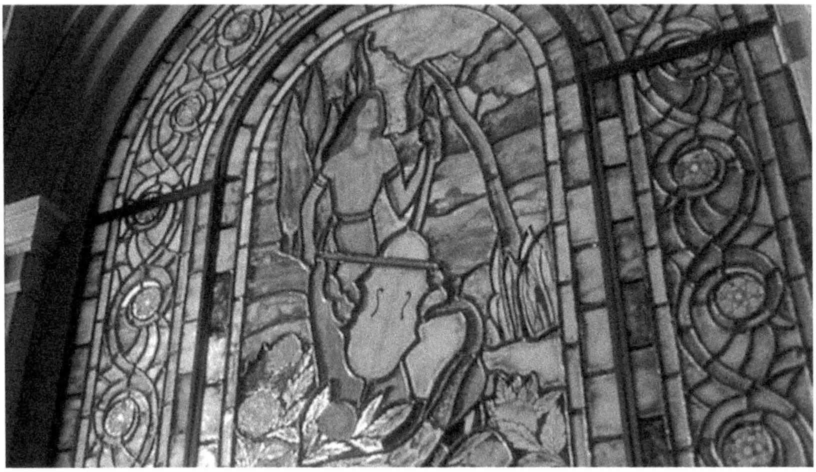

Figure 5.3 The viol/violoncello with violet frame.

conditions that led to the removal of the violation from speech whereby it was transmitted to Grace as unconscious knowledge.

The consistent confluence of issues involving madness and secrets suggests that madness itself is part of the secret drama encrypted within Grace's psyche and staged by her actions. Cryptic wordplay manifested in the hallucination scene as well as those that directly precede it concretely dramatize the obscured family history whose telltale traces are inscribed and readable within the film. The communion dress and hallucination scenes bring to the fore, literally and symbolically, the more deeply veiled aspect of the story. Haunted language, disguised lexical patterns, the means by which phantoms make their presence known, pervade these scenes as well as those that precede and separate them, and allow us to trace linguistic fragments back up toward their unspeakable signifying source or founding silence.

Charles Stewart's Return

Before we embark on this reading, however, it is important to note that the hallucination scene is one within a sequence of scenes that is bracketed by the arrival and departure of Charles Stewart. Grace did not find Father Legrand after she set out from the house, but she did come upon her children's father, who she assumes has finally returned from France. Her surprise, which is registered by her acknowledgment, "They said there was no hope. They said I should give you up for dead," also bespeaks some of the linguistic context of the circumstances that led to her psychotic breakdown. But Charles's enigmatic response, "They say a lot of things," injects a tone of ambiguity into the dialogue because it is not clear whether the referent for "they" is the one implied by Grace or, perhaps, is a cryptic reference to another context involving discussions of a death that has been elided from speech.

The ambiguity is magnified by Charles's reply to Grace's question about where he has been: "Out there, looking for my home." Given the specific and contained geography of Jersey Island, it is possible that Charles's statement does not refer to the physical location of the Stewart house per se but rather implies an extended sense of the term "home" to mean "the family or social unit occupying a house; a household" (*OED*). He does not elucidate why his household is difficult to find or identify, but his incongruous and bizarre utterance, "sometimes I bleed," as a rejoinder to Grace's observation that he is "so different" suggests that the reason might involve family lineage or bloodlines that are concealed. Indeed, the *OED* records that one meaning of the word "to bleed," namely, "to come to light," derives from the belief that that the body of a murdered man was supposed to bleed afresh when the murderer approached and thus reveal guilt. Embedded in Charles's comments are lexical fragments that connect to broader patterns and themes in the film: obscured family bloodlines, fear of enlightenment, and an unspeakable crime.

These three issues are tacitly underscored in a tense discussion between Grace and Anne that occurs immediately after Charles's return to the house and directly before the communion dress scene. Disappointment over Charles's absence at the lunch table—and his apparent apathy toward his family's excitement over his return—pervades the conversation; dialogue is initiated by Anne, who observes that her father had seen lots of dead men, and is punctuated by Grace's consistent attempts to stifle Anne's speech. Taken aback when Anne asks about what happens to people who die in the war, Grace invokes one's *identity* as a "goody" or a "baddy" as a decisive factor. But her vehement rebuff of Anne's request for clarification, which is followed by her categorical denial of the existence of the "intruders," notwithstanding her apparent acknowledgment of their presence the last time she and Anne were together, reveals a deep-seated anxiety about processes of identification. Contexts or conditions that require her to ascertain that a person is itself and not something else, a distinct impression presented to or perceived by others, in other words, are treated by Grace as needing to be shut out and excluded. This problem of identity ultimately catalyzes the disjunction that leads to Grace's vision of Anne's possession.

Hallucination of Anne's Possession

Anne's actions, which precede Grace's hallucination, display her assumption of a second identity, that of the Jewish "intruder." This duality is set up right in the beginning of the scene when Anne compares the reflection of her image in her communion dress with that of a bride. The sartorial overlap between the communion and wedding dresses is reflected linguistically as well: the word "communion" refers not only to the religious ceremony of receiving the Eucharist and thereby sanctifying a connection with Jesus, but it also more generally signifies a union between people, such as in the familial context of marriage. When Anne uses a French accent to invite an imaginary French man (*monsieur*) to dance, she acts out a drama of French courtship and marriage, a context that Anne fleshes out with her humming of a minuet tune.[19]

This is the same tune that Anne also hums when Grace sends her to the piano room, where she first encounters the "intruders." The suggestion that Anne's actions perform a temporally displaced scene that is implicated as a source of haunting is reinforced immediately following the marriage dance, when Anne faces the mirror and flips her veil over her face. Even if she did not emit the haunting noises, there is no doubt that she has converted herself into a ghost whose haunting derives from an act of concealment: Anne literally *veils* herself.[20] The motion of turning the veil, moreover, accentuates the sense of conversion. Anne's range of altered voices reveal the collective dimensions of the secret: from the French accent of the woman who initiates an invitation to dance; to the low-pitched response it elicits from a putative suitor; to the spectral "woooos" vocalized by the ghost; to the cackle that follows them, which, we soon discover, belongs to the repertoire of the medium who Grace hallucinates as possessing Anne. All of these voices point to an altered identity that was wrapped up in silence and transmitted transgenerationally.

The convocation of voices in Anne's speech evokes the context of a séance, which summons spirits to explain particular paranormal phenomena. Anne's language –both speech and actions translated into language—mimics the historicizing gesture of a séance. Séance, or, in French, *seoir*, refers to collective sittings, the arena in which spiritual communication may be conducted. Obscured by the overdetermined connotation of the word *seoir* as "spiritual sitting," is its connection to a lexical chain of words that denote processes of transformation, "becoming," as well as more precise notions of "fitting in," and "suiting up." The latter two connotations, which are sustained by semantic chains devolving on sewing, dresses, and dressing up, reveal how, by dressing Anne, Grace reenacts the means by which her ancestress camouflaged her Jewish identity. Grace's "suiting up" of Anne replicates how the ancestress layered and veiled her Jewish identity in her communion with a Catholic man. Anne "becomes" the hidden identity whose presence haunts Grace: She "suits up" to become an unknown Jewish bride.

If Grace's veiling of Anne as a bride unwittingly stages a commitment to concealing the "religious transvestism"[21] of her ancestress, her subsequent command for Anne "to take the dress off" unwittingly threatens its exposure. This explains why Grace hallucinated Anne's possession by the medium immediately thereafter: The phantom's emergence was triggered by this linguistic transgression. To understand why Grace was so susceptible to this fragmentation, it is helpful to contextualize more broadly the affective conditions that lead to Grace's delusion.

When Grace enters her daughter's room she is desolate over the emotional abandonment of her husband, from whom she has just come. This context is crucial for understanding why her vision of Anne triggers a psychotic fantasy. In an effort to encourage Charles to eat and engage more with her and the children, Grace sings to him a song entitled "I Only Have Eyes for You." Harry Warren and Al Dublin wrote the song for the 1934 Warner Brothers film *Dames*. Given Amenábar's attention to musical details as symbols pertaining to the silenced saga, we might expect this overdetermined quotation to be relevant in a similar way.

It is. *Dames* is about a family who, financially beholden to a rich uncle whose promise of an inheritance is contingent upon adherence to a specific moral code, does its best to hide the fact from him that a daughter is the lead in a so-called scandalous Broadway show. On the surface, the film's premise of a family's dealing with issues of inheritance, scandal, and deception certainly resonates with those of Grace's saga. But it is the surreal quality of Busby Berkeley's production of the "I Only Have Eyes for You" song-and-dance number, which theatrically acts out scenes of unconscious substitutions that bring even greater clarity to Grace's story.

Berkeley executes the act through the repetitious superimposition of an image of the head of the daughter—the person to whom the song is sung—on other women's heads, via placards that are held to conceal their real faces. The stage, full of multiple daughters, is arranged so that the placard-carrying girls ultimately form a gigantic headshot, an image that dissolves into a close-up of the eye out of which the "real" daughter rises. The scene's emphasis on the suspect nature of perspective, which is underscored by Berkeley's constant shifting of frames of reference, calls to mind the multiplicity of Annes reflected in the linguistic associations between Grace's and Anne's proper names and their relation to an intersubjective and intergenerational drama of Jewish matriarchy. While I do not mean to suggest that Berkeley's song-and-dance sequence should be interpreted as evidence that Berkeley's production points to a phantomatic dimension of *Dames*—although critics have examined the psychoanalytical implications of his work—the convergence of the song and a visual style evocative of unconscious processes of identity formation in the meta-theatrical production dovetails with several aesthetic dimensions of *The Others*.

This comparison is justified, I believe, by what appears to be a direct quote by Amenábar of Berkeley's cinematographic "sleight of hand" in his presentation of the hallucination scene. Specifically, to indicate Grace's awakening from her delusion of her daughter's possession, Amenábar uses a mirror to shift the frame of reference back from the object of Grace's gaze to Grace herself; this reflects Berkeley's abstract use of time and space and implicitly locates Grace's mental discontinuity in a source beyond herself.[22] The song that Grace sings in response to her husband's emotional abandonment can now be seen as a piece of the puzzle that prepares us to apprehend the scene that follows.

The words and images of the hallucination scene are all carriers of veiled lexical relationships that mutely articulate the shameful secret haunting Grace. Grace perceives Anne's disregard of her command to keep the dress "spotless" and not sit on the floor as a violation. The force of Grace's reprimand, which she utters when she first enters the room and sees Anne sitting on the floor, dramatically dissipates with the last three words: "What did I tell you about sitting on the floor ... Why can't you ever do as you're told ..." The camera reveals, via Grace's expression, that the source of this diffusion lies in something that Grace has seen. This vocal shift mirrors the ostensible shift from "sanity" to "fantasy." Careful examination of the images that comprise the object of Grace's vision during this shift reveals a particular pattern, which communicates a specific message when they are translated into language.

The first image that we see in Grace's line of sight is the marionette, whose haunting potential was foreshadowed in the eerie opening credit scenes. Amenábar uses a close-up shot to emphasize Grace's focus on the object. The puppet is in the form of an angel, which evokes a constellation of religious and psychoanalytical connotations. The angel is an iconographic religious symbol, "the arch mediator between absolute Otherness and humanity, between the creator and the creature."[23] Its role as a messenger, moreover, shores up faith in an omniscient and transcendent God, whose intentions can be discerned, notwithstanding the separation between the physical and metaphysical.

The angel's mediating significance is demonstrated through the language of puppetry, which embodies a concealed doubleness. The magic of the marionette puppet derives in part from the knowledge that there is significant separation between the agent of the puppet's movements and the puppet itself. It evokes the way a secret may be communicated silently from parent to child. The marionette epitomizes a position of being held or bound in a group dynamic constituted by adherence to a puppeteer's grammar. Just as the marionette is suspended by strings and controlled by someone's hand, so too does the presence of a phantom "hold the child (later the adult) ... in a silent partnership dedicated to preserving the secret intact."[24] The age and gender of the angel makes it clear just who that partner is: a Jewish ancestor who hid her identity, converted, and married into a Catholic family.

The shot following the close-up of the marionette reveals the gnarled hand of the old woman. Amenábar's slow pan of the camera underscores the narrative significance of the sequence: It points to the external source of Grace's haunting, the secret that was "handed" down to her thought the family as a silent psychic bequest.

The acoustic language that accompanies this visual sequence contributes to its uncanny quality. Anne's extended humming of the minuet tune is appropriately echoic of the context we have elucidated so far. Humming, singing without articulation, is associated with "hesitation, embarrassment or affectation" (*OED*). The idea of a collective psychology that is reflected in Anne's vocal alterations, and the séance, is also suggested in the connotation of the verb "to hum," namely, "to give forth an indistinct sound by the blending of many voices" (*OED*). Anne's murmuring thus reminds us to "hear" what Grace sees: The interlinguistic connection between the word "murmur" and *murmure* (from which "murmur" is derived) reminds us to listen in French.

At this point, it should not be a surprise that the object that triggered Grace's hallucination, the *marionette*, is a French word. According to the *OED*, the etymology of the term derives from the word *mariole* (Marie, the Virgin Mary), for "image of the Virgin Mary." *Marionette* represents a diminutive form of Maryam derived from Marianne, the Judeo-Aramaic form of (the Virgin) Mary. Marianne derived from Marie + Anne linguistically conflates Anne's (Mary's mother's) name with that of Mary's, and implicitly with that of Grace, because the Hebrew *Maryām* is thought to be derived from the Amorite word for "grace" or the "gift of God" (*OED*). The word *marionette* thus recapitulates the concatenation of transgenerational matrilineal experience that haunts Grace.

This context deepens the relevance of the film's overt references to the Virgin Mary. Grace demands that Anne ask for the Virgin Mary's forgiveness for her transgression of lying about the "intruders." Significantly, Anne's refusal to ask forgiveness leads her to reveal Grace's ineptitude with Catholic dogma. The Virgin Mary is thus implicated in a context of contesting truths. This context is extended to the realm of haunting in the second reference to the Virgin Mary, when Grace, finally convinced (temporarily) that there are "intruders," searches for them in a "junk room." The room is filled with objects that are shrouded with sheets—visually anticipating Anne's vision of ghostly bearings. Evidence of the "intruders'" presence is manifested aurally. What Grace hears is a dialogue between the old woman, the symbolic incarnation of Grace's ancestress; Victor Marlish, a young boy of the living family who inhabits the house and with whom Anne has interacted; and Mrs Marlish:

MEDIUM: She's here, she's here.
VICTOR: Mummy, she says she's here.
MRS. MARLISH: Shhhh.—She's what? She's what?
MEDIUM: (Groaning): Huh … Ooohhh …

Terrified by the ejaculation of the medium, which conveys fear and sadness, Grace backs away and bumps into the *hand* of an obscured figure, which she *unveils* to reveal a statue of the Virgin Mary, *mariole*. Shocked and frenzied, Grace continues to uncover a few more objects including, finally, a mirror, which stops her in her tracks. Grace's reflection shocks because she unconsciously sees herself as the Virgin Mary, a daughter of a Jewish woman who was (eventually) transformed into a Christian; Amenábar's meticulous camerawork with the mirror links this experience of unconscious awareness to her reaction to what she sees as Anne's possession.

When confronted with that image, the generational dissonance produced by the image of the woman's face and Anne's youthful voice, Grace becomes hysterical. This mismatch, or disorder, is perceived by Grace in terms of displacement. Her daughter is not where she should be: She screams, "You are not my daughter" and attempts to choke her, tearing the veil in the process (Figure 5.4).

Grace's reaction to Anne's displacement implies that her hallucination is linked to a family rearrangement. These associations are supported by lexical relationships in French, which connect the idea of being dismissed from a familial order or "rank," French *rang*, to "madness" *déranger*, "deranged." Anne's displacement is horrifying to Grace because what had been veiled—her disguised Jewish heritage—was brought to light. With Anne absent, Grace sees the unspeakable secret of her life: a woman whose religious mask has been exposed and brought to light (by the candle).

More details about this scenario emerge when we listen closely to the word "marionette." Pronounced in French, we can hear that concealed therein there are actually *two* French words: *mari* and *honnête*. The sound *mari* is homophonous with three other words that create a lexical chord of reverberating meanings that intersect with the film's symbolic patterns: *mari*, "husband"; *Marie*, "Mary"; and *marie*, "to marry" (as in the present tense, *je marie*, I marry); and finally *marri*, "to be aggrieved, distressed." When combined with the word *honnête*, the two words form the locution "honest husband."

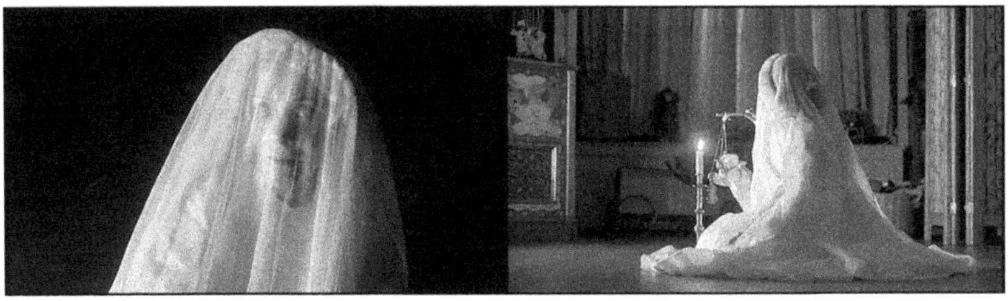

Figure 5.4 Anne's possession.

A veiled articulation of the source of Grace's psychic affliction is contained in this intralinguistic cryptonym. The vision of the marionette, coupled with the dissonance between image and sound, confronts Grace with the horrible scene of a Jewish woman whose concealed identity was exposed and the "honest husband" who would not lie to preserve her religious sham. If the marionette provokes in Grace a vision of displacement, it is because the ancestress' dishonor brought shame to the family. The opposite of an honest or "honorable husband," Grace's disgraced ancestor was *une femme déshonorée.*

In light of the interlinguistic quality of some of the film's wordplay, it is worthwhile to note that the French word for "shame," *honte*, rhymes with the English word "haunt"; Grace is indeed haunted by the shame suffered by an ancestress. Charles's dismissive treatment links him to her ancestor's husband who displaced her from her position in the family and abandoned her.

Although the film does not delineate in great detail why the French ancestress concealed her Jewishness nor the conditions that led to its discovery, several components do, nonetheless, point to a sociohistorical context: the emancipation of Jews in 1791, which allowed Jews to integrate into society in a way that blurred what had been clear identifiable markers of Jewish identity.[25] "Dressing up" or "suiting up" allowed people of Jewish heritage to move within Catholic circles without detection. This explains how Grace's French grandmother, who married above her born station or rank in life, might have concealed her Jewish identity. It also offers a possible explanation for how the ancestress' true identity might have been discovered: namely, if she had dressed the part of a convert to Catholicism but privately still adhered to Jewish rituals and customs.

The conflict played out between Grace and Anne, over what is a "true" truth and a lie, offers more perspective. We see how Anne's role as a truth-teller is the source of their contention. For example, right after Anne reads aloud the story of Abraham's sacrifice, just when Grace is made aware of the presence of unexplainable elements, Grace asks,

"Anne, tell me who's making that noise?"
"I can't tell you, mummy."
-"You tell me."
"I told you there was someone in the room and you punished me! Now I don't know what to say!"
"Anne, I want the truth!"

Of course what Grace wants is the version of truth that conceals the secret. Grace's extreme oscillation between acknowledging and denying the existence of the "intruders" is a symptom borne of the effect of a conscious lie perpetrated by someone else. Anne threatens to divulge deeds that are believed to be incriminating, while Grace, mummy, wants to keep them mum. Ultimately, Grace literally forces Anne to gag on the truth: She suffocates Anne to prohibit her from breathing a word about it.

Along these lines, Anne's superior grasp of Catholic dogma suggests that it was the daughter of the ancestress who exposed the secret of her mother's Jewish heritage. Recall that Anne revealed the "truth" of the day Grace "went mad" to her father; their rapport, separate and distinct from Grace, points to a possible alignment. In Grace's accusation that Anne is not her daughter, we hear the outrage of a mother toward the daughter who denounces her. The dynamic between Grace and Anne refines our perspective to the point that we are able to suggest that the agent of shame was the ancestress, but what haunts Grace and her children is the daughter's experience of it.

The film does not provide enough information to reconstruct with precision the processes by which the secret was generated. Nonetheless, it does yield a constellation of symbols that allow us to conjecture two more pieces of the puzzle. For example, the film intimates that either the ancestress or her daughter committed suicide by hanging: Thread motifs, such as Grace's needlework, her stitch work on the dress and veil, not to mention the broken-necked marionette strings, link her preoccupation to a concealed hanging. In addition, when Grace rips Anne's veil, she enacts a Jewish mourning ritual, *kriah*, a ritual that belongs to a broader practice of Jewish mourning known as *sitting shiva*; the tear represents a sorrowful heart rent by the loss of a love object.

Sitting shiva lasts seven days following the burial of a deceased loved one. The word "shiva" derives from the Hebrew word "seven," as does the name of the ritual of Shabbat, a day of rest. When Grace paraphrased God's creation of the world in the film's opening, she excised the part of Genesis that narrates the creation of humankind; this omission was accompanied by lacunae with regard to the number of days it took for God to create the world, and the day of rest, the cosmic origins of Shabbat practice. If we recall that the film's mimesis begins seven days after "that day,"[26] and consider the centrality of problematic mourning for Grace, it is likely that the aforementioned clues implicate the practice of Jewish rituals in a Jewish woman's suicide.

There is striking commonality between *The Others* and French narratives that are haunted by the inscription within them of secrets involving concealed Jewish identity. Esther Rashkin links the production of the phantom narratives to the emergence of secular forms of anti-Semitism that were catalyzed by French Jewish emancipation. Literary scholars who investigate the representation of Jews in European discourses attest to the catalyzing role played by the historical French Revolution, and its concomitant emancipation of the Jews, in shaping modern concepts of national identity. Scholars of the French Revolution are in consensus that the figure of the Jew was of special rhetorical significance during this period, even if there is division with regard to how to interpret it.[27] Michael Ragussis claims that the rhetorical inclination of the French (revolutionaries) to use the figure of the Jew as a discursive means to reconfigure what citizenship means in post-revolution France is also reflected in "figures of conversion" that permeate English national identity discourse. The trope of conversion, argues Ragussis, developed in the project of writing English nationalist history and was deployed to erase "racial and cultural difference."[28]

Ragussis argues that the source of spectral haunting in British gothic literature is a collective fear of Jewish assimilation. The trope of the converted Jew makes it clear that Jewishness is "an essential characteristic that may not be eradicated."[29] Grace's manic intention that the communion dress remain "spotless," along with the film's repetitive invocations of the Virgin Mary's "spotless" purity, bears traces of such stigmatization. British fear that Jewishness was a form of "disease that may contaminate Christian Britain"[30] is intimated in the film's representation of Anne and Nicholas's suffering from an "inherited disease," the contaminating source of which is revealed to be concealed Jewish identity.

Grace's Crypt

Now that we have reconstituted the secret, we are in a position to explain the film's ambiguity surrounding the conditions that triggered Grace's fatal actions. After Anne speaks with Charles about Grace's outburst, during which she also revealed information about when "mummy went mad," he demands to know from Grace what happened between them. Grace explains that something "came over" her that day as a result of the servants' craven departure the night before, when they knew that she would be unable to leave the house. Anne's account of what happened that day more simply refers to Grace's descent into madness; she makes no mention of the servants. Given Grace's earlier admission to Charles that she was urged to "give you up for dead," and given the new servants' awareness of their postmortem existence, which implies that said departed servants would also have been able to discriminate between people who are dead and alive, another possible chronology emerges: namely, that Grace apprehended the death of her husband, went mad, killed her children and then herself; the servants' departure was a *consequence*, and not the *cause*, of Grace's actions. Her inversion of the chronology must be viewed as symptomatic of her need to remain blind to—in fact deny—the true cause of her madness: the loss of her beloved husband.[31]

Although one could ascribe Grace's psychotic breakdown to the extreme shock of her loss, not to mention the acuteness of feelings of abandonment, especially after having survived the horrendous circumstances of Nazi occupation in full of anticipation of a reunion, the film's foregrounding of Grace's symptomatic blindness to her own death suggests that the same psychic structure that obstructs her awareness is in fact consequential of her blindness to Charles's death. Grace's use of the locution "something came over me" to describe her response to being abandoned conjures the arrival of a phantom.

Grace's discussion with Charles in the aftermath of her hallucination brings to the fore sheds more light on the link between her blocked mourning and the family drama of religious conversion that she must preserve. After her disclosure of what occurred "that day," Charles responds to Grace's request for forgiveness by telling her that he "just came back to say goodbye to his wife and children, now I must go." Incredulous that Charles plans to "go back to the front," Grace fiercely demands that he stay:

> You're not going, do you hear me? You left us once. You can't go! Why? Why did you go to that stupid war that had nothing to do with us? Why didn't you stay like the others? ... What were you trying to prove by going to war? Your place was here, with us. With your family.

As Grace gropes to understand Charles's motivation for leaving, she hints that there is something in her family story that essentially brought her to this point. In her diatribe, Grace links her experience of abandonment to actions related to the preservation of Jewish lives and identity. Her relationship with Charles thus emerges as a symbol of the unspeakable trauma involving her family. Consider, for example, that as a Stewart, a guardian, Charles, by virtue of his patronym, functioned for Grace—unconsciously—as life-preserving, someone whose family name identified him as an appropriate partner for the ensnared life that Grace must live as the inheritor of a phantom. She suggests as much a bit later in the dialogue when she speaks of how she could endure the prison-like house if only Charles were with her.

Grace emphasizes what she sees as the irrelevance of Charles's decision to go to a war "that has nothing to do with us."[32] This recalls an earlier conversation she has, with her son Nicholas, on the topic of their father's participation in the war. Grace, tucking the children into bed, tells him that his father "went ... he went ... because he wasn't prepared to let the Germans tell him what he had to do." She responds to Nicholas's follow-up question of "why" with only silence. What accounts for a gap in her speech surrounding Charles's rejection of German orders to persecute Jews that would also account for her claim that the war is irrelevant to them? Charles's unwillingness to stay with his family, and his insistent identification with an effort to defeat an enemy whose central concern was to *expose* and displace Jews from the *ranks* of society, strongly reverberates with Grace's unconscious knowledge of her ancestress' saga. In this aspect of Charles, Grace unknowingly sees the *honest husband* who abandons his wife for reasons related to Jewish identity.

This conversation sounds like one that Grace and Charles may have had before his initial departure to the war; the affective conditions may have triggered the return of a phantom. In this light, cognizance of his death put Grace in an impossible (unconscious) double bind: acknowledging his loss would mean having to acknowledge her resentment of having been abandoned by Charles to go to the war; this risked exposing the secret about the honest husband who abandoned his wife. Charles's return home can now be understood as a hallucination, produced to resist disrupting the psychic status-quo. Just as Su-mi's psyche deceives her into thinking that Su-yeon is still alive, so too does Grace sustain the fantasy that Charles's death has been psychically digested, in order to deny that it ever occurred. Grace's blindness to her existential status serves as a screen for her inability to psychically bury Charles. The film implies that the question of who is dead and alive is not metaphysical but metapsychological: In *The Others*, the dead are the psychically unburied.

In the film's final mise-en-scène the Stewarts' language exhibits a specific speech pattern, which Nicolas Abraham and Maria Torok have claimed is characteristic in people who suffer blocked mourning catalyzed by preservative repression. The pattern refers to the way a word's meaning is truncated in order to support the psyche's denial that a loss has occurred. The process is decontaminative; it drains words of negative affects by circumscribing the metaphoric scope of their denotative force. Negative words become positive; excrement becomes delicious.[33] We see this occur when Grace, Anne, and Nicholas's apprehend the truth of their deaths. For example, Anne and Nicholas's newfound capacity to withstand sunlight without harm, drains from the word "sun" another possible, metaphorical, connotations, such as "enlightenment." Likewise, the palpable reassurance derived from the Stewarts' mantra-like repetition of the phrase "this house is ours" derives from draining "house" of its capacity to connote family lineage.

I will demonstrate how these lexical patterns of avoidance derive from collective rhetorical antecedents that bore directly on processes of English collective memory formation. Amenábar himself signals a shift in focus from Grace's saga to a broader allegorical perspective in his penultimate shot of the film. First, Amenábar establishes a master long shot from outside the house; it shows us the family standing by a window, looking outward and chanting. Shortly thereafter, Amenábar pans slowly to establish a point-of-view shot from Victor's perspective. Because we know that Grace and her children are apparitions, the transfer to Victor's point of view indicates that Grace's story, that is, her saga and crypt (the dead but alive people who inhabit it), is actually a construct of his psyche. An earlier comment made by Mrs Marlish reinforces this idea. Rejecting her husband's assurance that Victor had not suffered from the impact of haunting Mrs Marlish claims, "Yes there is [something wrong with Victor], he has nightmares and he has seen the girl." Indeed, Grace's defiant assertion that "no one will ever make us leave" intimates that her saga is an intractable dimension of Victor's selfhood.

Historical Extension

The film's idiom proves a useful guide for reconstructing the sociohistorical and political conditions that are the absent complements of the film. Victor's proper name, which is also a noun meaning "one who overcomes or vanquishes an adversary" (*OED*), offers a promising starting point for the exploration of concealed national experience. Given the film's setting in post-occupation Jersey, Victor's name may understandably be read as a metonym for England, victorious in its fight with Nazi Germany. While the Nazi occupation of Jersey does establish a context for unspoken historical secrets regarding Jewish identity, the film's clear depiction of Victor, or England, as haunted by the *Stewart* family's shameful secret, suggests a different interpretive position: namely, that Grace's private tale inscribes within it traces of a shameful English collective trauma related to religious oppression during the life of another Stuart, King Charles I (r. 1626–1649). I will suggest that his reign, and the traumatic conditions that lead to his death, catalyzed an obstacle to national self-fashioning, and I will demonstrate how the legacy of this blockage intersects with Grace's phantom. This will allow us to explain why Victor, at that particular moment, was haunted by Grace's family drama.

Reinforcement for this interpretative gesture is found in a highly determined yet ciphered reference, in *The Others,* to King Charles I. The allusion appears in the form of a detail of a celebrated painting, William Shakespeare Burton's *The Wounded Cavalier* (1855), a copy of which is stored in the junk room that Grace searches for evidence of the intruders. Prized for its naturalism and realism, Burton's painting was seen from its inception as freighted with historical, nationalistic, and religious significance: It is an allegorical portrait of the Civil War (1642–1652), the repercussions of which still reverberate in representations of English national consciousness. I will illustrate in more detail the implications of Amenábar's artistic citation for our understanding of English collective memory formation but, first, some context.

The century preceding Charles Stuart's reign was marked by complex and traumatic social transformations. The story starts with Henry VIII's (r. 1509–1547) wish to abandon his first wife. Because divorce was not sanctioned by the English Church, which had adhered to the rules of the See of Rome for almost a millennium, Henry generated legislative acts to establish a Church of England.[34] He desired that this Church sanction his marriage to an English-born woman and annul his marriage to Queen Catherine of Aragon, the daughter of Isabelle I and Ferdinand II, who established the Spanish Inquisition.[35] The legislative acts made Catholic worship impractical if not dangerous; they established a new grammar for spiritual practice with violent repercussions for families who did not adhere. The imposition of a new religious grammar required that English subjects abandon symbolic systems of signification that had structured collective consciousness. Catholic religious rituals had provided schemata for making sense of existence; our interest is in tracing the affective impact of this epistemological change on collective memory formation.

Henry VIII's religious transformation was instigated by a *violation* of Roman Catholic authority. English historian Robert Ashton, who observes "Henry VIII had no real intention of reforming the Church but rather intended only to secure the succession by a divorce which he could only ensure if he controlled the necessary machinery of the Church of England," situates his religious violation in the context of a family drama about abandoning a wife.[36]

As is the case when new epistemological and semiotic systems are imposed by fiat on a collective, there are limited opportunities for that collective to grieve the loss of what was displaced. Such was the case of the eradication of Catholicism by the Church of England. The repression extended to language that mourned the displacement of Queen Catherine, whose renowned religious devotion may be one reason that she was an object of collective affection. Her religious zeal counteracted Henry's violation of the Catholic Church; discussions about her became taboo lest they were misunderstood as challenges to the Church of England's spiritual authority. In short, Henry's religious legislation rendered affection for Catholic rituals, rites, and Queen Catherine, retroactively clandestine. These conditions inhibited the possibility of naming what was lost and thus mourning it.

The components of Henry VIII's family drama—which concerns an abandoned wife, problematic religious identity, shame, and blocked mourning—resonate with the central elements of Grace's secret. It suggests that Grace's secret refracts a national drama that was catalyzed by one monarch's family saga. But notwithstanding the remarkable overlaps between the themes of Grace and Henry's family sagas, Amenábar's citation of *The Wounded Cavalier* within the context of Grace's haunting tells us that the collective memory of Charles Stuart's reign specifically is what haunts England.

Burton's *The Wounded Cavalier* evokes the conflict generated by dilemmas of loyalty during the Civil War, when those loyal to King

Charles, the Royalists, represented by the Cavalier, fought against the Parliamentarians, represented by the Puritan, over issues of royal prerogative.[37] The painting depicts a scene from the English Civil War, in which a Puritan woman comforts a Royalist while her lover looks on. The painting appears in the scene in which Grace, still searching for the intruders, finds herself in a room full of furniture and photos that belonged to the former inhabitants of the house. This scene directly follows the extended illumination of the stained-glass violoncello, a symbol of religious violation and transgression. Breathing heavily, Grace enters the room holding a gas lamp, which she places on a table. As she turns to open the curtains, the image of a heavily shadowed face appears to look over her shoulder. Amenábar uses the same illuminating technique that he deployed to draw attention on the violoncello to bring definition to the amorphous facial image; once illuminated, the image resolves into a painting on the wall. The narrow focus of the lens reveals a close-up of the Puritan lover. This overdetermined bracketing implores us to unpack the symbols that connect the film, Burton's painting, and a particular shameful collective experience involving the Stewart family (Figure 5.5).

As an allegorical portrait of the Civil War, the death of the Royalist refers to the death of the object of Royalist devotion, the monarch Charles Stuart. The invocation of the word "cavalier" (equestrian) not only denotes the Royalist political position, but it also evokes the "predominant leitmotif of the reign of Charles I," which was established in a series of portraits by his court painter, Sir Anthony Van Dyck.[38] The term "Cavalier" was applied derogatively in 1642 to refer to the professional soldiers that the king was gathering as his armed following. It was

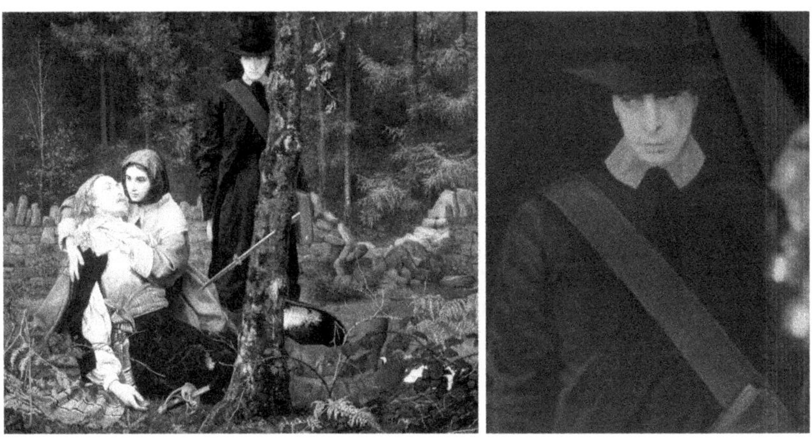

Figure 5.5 William Shakespeare Burton's "The Wounded Cavalier"; courtesy of HIP/Art Resources, NY; juxtaposed with Amenábar's detail of the Puritan.

Spanish [read Catholic] for "horseman" or "soldier." The term implied that these men were the enemies of the godly people of Protestant England. The depiction of the imminent death of the Cavalier in Burton's painting, therefore, is a commentary on the Regicide.[39]

The scowling image of the Puritan meshes with Grace's shameful drama of religious approbation and serves an analogous purpose in Burton's painting. Terry Boardman has shown how Burton's depiction of the Puritan, who holds a Bible, implies that he is the source of the Cavalier's death—through the spatial contiguity of the broken blade of the sword that caused the fatal blow. He notes too the level of the Puritan's hand, which appears as if the Puritan is holding a sword that proceeds from the Bible down diagonally toward the Cavalier's wound.[40] Implicating the Puritan as perpetrator of the death of the Cavalier tacitly condemns the English Church as an accomplice in the Regicide. The Puritan's distrustful visage reflects suspicion of King Charles's policies, which had Catholic inflections. One such accent is emblematized by the Cavalier's sartorial elegance, which mirrors favored ritual practices associated in the popular mind with Roman Catholicism: Some scholars refer to this political feature as crypto-Catholicism.[41] The Puritan's expression conveys a position that views the cavalier's existence as an explicit attack on the reformed Church of England.

Charles Stuart's crypto-Catholic policies themselves have been viewed as a symptomatic response to the excesses of Henry VIII's legislative acts to break from the authority of the Pope and the Roman Catholic Church.[42] Historians have viewed the marriage between Charles I and his wife, Henrietta Maria, who was French Catholic, as a contributing factor to his proclivity toward Catholic-inflected rituals to assert his royal prerogative.[43] His idiom of rule, his preference for a political aesthetic replete with emotional associations reminiscent of French Catholic rituals, may have brought to the surface political and religious affective continuities with medieval English Catholicism that English Protestantism sought to belie.[44] Burton's painting brings to the fore the persistent presence of an anxiety over a national identity that devolves on the "antithesis between continental Catholicism and insular Protestantism."[45] The artist's realist aesthetic viscerally portrays this widely acknowledged political drama of religious intolerance. But his painting "complicates matters" by introducing into a visual allegory of religious division an implication of "the possibility of an amorous attraction between the cavalier and the Puritan lady who is nursing him."[46]

The complication is conveyed through Burton's compositional strategy. The canvas is divided by the standing Puritan, whose position in the center of the painting—behind the trunk of a birch tree—vertically cuts the scene in half; the bisection reflects the divisive impact of Puritanism during King Charles's reign. The axial position of the Puritan, which suggests an authoritative status, however, is in fact undermined by the compelling interest of the rich human saga that occupies the left part of the painting. This paradoxical position functions as a linchpin around which notions of national and religious identity first coalesce but then break down.

Burton's composition implies that the source of the breakdown of national and religious identity is connected to what transpires between the Cavalier and the Puritan woman. Terry Boardman notes the artist's painstaking detail with regard to the accouterments of the dying chevalier that "litter" the sparse space, such as the hat on the ground; his boots, no longer of use; and a playing card with a single heart on it lying among the brambles, all silently speak of what has not been shown: how the couple happened upon the Cavalier, what occurred in the course of the fight, not to mention the nature of the relationship between the woman and the dying man. If the Puritan's clenched jaw and piercing glare reflect jealousy, it also conveys a discomfort triggered by the Puritan woman's sentimental attachment to the Cavalier, whose disarrayed artifacts by extension represent the cultural sensibility and religious milieu of Continental Catholicism. Indeed, the emotional tension of the painting is enhanced by the possibility that the Puritan woman's attraction to the wounded soldier is the unsettling, yet invigorating stimulus that the Chevalier's aesthetic exerts on a romantic spirit obliged to fulfill religious loyalties.[47]

Burton's Puritan woman "unwittingly challenges the claims to national and religious distinctiveness and superiority."[48] In this vein, the Puritan man's emotional unrest may derive from what he perceives as an ineradicable intimacy between England and its Catholic past. The affective attachment to Catholicism taints and thwarts Protestant projections of English national consciousness. The Puritan woman's position expresses a fervor (of pre-Reformation England) that cannot be disguised by her Puritan garb. Her attraction to the Cavalier allows the viewer to look back onto the Catholic England of old, to see an image of England where affective sensibilities were the lifeblood of social and religious life. The Puritan's visage reveals how he sees in this gesture an "unwelcome, ghostly reminder of an erstwhile English self."[49]

Burton's romantic context exposes an omission in the narrative of England's religious history advanced by the Puritans responsible for King Charles's death. This narrative "ignores the complex, violent reality of coercion and resistance, of torture and martyrdom, and of reverses and compromises that often drove the process of religious reform."[50] Burton's painting reflects a collective memory agitated by the incompatibility of a triumphalist perspective of English religious unity and the reality of England's Catholic origins. The incompatibility of two different relationships with England's Catholic past is the affective precondition of the English Civil War. The discordance manifested itself in the execution of

Charles I; this led to problematic collective mourning, which effectuated what one scholar has called "cultural amnesia."[51]

Studies of literary trends that emerged in the wake of the Regicide attest to its traumatic impact on collective memory formation processes.[52] Many scholars acknowledge the general desire to repress "'the Fatal day' that [the Parliamentarians] asked to be 'from time … blotted quite'";[53] the Regicide "created a rupture within the collective psyche"[54] that had a haunting effect. The desire to exempt the collective from having to psychically process the experience is manifested linguistically in lexical patterns that reveal obstacles to expression in contemporary writings. Especially challenging was the inaptness of "the old mold of the organic analogy," which linked the king's body to the body politic. The origin of this linguistic vacuum has been explained in terms of trauma.[55] The linguistic inadequacy was also an index of a resistance against master historical narratives promoted by the Parliamentarians, which lacked impartial historical accounts of the event.[56]

Alex Garganigo invokes Abraham and Torok's theory of preservative repression to explain the breakdown in significations regarding King Charles I's death.[57] He cites a poem ostensibly written to celebrate Oliver Cromwell, a signatory of King Charles's death warrant, who ruled the short-lived Commonwealth of England as a member of the Parliament (1649–1653). In the poem, however, King Charles's "severed head pops up like a repressed memory to sabotage the whole [honorific] enterprise." Garganigo interprets the salience of allusions to Charles's decapitation pressed between the lines of the paean to Cromwell's commonwealth, as examples of rhetorical impoverishment that results when language is drained of its metaphoric range; the trauma, Garganigo argues, rendered the metaphor of the body politic inadequate for naming Cromwellian rule.[58]

Garganigo notes that representations of the king's bloody decapitated body are frequently expressed in terms that eroticize it and make it desirable; he claims that this linguistic pattern vitiates the memory of the trauma in its apparent denial of grief and loss.[59] But, according to Abraham and Torok, these linguistic processes are triggered not simply by a trauma but a trauma that involves the preservation of a *shameful* secret. Garganigo's analysis does not identify the collective secret that would account for the truncating of language's metaphorical range seen in the literary texts. To confirm that such lexical patterns point to the presence of a secret, we would need to approach the eroticized expressions as textual fragments that symbolize with a concealed shameful experience.

While this is not something I can pursue here, Garganigo's insights about literary trends triggered by the Regicide reinforce the idea that collective mourning of King Charles's death was problematic. I submit that the eroticization of King Charles I anticipates William Shakespeare Burton's complex portrait of a Puritan woman, whose attraction to the Cavalier imbues her with an eroticized sensibility. Charles's Cavalier ruling idiom agitated a collective memory that had repressed its attachment to England's Catholic origins as a result of violent processes of religious reform. Just as Grace's mourning of Charles was obstructed because it threatened the revelation of her shameful family saga of religious differences, so too were collective mourning processes thwarted in the wake of Charles I's execution; language was unavailable for collective communication because acknowledging his death would require acknowledging the secret of England's Catholic origins, which had fatal implications in a society organized and ruled by a triumphalist perspective of English religious unity.

Thus, King Charles lives dead but alive in the texts written about the Commonwealth. *The Others* suggests that such is the case in collective memory as well: Because the affective charge of King Charles's death could not be named, processed, and therefore memorialized, he lives, encrypted in collective memory, to exert a silent but traceable influence on English self-fashioning processes. Amenábar's film is thus about more than Grace's unmourned loss and an unspeakable secret of religious transgression that lives buried alive in an intrapsychic crypt; it is also about the collective trauma experienced at the death of another Charles Stuart at the hands of Puritan oppressors and the impossibility of mourning this loss.

Returning to Victor, in whose psyche the crypt of the Stewart family secret is concealed, will allow us to uncover the film's implicit metahistorical commentary. The association between the Stewart family and the Royal House of Stuart allows us to interpret Victor's character as a contemporary (1945) incarnation of the national psyche. If Victor is susceptible to haunting by the Stewart family in their house on Jersey Island right after the end of the war, it must be because something about England's self-fashioning as "the Victor" resonates with a shameful secret of a national identity stained by the shame of its repression of its Catholic origins.

England's War Strategy and Collective Haunting

The relationship between the House of Stuart and Jersey Island, to which the son of King Charles I fled when his father was captured by Parliamentary forces in 1642, offers historical context for Victor's haunting. Not only were Jersey subjects loyal to Charles II (r. 1662–1685), when he was in exile, before he was called back to London to restore the monarchy in 1660, but as the site where he commemorated the first anniversary of the death of his father after the Regicide, the island is particularly connected to collective mourning processes as well. The son's fastidious attention to ritualized eating behavior—making it a public spectacle during his three-year stay on Jersey immediately after the Regicide—attests to the feast's symbolic function for reconsolidating power.[60]

Charles II's emphasis on feasting rituals may be read metaphorically as representing his need to initiate self-fashioning processes of mourning in the face of changes in the psychological, emotional, relational, and political landscape. In light of the fact that the Civil War was ongoing, and that the divisiveness over loyalty had made his own situation very precarious, Charles II's fastidiousness with regard to its performance, and the spectacular dimension of the feasts, suggests an intention to transcend obstacles that thwart his self-fashioning. The extravagance calls to mind the concealed reverence for the sensuality of Catholic rituals; it is a gastronomic analogue of Charles I's Cavalier aesthetic. Even more, spectacles of sumptuous feasting stage that the royal House of Stuart *can swallow* and *digest* this aesthetic, all the while it conceals from the psyche that a devastating loss poses a problem to self-fashioning.

These associations find expression in *The Others*, when the Stewart family on Jersey Island eats its Sunday dinner right after Charles has returned from the war. The table has been laid out formally in anticipation of Charles joining them, but he stays absent, much to their disappointment. Grace is discomfited by her children's questions about the loyalties of their father and is unable to clearly articulate the standards by which such positions are established. The queries, voiced by Anne, implicitly link Charles Stuart's withdrawal from eating to issues of loyalty and death. It suggests that he can't swallow the truth about these issues.

The saga that haunts the Stewart house in Jersey allegorizes England's haunting by a history of religious repression and forced assimilation. Parallels between Grace's house and the Scotch-Anglo royal *house* of the Stuarts, who were most influential in the seventeenth and eighteenth centuries, reinforce these links. This era witnessed radical rearrangements of churches—often to the dismay of congregations—which was driven by an obsession with "intruders."[61] The intersection of the lines of royal Stuart family rule and Grace's experience on Jersey encapsulates the religious schisms haunting England.

The Film's Contemporary Context

The 1936 saga of King Edward VIII's abdication in order to marry American divorcée, Mrs Wallis Simpson, brings to focus the path by which the collective crypt of Charles Stewart's regicide continues to impact English self-fashioning. Consider the resonance between the source of this constitutional crisis and that associated with the Regicide, which include the convergence of conjugal desire (for a foreign wife), religion, and monarchical authority. The opposition to the marriage, which reflected societal, religious, legal, moral, and nationalistic concerns, evoked anxieties that trace directly to the problematic schism of national identity that we have discussed.

The abdication crisis became a catalyst for the expression of anxieties about the "relationship between private life and public responsibility and about the disputed claims of human feelings on national and imperial affairs."[62] Insofar as the abdication of Edward VIII reflected on a major crisis of national self-consciousness, these anxieties concerned more than support for or opposition to Edward VIII's marriage; they also reflected issues of English identity that lay beneath multiple layers of concealment and denial that centered on the behavior of the sovereign. Political interpretations that "cast the King's reign as an irregular interlude in the crystallization of a specifically British tradition of sovereignty that is both conscientious and popular"[63] reflect a discomfort with the possibility that Edward VIII's actions tacitly point to a historical legacy that was silenced and repressed.

That the crisis may have resonated unconsciously with the shameful trauma of the Regicide is suggested by the threat of disintegration posed by the king's disregard for the will of Parliament, which echoed the actions of Charles I. This idea is reinforced linguistically when one considers the media's and opposition's invocation of the term "royalist" to describe Winston Churchill's support of the king's wish to marry Simpson, up until his abdication. Moreover, the simultaneity of the crisis with growing religious intolerance both domestically and abroad evokes the memory of a nation badly damaged by religious upheaval. The interconnectedness of these two themes found expression in German diplomatic writings; the documents reveal how they saw the crisis in terms of Anglo-German relations: They saw the breach between Parliament and the king as consequent to Edward VIII's desire to maintain friendly Anglo-German relations in the face of a hawkish Parliament.[64] There is some evidence to support the view that the king was anti-Semitic, including photographs of a highly publicized tour of Germany that he took after he abdicated and married Wallis Simpson; one photo records when Edward and Wallis Simpson met and were entertained by Adolph Hitler.

This perspective of King Edward is not incidental. There was a significant resurgence of anti-Semitism in Britain during World War II, and the government's position, as reflected in domestic policy in the 1930s and 1940s, was ambiguous at best. Aaron Goldman has argued that while ostensibly anti-Nazi, British government policies, such as "obstructing large-scale Jewish immigration, continued during the war when millions of Jews were being murdered." The reluctance of British authorities to formally recognize the systematic killing of Jews, which happened only in 1942, despite widespread evidence that they were aware of this much earlier, suggests a more ambivalent position.[65] This "curious" focus has been explained in terms of Britain's war priorities: first and foremost, winning the war, and second, strategizing policies with an eye toward enhancing postwar strength.

Amenábar's film offers a different context for understanding the ambivalent language that marked England's confrontation of Jewish persecution. His substitution of an image of Spanish actor Eduardo Noriega's face for that of the Puritan depicted in Burton's painting recalls the role played by Spain during the traumatic transformations we have sketched out. Recall that Queen Catherine, Henry's abandoned wife, and devoted Catholic, was Spanish, and English history is replete with examples of how Spain's devotion to the papacy created domestic problems for the English.[66] Noriega's face retains the affective countenance and garb of the Puritan to evoke a specter of Popery[67] in the (disguised) form of a Spanish Inquisitor.[68] Here, Amenábar links the crypto-religious identities forged by the Spanish Inquisition to the context of the English Civil War.[69] The potency of Noriega's haunting derives from its representation of the dangers that Popery posed to England and the potential for it to "be reimposed by foreign powers."[70]

At the same time, Amenábar's substitution cryptically points to an anxiety over the "conversion" of England from Catholicism to Protestantism; this of course is the unrecognized drama of conversion whose concealment accounts for the problematic collective mourning of King Charles. Inserting Noriega's face tacitly parallels the insertion of the figure of the converted Jew into English national discourse as a means to disguise England's own unutterable conversion. In this way, we may extrapolate Grace's shameful saga of a Jew's hidden conversion as a disguised account of England's shameful origins.[71] Nineteenth-century English cultural artifacts reveal deep-seated Protestant anxiety provoked by the continued existence of Jews beyond what was established as a providential temporal change; this was perceived as transgression of temporal boundaries. Jews continued existence "intruded" into and thereby advanced an affront to Christian identity. Jewish identity became a figure of temporal and spatial transgressions and thus an apt figure for a phantom.

The vivid image of Nicholas, dressed in striped pajamas resembling the uniforms of Nazi prisoners, right at the point when he apprehends the "ghosts" among the tombstones and crypts of the House of Stewart, connects Nazi oppression and a haunting British history. Although history is written by the [V]ictor, to quote Winston Churchill, the prime minister during World War II, *The Others* suggests that the history of England's participation in World War II was shaped by concealed dramas of religious exclusion that will continue to inform English self-fashioning. Bertha Mills says as much when she explains to Grace, "The 'intruders' are leaving, but others will come. Now, sometimes we'll sense them and other times we won't. But that's the way it's always been." Ultimately, *The Others* comments on the haunting effects wrought by religious intolerance in England and reflects on the implications of a legacy of unspeakable mourning on domestic and international war policy.

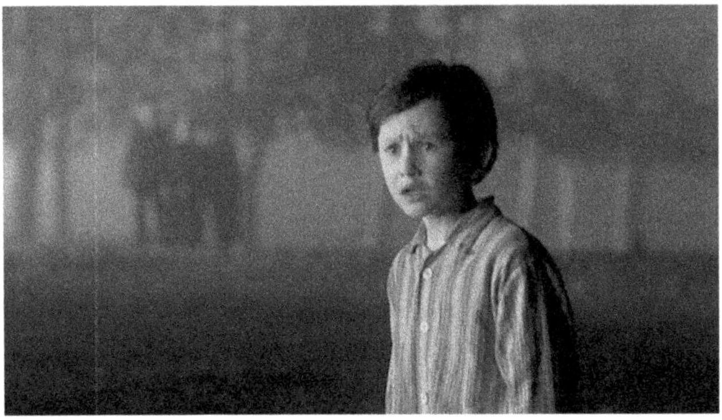

Figure 5.6 Nicholas's pajamas.

The film suggests that unless acknowledged and worked through, this traumatic history will repeat itself. As Charles Stewart claims, "The war is not over" (Figure 5.6).

Notes

1 "Alejandro Amenábar," *Box Office Mojo*, IMBD, August 10, 2001.
2 James Beradinelli, "Review. The Others," *ReelViews*, August 14, 2001.
3 See George Mott, "The Vanishing Point of the Sexual Subject: The Closet, Hedwig and the Angry Inch, LIE, the Sixth Sense, the Others, Y Tu Mamá También," *The Psychoanalytic Review* 91.4 (2004): 607–614; Aviva Briefel, "What Some Ghosts Don't Know: Spectral Incognizance and the Horror Film," *Narrative* 17.1 (2009): 95–108; Susan Bruce, "Sympathy for the Dead: (G)hosts, Hostilities and Mediums in Alejandro Amenábar's *The Others* and Postmortem Photography," *Discourse* 27.2 (2005): 21–40.
4 Anabel Altermir and Ibanez Rosales, "Otherness in the Others" in *Roman Catholicism in Fantastic Film: Essays on Belief, Spectacle, Ritual and Imagery,* ed. Regina Hansen (Jefferson, NC: McFarland & Co., 2011), 275.
5 A. O. Scott, "Film Review; Now, Which of You Are Dead?," *New York Times,* October 8, 2001, questions if Grace's affliction is supernatural or psychological.
6 Michelle Massé, "Gothic Repetition: Husbands, Horrors, and Things That Go Bump in the Night," *Signs: Journal of Women in Culture and Society* 15.4 (1990): 679–709.
7 Esther Rashkin, *Unspeakable Secrets and the Psychoanalysis of Culture* (Albany, NY: SUNY Press, 2008), 9.
8 According to Reverend Alban Butler's *Lives of the Fathers, Martyrs, and Other Principal Saints*, 12 vols. (Dublin, OH: James Duffy, 1866; Bartleby.com, 2010) vol. VIII: August, Justus, and Pastor's persecution was executed by Dacian, a Roman governor of Spain in 304.
9 www.bbc.co.uk/schoolradio/subjects/history/britainsince1930s/media/listen_with_mother.
10 "This story started many thousands of years ago... but it was all over in just days. All that long, long time ago, none of the things we can see now...the

sun, the moon, the stars, the earth, the animals and plants...none existed. Only God existed...and so only He could have created them. And He did."

11 See Victor P. Hamilton, *The Book of Genesis, Chapters 1–17* (Grand Rapids, MI: Wm. B. Eerdmans, 1990).

12 "Therefore the Lord God sent him forth from the garden of Eden...to till the ground from whence he was taken. So he drove out the man: and placed at the east of the garden of Eden Cherubims ... and a flaming sword to keep the way of the tree of life." This section can be found in Genesis 3:24.

13 "And Abraham took the wood of the burnt offering ... and laid it upon Isaac, his son. And he took the fire in his hand ... and a knife; and they went both of them together. And Isaac spoke unto Abraham his father, and said ... My father: and he said, Here am I, my son. And he ..." (voice trails off). Anne's reading KJB, Genesis 22:15.

14 Rashkin, *Unspeakable Secrets*, 30.

15 W. A. Meeks, *The First Urban Christians. The Social World of the Apostle Paul* (New Haven, CT and London: Yale University Press, 1983), 62. Cf. Meeks's suggestion that the emergence of "Christian 'cells' where a new social reality with a distinctive 'set of beliefs' is related to the psychosocial consequences of vulnerability, anxiety and loneliness," ibid., 104–191.

16 Ibid., 62.

17 Jersey lay "in the French diocese of Coutances, and later of Nantes, until the time of the Reformation and, even, then, clergy were either French, Huguenots or Channel islanders trained in France." See Anthony Liddicoat, *A Grammar of the Norman French of the Channel Islands: The Dialects of Jersey and Sark* (Berlin and New York: Mouton de Gruyter, 1994), 6.

18 "Mrs. Mills, our father is fighting in a war in France, you know."—It's the World War.—I know, but he's in France."

19 Julia Sutton, "The Minuet: An Elegant Phoenix," *Dance Chronicle* 8, no. 3/4 (1985): 120, identifies the minuet as a "courtly and courting social dance for one couple at a time."

20 Cf. Anne's definition of a ghost as a white-robed entity when she and Nicholas discuss a ghost's form.

21 I borrow this evocative term from Esther Rashkin, "Religious Transvestism and the Stigma of Jewish Identity," *Unspeakable Secrets,* 113–136.

22 Describing the concluding shot of the "I Only Have Eyes for You" song and dance sequence, Jeffrey Spivak notes, "Another Berkeley sleight of hand has Ruby posted on the backside of a handheld mirror. As the mirror turns toward the camera, the frame of reference shifts back to the 'reality' of the subway car, where Ruby and Dick awaken from their nap realizing they've come to the final stop in the line." See Jeffrey Spivak, *Buzz: The Life and Art of Busby Berkeley* (Lexington: University Press of Kentucky, 2010), 108.

23 Sandra Gorgievski, *Face to Face with Angels: Images in Medieval Art and in Film* (Jefferson, NC: McFarland & Company, 2010), 7.

24 Ibid.

25 See Rashkin, "Religious Transvestism," 113–136.

26 Simcha Paull Raphael, "Grief and Bereavement" in *Jewish Pastoral Care: A Practical Handbook from Traditional and Contemporary Sources,* eds. Rabbi Dayle A. Friedman (New York: Jewish Lights, 2001), 400.

27 Shmuel Trigano, "The French Revolution and the Jews," *Modern Judiasm* 10.2 (1990): 171–190; Ronald Schechter, *Obstinate Hebrews: Representations of Jews in France, 1715–1815,* vol. 49 (Berkeley: University of California Press, 2003).

28 Michael Ragussis, *Figures of Conversion: "The Jewish Question" & English National Identity* (Durham, NC: Duke University Press), 93.

29 Carol Davison, *Anti-Semitism and British Gothic Literature* (London: Palgrave Macmillan, 2004), 86.
30 Ibid.
31 This inversion aligns with Grace's initial attempt to deny to Charles that anything at all had occurred: her initial response to his question about what happened that day claimed "I don't know what you are talking about." Cf. the interpolation of the scene in which Nicholas asks Anne what happened and she says, "She hit me, she went mad, just like that day, do you remember?" to which Nicholas vehemently says "No."
32 Grace's vehemence may derive from the timing of Charles's war venture, which, Grace tells Bertha was "a year and a half ago." Charles's departure was thus not undertaken when the majority of Channel Islanders had the opportunity to evacuate right before England demilitarized the islands in 1940, which is when Grace's family left. Rather, he must have been one of the few men who escaped the island in 1943 or 1944 to join the British forces. According to one scholar, the number of men joining the British forces increased after D-Day (June 6, 1944), which inspired desire to join in the liberation of Europe.
33 Rashkin, *Unspeakable Secrets*, 43, citing Abraham and Torok, *The Shell and the Kernel*, 132. Abraham and Torok call this psycholinguistic process "demetaphorization."
34 King Henry VIII broke with the Papacy in 1543. The leadership of the Church in England then became progressively more Protestant in its outlook, culminating in the introduction of the 1552 prayer book under his son Edward VI (1547–1553).
35 This occurred in 1469; the Inquisition was formally initiated in 1488. See Henry Kamen, *The Spanish Inquisition: A Historical Revision* (New Haven, CT: Yale University Press, 2014), 64.
36 Robert Ashton, "Popular Entertainment and Social Control in Later Elizabethan and Early Stuart London," *The London Journal: A Review of Metropolitan Society Past and Present* 9.1 (1983): 3.
37 Robert Ashton, *The English Civil War* (London: Weidenfeld & Nicolson, 1989), provides a detailed, thematic examination of the background to the war.
38 For Van Dyck's representation of Charles as a Cavalier, see John Moffit, "'Le Roi à La Ciasse'? Kings, Christian Knights and Van Dyck's Singular 'Dismounted Equestrian-Portrait' of Charles I," *Artibus et Historiae* 4.7 (1983): 79–99.
39 The idea that artistic iconography is a rich source for historical commentary on a "particular obsession" with the Civil War is the premise of scholars such as Roy Strong, who examines the legacy of this obsession within the context of Victorian iconography: *And When Did You Last See Your Father?: The Victorian Painter and British History* (London: Thames, 1978). See also Martin Meisel, "For King or Parliament?: Attitudes of Nineteenth Century Painters to the Civil War," which appears in a catalog to an exhibition mounted in 1978–1979 by the Wolverhampton Art Gallery, Wolverhampton, and the Mappin Art Gallery, Sheffield.
40 Terry Boardman, "'The Wounded Cavalier' as a Key to Understanding British History," *Threeman.org*. WordPress, July 17, 2012.
41 For the perception that the royal court was crypto-Catholic, see Anthony Milton, *Catholic and Reformed: The Roman and Protestant Churches in English Protestant Thought, 1600–1640* (Cambridge: Cambridge University Press, 2002); John Morrill, *Stuart Britain: A Very Short Introduction* (Oxford: Oxford University Press, 2000). Interestingly, it is within the

context of anti-Calvinist reforms, which sought to enforce religious uniformity by substituting nonconformist preachers with those more aligned with the Crown, that the term "intruder" acquired its specific religious connotation. Colin Haydon, *Anti-Catholicism in Eighteenth-Century England, C. 1741–80: A Political and Social Study* (Manchester: Manchester University Press, 1993), 3, emphasizes how the Reformation ultimately devolved on issues of loyalty.

42 King Henry VIII broke with the Papacy in 1543. The leadership of the Church in England then became progressively more Protestant in its outlook, culminating in the introduction of the 1552 prayer book under his son Edward VI (1547–1553).

43 R. Malcolm Smuts, "The Puritan Followers of Henrietta Maria in the 1630s," *The English Historical Review* 93.366 (1978): 26, suggests that the view of Henrietta Maria as a "vivacious but irresponsible papist queen, cajoling her uxorious husband to defy his subjects" is too exaggerated, but his essential argument that her objective to stress forms of Catholic piety, believed to be broadly acceptable to Protestants, in hopes of gradually drawing them closer to Rome, still reflects her important role in court politics.

44 David Newcombe, *Henry VIII and the English Reformation* (London: Routledge, 1995), 2, critiques the traditional Protestant interpretation of the Reformation as oriented toward a desire to separate from "an old and decrepit Church, riddled with abuses of all kinds and controlled by an Italian princeling whose only concern was to sap England's wealth for his own temporal ambitions." His conclusion that the English Reformation must be construed as an act of state and not an act of faith is nuanced by his observation that the Church of England managed to maintain an essentially orthodox religious structure.

45 David Salter, "Remembering the Catholic Middle Ages: The Franciscans, English National Identity, and William Hogarth's the Roast Beef of Old England," *Logos: A Journal of Catholic Thought and Culture* 16.4 (2013): 99–123.

46 Boardman, "The Wounded Cavalier."

47 Boardman, "The Wounded Cavalier."

48 Salter, "Remembering the Catholic Middle Ages," 103.

49 Ibid., 117.

50 Ibid.

51 Ibid.

52 See Alex Garganigo, "Mourning the Headless Body Politic: The Regicide Elegies and Marvell's 'Horatian Ode'," *Exemplaria* 15.2 (2003): 509–550; Nancy Klein Maguire, *Regicide and Restoration: English Tragicomedy, 1660–1671* (Cambridge: Cambridge University Press, 1992); Anne Elizabeth Carson, "The Hunted Stag and the Beheaded King," *Studies in English Literature 1500–1900* 45.3 (2005): 537–556.

53 Andrew Marvell's "Horatian Ode" (1650), cited by Garganigo in "Mourning the Headless Body Politic," 512.

54 Maguire, *Regicide and Restoration*, 1–12.

55 Ibid., 538.

56 The term "Party Spirit" was used by Daniel Defoe to decry the lack of impartial historical work. See Nicholas Seager, "'A Romance the Likest to Truth That I Ever Read': History, Fiction, and Politics in Defoe's Memoirs of a Cavalier," *Eighteenth Century Fiction* 20.4 (2008): 481.

57 Garganigo, "Mourning the Headless Body Politic," 534. Deployment of the discourse of the body politic "was more than just a residual paradigm after 1649: it was an obsession."

58 Ibid., 538.
59 Ibid., 535.
60 See Esther Rashkin, "A Recipe for Mourning: Isak Dinesen's 'Babette's Feast'," *Style* 29.3 (Fall 1995): 369.
61 Alasdair Raffe, *The Culture of Controversy: Religious Arguments in Scotland, 1660–1714*, vol. 28 (Woodbridge: Boydell Press, 2012), 55, 193–194.
62 Frank Mort, "Love in a Cold Climate: Letters, Public Opinion and Monarchy in the 1936 Abdication Crisis," *Twentieth Century British History* 25.1 (2013): 30–62.
63 Ibid., 33. Cf. Mort's discussion of scholarship that views the reign of Edward VIII as a "pathological moment."
64 Philip Ziegler, *King Edward VIII: A Biography* (New York: Alfred A. Knopf, 1991).
65 Aaron Goldman, "The Resurgence of Antisemitism in Britain during World War II," *Jewish Social Studies* 46.1 (1984): 38.
66 Simon Adams, "Spain or the Netherlands? The Dilemmas of Early Stuart Foreign Policy," *Before the English Civil War* (Macmillan Education UK, 1983), 79–101. Howard Tomlinson, *Before the English Civil War: Essays on Early Stuart Politics and Government* (Macmillan, 1983).
67 Cf. Colin Haydon's discussion of the "'No Popery' Troubles" that characterized the Stuart era, *Anti-Catholicism*, 2.
68 John Miller, *Religion in the Popular Prints, 1600–1832* (Cambridge: Cambridge University Press, 1986), 38 claims that it is Popery as opposed to Catholic theology that is the object of most anti-Catholic images. Colin Haydon, *Anti-Catholicism in Eighteenth-Century England*, 46, identifies "the Papist in disguise" as the "most hysterical anti-Catholic obsession of the eighteenth century."
69 Scholars of anti-Catholicism in England also cite "Popish atrocities" and persecution of heretics during the Inquisition as a generative source of its expression in cultural products, which were meant to convey "the message that 'Popery is always the same.'" Colin Haydon, *Anti-Catholicism in Eighteenth-Century England*, 45.
70 Ibid.
71 Michael Ragussis, "The 'Secret' of English Anti-Semitism: Anglo-Jewish Studies and Victorian Studies, Review Essay," *Victorian Studies* 40.2 (1997): 296.

Bibliography

Achinstein, Sharon. "John Foxe and the Jews." *Renaissance Quarterly* 54.1 (2001): 86–120.

Adams, Simon. "Spain or the Netherlands? The Dilemmas of Early Stuart Foreign Policy." *Before the English Civil War*. Macmillan Education UK, 1983. 79–101.

"Alejandro Amenábar." *Box Office Mojo*. IMBD, 10 August 2001.

Altermir, Anabel and Ibanez Rosales. "Otherness in the Others." Ed. Regina Hansen. *Roman Catholicism in Fantastic Film: Essays on Belief, Spectacle, Ritual and Imagery*. McFarland, 2011. 275–286.

Ashton, Robert. "Popular Entertainment and Social Control in Later Elizabethan and Early Stuart London." *The London Journal* 9.1 (1983): 3–19.

———. *The English Civil War*. Weidenfeld & Nicolson, 1989.

Briefel, Aviva. "What Some Ghosts Don't Know: Spectral Incognizance and the Horror Film." *Narrative* 17.1 (2009): 95–108.

Bruce, Susan. "Sympathy for the Dead: (G)hosts, Hostilities and Mediums in Alejandro Amenábar's *The Others* and Postmortem Photography." *Discourse* 27.2 (2005): 21–40.

Boardman, Terry. "'The Wounded Cavalier' as a Key to Understanding British History." *Threeman.org*. WordPress, 17 July 2012.

Butler, Alban and Paul Burns. *Butler's Lives of the Saints: August*. Vol. 8. Burns & Oates, 1998.

Carson, Anne Elizabeth. "The Hunted Stag and the Beheaded King." *Studies in English Literature 1500–1900* 45.3 (2005): 537–556.

Davison, Davison. *Anti-Semitism and British Gothic Literature*. Palgrave Macmillan, 2004.

Frankel, Ellen, and Betsy Platkin Teutsch. *The Encyclopedia of Jewish Symbols*. Rowman & Littlefield, 1992.

Garganigo, Alex. "Mourning the Headless Body Politic: The Regicide Elegies and Marvell's 'Horatian Ode'." *Exemplaria* 15.2 (2003): 473–508.

Goldman, Aaron. "The Resurgence of Antisemitism in Britain during World War II." *Jewish Social Studies* 46.1 (1984): 37–50.

Gorgievski, Sandra. *Face to Face with Angels: Images in Medieval Art and in Film*. McFarland, 2010.

Hamilton, Victor P. *The Book of Genesis, Chapters 1–17*. Wm. B. Eerdmans 1990.

Hansen, Regina. Ed. *Roman Catholicism in Fantastic Film: Essays on Belief, Spectacle, Ritual and Imagery*. McFarland & Co., 2011.

Haydon, Colin. *Anti-Catholicism in Eighteenth-Century England, C. 1741–80: A Political and Social Study*. Manchester, 1993.

Kamen, Henry. *The Spanish Inquisition: A Historical Revision*. Yale University Press, 2014.

Lacey, Andrew. *The Cult of King Charles the Martyr*. Boydell & Brewer, 2003.

Liddicoat, Anthony. *A Grammar of the Norman French of the Channel Islands: The Dialects of Jersey and Sark*. Mouton de Gruyter, 1940.

"Listen with Mother." *Learning School Radio. Audio Resources for Primary Schools*. BBC.

Maguire, Nancy Klein. *Regicide and Restoration: English Tragicomedy, 1660–1671*. Cambridge, 1992.

Massé, Michelle. "Gothic Repetition: Husbands, Horrors, and Things That Go Bump in the Night." *Signs: Journal of Women in Culture and Society* 15.4 (1990): 679–709.

Meeks, W. A. *The First Urban Christians. The Social World of the Apostle Paul*. Yale University Press, 1983.

Meisel, Martin. *Realizations: Narrative, Pictorial, and Theatrical Arts in Nineteenth-Century England*. Princeton University Press, 1983.

Miller, John. *Religion in the Popular Prints, 1600–1832*. Chadwyck-Healey, 1985.

Milton, Anthony. *Catholic and Reformed: The Roman and Protestant Churches in English Protestant Thought, 1600–1640*. Cambridge University Press, 2002.

Moffit, John. "'Le Roi à La Ciasse'? Kings, Christian Knights, and Van Dyck's Singular 'Dismounted Equestrian-Portrait' of Charles I." *Artibus et Historiae* (1983): 79–99.

Morrill, John. *Stuart Britain: A Very Short Introduction.* Oxford, 2000.
Mort, Frank. "Love in a Cold Climate: Letters, Public Opinion and Monarchy in the 1936 Abdication Crisis." *Twentieth Century British History* 25.1 (2013): 30–62.
Mott, George. "The Vanishing Point of the Sexual Subject: The Closet, Hedwig and the Angry Inch, LIE, the Sixth Sense, the Others, Y Tu Mamá También." *The Psychoanalytic Review* 91.4 (2004): 607–614.
Newcombe, David. *Henry VIII and the English Reformation.* Routledge, 1995.
Raffe, Alasdair. *The Culture of Controversy: Religious Arguments in Scotland, 1660–1714.* Vol. 28. Boydell Press, 2012.
Ragussis, Michael. *Figures of Conversion: "The Jewish Question" & English National Identity.* Duke, 1995.
———. "The 'Secret' of English Anti-Semitism: Anglo-Jewish Studies and Victorian Studies, Review Essay." *Victorian Studies* 40.2 (1997): 295–307.
Raphael, Simcha Paull. "Grief and Bereavement." *Jewish Pastoral Care: A Practical Handbook from Traditional and Contemporary Sources.* Ed. Rabbi Dayle A. Friedman. Jewish Lights, 2001. 400–433.
Rashkin, Esther. "A Recipe for Mourning: Isak Dinesen's 'Babette's Feast'," *Style* 29.3 (1995): 356–374.
———. *Unspeakable Secrets and the Psychoanalysis of Culture.* SUNY Press, 2008.
———. *Family Secrets and the Psychoanalysis of Narrative.* Princeton University Press, 1992.
Salter, David. "Remembering the Catholic Middle Ages: The Franciscans, English National Identity, and William Hogarth's the Roast Beef of Old England." *Logos: A Journal of Catholic Thought and Culture* 16.4 (2013): 99–123.
Scott, A. O. "Film Review; Now, Which of You Are Dead?" *New York Times,* 8 October 2001.
Schechter, Ronald. *Obstinate Hebrews: Representations of Jews in France, 1715–1815.* Vol. 49. University of California Press, 2003.
Seager, Nicholas. "'A Romance the Likest to Truth That I Ever Read': History, Fiction, and Politics in Defoe's Memoirs of a Cavalier." *Eighteenth Century Fiction* 20.4 (2008): 479–505.
Smuts, Malcolm R. "The Puritan Followers of Henrietta Maria in the 1630s." *The English Historical Review* 93.366 (1978): 26–45.
Spivak, Jeffrey. *Buzz: The Life and Art of Busby Berkeley.* Kentucky, 2010.
Strong, Roy. *And When Did You Last See Your Father?: The Victorian Painter and British History.* Thames, 1978.
Sutton, Julia. "The Minuet: An Elegant Phoenix." *Dance Chronicle* 8.3 (1985): 119–152.
The Others. Dir. Alejandro Amenábar. Lionsgate 2001. DVD.
Thomas, Robert. "Civil Society and the English Civil War." *Historical Notes* No. 20 (1992).
Tomlinson, Howard. *Before the English Civil War: Essays on Early Stuart Politics and Government.* Macmillan, 1983.
Trigano, Shmuel. "The French Revolution and the Jews." *Modern Judaism* 10.2 (1990): 171–190.
Ziegler, Philip. *King Edward VIII: A Biography.* Knopf, 1991.

6 Epilogue

We have seen how uncovering a lineage secret may entail the reconstruction of a collective psychology: on the first level, the psychology of a subject's ancestors; on a deeper level, the psychology of the society at the moment the lineage secret was generated. The lexical strategies of avoidance that enable us to reconstruct a silenced secret are historical evidence that a lineage's linguistic surround was pruned in order to preserve it. In the preceding chapters, I have approached resulting excisions as portals through which can be explored a dense matrix of human interaction, collective memory, and their representation in cultural objects such as film. Here, I offer a few reflections and some deeper historical principles that emerge when individual interpretations of the national films are considered together.

All four of these films are marked by links to the reigns of sixteenth- or seventeenth-century monarchs. This was an era rife with conflicts about the limits of monarchy, although the emphases of individual historians differ. For example, Immanuel Wallerstein links the rise of absolute monarchy in Western Europe to the emergence of a European world economy, which, in his view, figured largely as a mechanism in the "creation of [state] legitimacy."[1] Christopher Bayly notes a long-term transformation from nomadism to intensive agrarian exploitation, which engendered political and cultural uniformity and established the basis of modern social, economic, and political patterns, including monarchism.[2] Perry Anderson argues that the sixteenth-century Absolutist state was a refashioning of an old political framework that protected the domination of the nobility, which had eroded as feudal modes of production did.[3]

Phantom films focus us on the way unarticulated prehistories—especially the histories of lineage on which absolute monarchies depend for their legitimacy—may resonate in individual experience for generations and even centuries. All four of my examples implicate as the catalyst for secret formation the advent of new sociopolitical grammars established to bolster the claim for sovereignty of a reigning monarch and his family.[4] The *legitimacy* of such claims, according to the *Oxford English Dictionary*, depended on "the fact of a sovereign's title being derived by regular descent" (*OED*). The purity of the genealogical line was essential for a family's claim to royal status; this may account for the intense preoccupation with the context of conception revealed in these films. Three of the four secrets involve illicit sexual encounters; the other reflects a marriage construed as illicit because of religious differences.[5] The secrets betray the anxiety over genealogical legitimacy that suffused the ruling idioms of Isabella I and Ferdinand II, Ivan the IV, Yŏngjo, and Charles I. Unarticulated prehistories relating to illicit conjugal relations and conceptions clearly shaped the way these monarchs self-fashioned themselves and, by extension, the language surround of the societies they controlled.

Daniel Lord Smail, who has advanced a neurohistorical approach to historical analysis, investigates the social and political consequences of chronic stress. He concludes that manipulation of stress and prestige is endemic to "human behavioral patterns"[6] and that one of the state's means of ensuring compliance by the collective is through "systems for delivering stress, in the form of pillories, shaming rituals, [and] public spectacles."[7] He connects the emergence and endurance of monarchical institutions to a state's effectiveness in commandeering these systems of social control.[8] Specifically, he argues that whereas stress transactions had hitherto been used primarily to enforce (private) concerns about honor and justice, the new monarchies used them in the interest of the state's need to legitimize itself. My own historical inquiries lead me to wonder to what extent this shift might have to do with the presence of lineage secrets among the rising families; in other words, whether preservative repression is a heretofore unexamined agent in the establishment of monarchies.

Phantom films magnify historical experience at many different levels and on many different scales—the individual, the collective, the societal, and the cultural. Smail argues that historical experience for human beings is actually a "dialogue between an organism and its environment." This is a central tenet of the concept of the theory of "coevolution,"[9] which explains human behavior as a product of interacting yet distinct evolutionary processes; genetics and culture form an ecosystem wherein changes to one process influence the other.[10] Smail cites studies of rats that show that stress is heritable and how gene expression cannot be divorced from the social, cultural, and individual life circumstances of a descendant.[11]

A phantom travels across generations and across cultures. It is quiescent as long as its secret remains secure, and emerges when its secret is threatened; it can lie dormant for generations, or haunt generations consecutively. Indeed, latent in Nicolas Abraham and Maria Torok's work is an evolutionary axiom: even as human lives are shaped by their interaction with their lived environments, they are always adaptations of their ancestors' sagas.[12] Abraham and Torok's theory of self-fashioning is, in essence, a genetic principle in which linguistic mechanisms transmit an emotional DNA. Their metapsychology is an affective corollary to the theory of language evolution proposed by cognitive psychologist Merlin Donald, a leader in the field. Donald argues that language is "not a feature of the brain per se." It is a "cognitive epiphenomenon, a social construction"; language is a product of a turn in human cognitive evolution toward a "*collective* direction" (original emphasis).[13] The collective orientation, he suggests, followed major advancements in primate motor learning capacity that enabled the deliberate modification of procedural memories. This important advance had implications that went far beyond the manufacture of stone tools. It established a key precondition for the future evolution of more sophisticated expressive systems, and the capacity to refine and rehearse skill sets. It also started, however modestly at first, a hominin process of externalizing memory, that is, using the material cultural products of skill to build a record of past achievements and knowledge that could exist external to the brain, and be carried forward for future generations.

Donald concludes that

> [l]anguage has its origin in a distributed cognitive system, while it is performed by a local cognitive system, that is, the brain of an individual. It is the child of an interactive cultural imagination, that is, of groups of brains in collision.[14]

Gradual cognitive expansion catalyzed processes by which groups "distributed and shared system[s] of thought and memory."[15] In this way, language itself is an artifact that externalizes the collective memory of a group's self-fashioning processes; it is the symbolic analogue of the material culture, and like flint tools or fire pits, language systems point to the (affective) collective conditions that lead to their production.

This idea, that the intricacies of language, "including even such exquisite phenomena as syntax,"[16] were *responses* to early changes in the primate cognitive repertoire, strongly reverberates with Abraham and Torok's psychoanalytic concept of self-fashioning and symbol production. Donald's orientation, however, does not allow for the possibility that the distributive cognitive system might be connected to the function of emotion in human evolution, even though he acknowledges that the system is based on nonlinguistic (and likely affectively charged) mimetic practices.[17] Abraham's conception of the symbol as a trace of (intrapsychic) collective conflict helps to fill out Donald's theory, which passes over the role language plays in constructing emotional life.

Stephen Pinker, an expert in psycholinguistics, hypothesizes that emotion evolved as a "credible deterrent" of social defiance or other trespasses that could threaten the survival of a family or extended collective. This idea provides a context for the cognitive and affective evolution of shame as language developed.[18] Psychic repression triggered by shame would have great power in sociocultural environments where issues of inclusion or exclusion were at stake.[19] The capacity of the psyche to displace words contaminated by unutterable shameful experience into lexical and phonetic fragments suggests that such expressive linguistic hiding benefited human continuity.[20] Preservative repression may have developed as a "fast and frugal," as Brian Boyd puts it, way of compacting dangerous facts and feelings into safe little packets at a time in human linguistic and cognitive evolution when new social and environmental demands for cooperation were increasing the need for economical information transmission.[21]

The survival benefits of cooperation thus shaped linguistic behavior to ensure that language continues the conditions that maintain it. The structure of phantoms is a vestige of intragroup conflicts experienced in the early stages of human self-fashioning, when spoken language was evolving. It reflects the regulatory role of shame in a culture's survival strategy. The endurance of such historically derived group "structures of mind" may shed light on the relationship between literature and human evolution, exemplifying as they do the operation in unison of emotion, language, and form.[22]

Donald, who acknowledges, "To a cognitive scientist, art represents a singular, rather peculiar way of knowing the world," views art as the evolutionary end product of a slow cumulative progression of cognitive expansion.[23] Social products, such as storytelling, derive from ancient patterns that evolved from the human capacity to reenact "events in a nonverbal, gestural, fuzzy, quasi-symbolic manner."[24] Donald advances a genealogy of artistic forms based on the evolution of pantomime gestures to vocal mimetic expression, to whole-body and vocal mimetic expression, which he identifies as the basic elements of "most rituals."[25] Thus, he categorizes oral storytelling, epic poetry, and other narrative forms as the linguistic offspring of rituals, whose formation and affective value are the very founding blocks of human culture.

Steven Pinker claims that "connecting literary analysis with evolutionary psychology is an idea whose time has come," because fictions reflect "our species' obsessions, and provide an ecologically valid source of data about what matters to us."[26] But he warns against evolutionary explanations of literature that are limited to metaphors inspired by group selection (bonding, social cohesion, and so on)," because, they "don't do justice to the ambivalent mixture of selfish, nepotistic, strategic, and self-advertising motives that really animate a person's feelings toward his or her group, and that fiction deliciously plays out for us." Citing John Updike, Pinker suggests that the evolutionary explanation for why people like to tell stories is in the "groping" way "fiction is drawn to those moments of discomfort when society asks more than its individual members can, or wish to, provide."

The centrality of fantasy in cinematic expressions of haunting suggests an explanation for the production and endurance of fictional forms. Social groups depended on cognitive (and affective) distributive networks to survive, but how did they deal with difficult conflicts and still remain able to cooperate with others who are implicated in them? For example, consider sexual jealousy; Pinker suggests this emotion is "presumably an adaptation against the evolutionary disaster of cuckoldry."[27] Fantasy, produced to exempt subject(s) from the painful process of reorganization and thereby preserve the status quo, may have evolved as a means for a collective to externalize while also concealing memories of shameful intrapersonal and intragroup conflicts, that is, as a by-product of preservative repression. Along these lines, the evolution of the literary forms that so enchant and transport us may perhaps be understood as epigenetic descendants of fantasy.

Phantoms conceal and transmit collective memories related to a lineage's survival; we may construe them as disguised, whispered injunctions for family preservation. The link between preservation and injunction may account for the prominence of religious symbolism in my four phantom films. Royal families in Spain, Russia, Korea, and Britain all invoked religious symbols and doctrine to justify their attempts to expand and define their political authority, and in the films, these invocations are both repressed and preserved. Studies investigating the relationship between monarchic authority and imagery emphasize how a regime's power is enhanced by the religious symbolic system in which it is framed.[28]

Some early monarchs, for instance, used the "sacral presence" of Christian symbols both as a screen to hide the vulnerability of ordinary personhood and as a fount of the transcendent power that supported their claims to legitimacy.[29] Religious symbols are deployed similarly in phantom films to occlude the ancestor whose shameful experience was silenced, but the veiled lexical networks that they encrypt point to the very part of the family's prehistory that had to be hidden. Given the transcultural dominance of the Old Testament as a paradigm of family narrative, it is not surprising that Genesis figures so significantly in the cinematographic idioms of the European films. Kim Jee-woon's film is built on an analogous framework of Confucian familial norms.

All of this raises the possibility of an affiliative relationship between phantom structures and religious discourse. That is, if religious symbolism makes it possible to hear what had to be silenced in a protagonist's family history, it may be because religious discourse itself was borne out of a family's unutterable secret. *The Return* especially highlights the metapsychological (as opposed to the metaphysical) implications of religious symbols; we have noted how the transcendent dimension of a discourse that presumes to represent hidden (spiritual) truths resonates with structure of phantom films and the secret truths they hide within their own discursive form.[30] It will be a long time before Abraham and Torok's deep and rich concept of preservative repression, and the tools they offered for analyzing it, has been exploited to the full. In the meantime, however, this small study affirms one aspect of their work: The heuristic potential of shame in explorations of human behavior.[31] Phantom films represent disturbances undermining the foundations of emotional and linguistic organization; the process they delineate is simultaneously specific to the characters portrayed and generalizable to humanity at large. Like a Rembrandt painting that visualizes the "marks left by the bite of worldly experience, the pits and pocks; the shame and shams, to render human subjectivity as a matter for close and empathic inspection,"[32] phantom films implore us to consider what it means to us when the foundational dramas of our lives are blocked from our view. Phantom structures are vestiges of human cognitive evolution forged by the dynamic between experiential shame and social environments. They are archival, permeated with linguistic data that have much to reveal not only about a shameful secret itself but also about the psychogenetics of cultural production and of aesthetic experience. The endurance of phantom structures across cultures and centuries and genres derives from their extraordinary capacity to communicate affective experiences between individuals and among collectives; phantom films, which give voice to unarticulated yet ever-present prehistories, not only exemplify film's power to represent unconscious dimensions of human suffering but also provide tools for collective mitigation of their haunting effect.

Notes

1 Immanuel Wallerstein, *The Modern World-System I: Capitalist Agriculture and the Origins of the European World-Economy in the Sixteenth Century* (Berkeley: University of California Press, 1974), especially the chapter on "The Absolute Monarchy and Statism."

2 Christopher Bayly, *The Birth of the Modern World 1780–1914: Global Connections and Comparisons* (Oxford: Blackwell, 2004).

3 Perry Anderson, *Lineages of the Absolutist State* (London: Verso, 1979), 11–20.

4 Jeroen Deploige and Gita Deneckere, "Introduction," idem., eds., *Mystifying the Monarch: Studies on Discourse, Power, and History*, (Amsterdam: Amsterdam University Press, 2006), 10:

> There is a remarkable link to be observed between the institution of monarchy – which, of course, has not remained untouched by the finger of time but nonetheless has endured – and the symbolic, discursive order in which it is framed. In spite of the fundamental processes of modernization, secularization, and bureaucratization of power, the affective, archaic, and almost timeless relationship between sovereigns and their 'subjects' still prevails today.

5 Esther Rashkin finds a similar cluster of concerns with illegitimacy in eighteenth- and nineteenth-century French and English short stories. Rashkin,

Family Secrets and the Psychoanalysis of Narrative (Princeton: Princeton University Press, 1994).

6 Daniel Lord Smail, "Neuroscience and the Dialectics of History," Análise Social 47.4 (2012): 895.

7 Ibid., 899.

8 Ibid., 895.

9 Ibid., 900. For concise explanations of epigenetic research and conclusions, see Frances A. Champagne, "Epigenetic Mechanisms and the Transgenerational Effects of Maternal Care," *Frontiers in Neuroendocrinology* 29.3 (2008): 386–397; Tie-Yuan Zhang and Michael J. Meaney, "Epigenetics and the Environmental Regulation of the Genome and Its Function," *Annual Review of Psychology* 61 (2010): 439–466.

10 Daniel H. Janzen, "When Is It Coevolution," *Evolution* 34.3 (1980): 611–612.

11 Karina L. Walters et al., "Bodies Don't Just Tell Stories, They Tell Histories," *Du Bois Review: Social Science Research on Race* 8 (2011): 179–189; and Jörg Niewöhner, "Epigenetics: Embedded Bodies and the Molecularisation of Biography and Milieu," *BioSocieties* 6 (2011): 279–298.

12 Esther Rashkin, *Family Secrets*, 18.

13 Merlin, Donald, "Key Cognitive Preconditions for the Evolution of Language," *Psychonomic Bulletin & Review* 24.1 (2017): 205.

14 Ibid., 207.

15 Ibid.

16 Ibid., 205.

17 Ibid., 204.

18 Steven Pinker, "How the Mind Works," *Annals of the New York Academy of Sciences* (1999): 127. Pinker explains the evolutionary function of emotion in human behavior as "the neural equivalents of laws and contracts."

19 Robert Boy and Peter J. Richerson, "Culture and the Evolution of Human Cooperation," *Philosophical Transactions of the Royal Society of London B: Biological Sciences* 364.1533 (2009): *3286*, suggest that shame emerged in a "new social world, created by rapid cultural adaptation, [which] led to the genetic evolution of new derived social instincts." They surmise that

> [g]roups which developed traditions of punishing selfish behavior detrimental to the group as a whole may well have been more successful than groups which tolerated more individualistic behavior. Genes which facilitate cooperation could have arisen in such groups because the cultural environment would have favored individuals who were more docile and willing to behave in accordance with cultural norms. Repeated coevolutionary cycles could eventually drastically modify the psychological mechanisms that influence human social interaction. Ibid.

20 Leda Cosmides and John Tooby, "Cognitive Adaptations for Social Exchange" in Jerome Barkow, Leda Cosmides, and John Tooby, eds. *The Adapted Mind: Evolutionary Psychology and the Generation of Culture* (Oxford: Oxford University Press, 1992); Boy and Richerson, "Culture and the Evolution of Human Cooperation," 3281–3288.

21 Brian Boyd, "Getting It All Wrong: Bioculture Critiques Cultural Critique" in Brian Boyd, Joseph Carroll, Jonathan Gottschall, eds., *Evolution, Literature, and Film: A Reader* (New York: Columbia University Press, 2010), 201.

22 Daniel Nettle, "What Happens in Hamlet? Exploring the Psychological Foundations of Drama" in Jonathan Gottschall, David Sloan Wilson, eds.,

The Literary Animal: Evolution and The Nature of Narrative (Evanston: Northwestern University Press, 2005); Brian Boyd, "Literature and Evolution: A Bio-Cultural Approach," *Philosophy and Literature* 29.1 (2005): 1–23; Joseph Carroll, "An Evolutionary Paradigm for Literary Study," *Style* 42.2–3 (2008): 103–134.

23 Merlin Donald, "Art and Cognitive Evolution," Mark Turner, ed., *The Artful Mind: Cognitive Science and the Riddle of Human Creativity* (Oxford: Oxford University Press, 2006), 13.

24 Ibid., 16.

25 Ibid., 9.

26 Steven Pinker, "Toward a Consilient Study of Literature," *Philosophy and Literature* 31.1 (2007): 163.

27 Ibid., 169.

28 See, for example, the exciting and wide range of studies collected in Jeroen Deploige and Gita Deneckere, *Mystifying the Monarch: Studies on Discourse, Power, and History.*

29 Ibid., "Introduction," 10, 12, 13, 14.

30 Kelly Besecke, "Seeing Invisible Religion: Religion as a Societal Conversation about Transcendent Meaning," *Sociological Theory* (2005): 179–196, critiques trends that dichotomize religion along institutional or individual lines, to conceptualize religion as an evolving societal conversation about transcendent meaning.

31 William Reddy, *The Navigation of Feeling: Framework for the History of Emotions* (Cambridge: Cambridge University Press, 2001), and Barbara H. Rosenwein, "Worrying about Emotions in History," *American Historical Review* 107 (2002): 821–845. These works are discussed in Ruth Leys, "The Turn to Affect: A Critique," *Critical Inquiry* 37.3 (2011): 434–472.

32 Simon Schama, *Rembrandt's Eyes* (New York: Knopf, 1999), 13.

Bibliography

Abraham, Nicolas and Maria Torok. Trans. Nicholas T. Rand. *The Shell and the Kernel: Renewals of Psychoanalysis.* Vol. 1. University of Chicago Press, 1994.

Anderson, Perry. *Lineages of the Absolutist State.* Verso, 1979.

Bayly, Christopher. *The Birth of the Modern World 1780–1914: Global Connections and Comparisons.* Blackwell, 2004.

Besecke, Kelly. "Seeing Invisible Religion: Religion as a Societal Conversation About Transcendent Meaning." *Sociological Theory* (2005): 179–196.

Boy, Robert, and Peter J. Richerson. "Culture and the Evolution of Human Cooperation." *Philosophical Transactions of the Royal Society of London B: Biological Sciences* 364.1533 (2009): 3281–3288.

Boyd, Brian. "Getting It All Wrong: Bioculture Critiques Cultural Critique. 2006." Eds. Brian Boyd, Joseph Carroll and Jonathan Gottschall. *Evolution, Literature, and Film: A Reader.* Columbia University, 2010. 197–210.

———. "Literature and Evolution: A Bio-Cultural Approach." *Philosophy and Literature* 29.1 (2005): 1–23.

Carroll, Joseph. "An Evolutionary Paradigm for Literary Study." *Style* 42.2–3 (2008): 103–134.

Champagne, Frances A. "Epigenetic Mechanisms and the Transgenerational Effects of Maternal Care." *Frontiers in Neuroendocrinology* 29.3 (2008): 386–397.

Cosmides, Leda, and John Tooby. "Cognitive Adaptations for Social Exchange." *The Adapted Mind: Evolutionary Psychology and the Generation of Culture.* Eds. Jerome Barkow, Leda Cosmides, and John Tooby. Oxford University Press, 1992: 163–228.

Deploige, Jeroen, and Gita Deneckere. Eds. *Mystifying the Monarch: Studies on Discourse, Power, and History.* Amsterdam University Press, 2006.

Donald, Merlin. *The Origins of the Modern Mind.* Harvard, 1992.

———. "Art and Cognitive Evolution." Ed. Michael Turner. *The Artful Mind: Cognitive Science and the Riddle of Human Creativity.* Harvard, 2006. 3–20.

———. "Key Cognitive Preconditions for the Evolution of Language." *Psychonomic Bulletin & Review* 24.1 (2017): 204–208.

Gottschall, Jonathan, and David Sloan Wilson. Eds. *The Literary Animal: Evolution and the Nature of Narrative.* Northwestern University, 2005.

Janzen, Daniel H. "When Is It Coevolution." *Evolution* 34.3 (1980): 611–612.

Leys, Ruth. "The Turn to Affect: A Critique." *Critical Inquiry* 37.3 (2011): 434–472.

Nettle, Daniel. "What Happens in Hamlet? Exploring the Psychological Foundations of Drama." *The Literary Animal: Evolution and the Nature of Narrative.* Jonathan Gottschall, David Sloan Wilson. Eds. Oxford, 2005. 56–75.

———. "Language: Costs and Benefits of a Specialized System for Social Information Transmission." Eds. Jonathan CK Wells, Simon Strickland, Kevin Laland. *Social Information Transmission and Human Biology.* Taylor and Francis, 2006. 137–152.

Niewöhner, Jörg. "Epigenetics: Embedded Bodies and the Molecularisation of Biography and Milieu." *BioSocieties* 6 (2011): 279–298.

Pinker, Steven. "How the Mind Works." *Annals of the New York Academy of Sciences* (1999): 119–127.

———. "Language as an Adaptation to the Cognitive Niche." Eds. Morten H. Christiansen and Simon Kirby. *Language Evolution.* Oxford, 2003. 16–37.

———. "Toward a Consilient Study of Literature." *Philosophy and Literature* 31.1 (2007): 162–178.

Rashkin, Esther. *Family Secrets and the Psychoanalysis of Narrative.* Princeton, 1992.

Reddy, William. *The Navigation of Feeling: Framework for the History of Emotions.* Cambridge, 2001.

Rosenwein, Barbara H. "A History of What Has Not Yet Happened." *Rethinking History* 4.2 (2000): 183–192.

———. "Worrying About Emotions in History." *American Historical Review* 107 (2002): 821–845.

Schama, Simon, and Rembrandt Harmenszoon van Rijn. *Rembrandt's Eyes.* Alfred A. Knopf, 1999.

Shryock, Andrew, and Daniel Lord Smail. *Deep History: The Architecture of Past and Present.* University of California Press, 2011.

Smail, Daniel Lord. "Neuroscience and the Dialectics of History." *Análise Social* 47.4 (2012): 894–909.

Wallerstein, Immanuel. *The Modern World-System I: Capitalist Agriculture and the Origins of the European World-Economy in the Sixteenth Century.* University of California, 1974.

Walters, Karina L., Selina A. Mohammed, Teresa Evans-Campbell. "Bodies Don't Just Tell Stories, They Tell Histories." *Du Bois Review: Social Science Research on Race* 8 (2011): 179–189.

Wells, Jonathan C. K., Simon Strickland, and Kevin Laland. Eds. *Social Information Transmission and Human Biology*. Taylor & Francis, 2006.

Zhang, Tieyuan, and Michael J. Meaney. "Epigenetics and the Environmental Regulation of the Genome and Its Function." *Annual Review of Psychology* 61 (2010): 439–466.

Index

www.ingramcontent.com/pod-product-compliance
Ingram Content Group UK Ltd.
Pitfield, Milton Keynes, MK11 3LW, UK
UKHW022001180926
475701UK00003B/138
* 9 7 8 0 3 6 7 5 9 3 0 3 2 *